Vitamin C and Cancer

Mechanisms and Therapeutic Synergies

Medicine & Health
www.novapublishers.com
New York

Cancer Etiology, Diagnosis, and Treatments

More information about this series can be found at

Nutrition and Diet Research Progress

More information about this series can be found at

Lunawati L. Bennett

Vitamin C and Cancer

Mechanisms and Therapeutic Synergies

nova
Medicine & Health
www.novapublishers.com
New York

DOI: https://doi.org/10.52305/PHTR7486

Library of Congress Cataloging-in-Publication Data

ISBN: 979-8-90134-231-2 (Hardcover)
ISBN: 979-8-90134-292-3 (eBook)

Published by Nova Science Publishers, Inc. † New York

To my Lord and Savior, Jesus Christ
YOU placed the calling in my heart and gave me the strength to finish it.
This work is for YOUR glory alone.

Every good and perfect gift is from above - James 1:17

"Vitamin C and Cancer: Mechanisms and Therapeutic Synergies" is a much needed and insightful contribution to the growing body of literature on cancer therapeutics. Dr. Lunawati Bennett combines rigorous scientific research with a clear, accessible presentation of how high-dose vitamin C can act as a pro-oxidant to selectively kill cancer cells and synergize with existing chemotherapies. The book bridges the gap between historical controversies and exciting new findings, offering a balanced and evidence-based perspective.

As a cancer researcher, I find this work particularly valuable because it not only reviews the foundational studies of vitamin C but also presents original research across a wide range of cancer models, from osteosarcoma and neuroblastoma to breast, liver, and lung cancers. By exploring the molecular mechanisms - ROS generation, caspase activation, signaling pathways - Dr. Bennett highlights both the challenges and opportunities of integrating vitamin C into cancer treatment strategies.

This book will be an excellent resource for scientists, physicians, pharmacists, and healthcare providers who are seeking new therapeutic insights. It underscores the importance of looking beyond conventional approaches and revisiting familiar molecules in new contexts.

I strongly recommend Vitamin C and Cancer: Mechanisms and Therapeutic Synergies to anyone committed to advancing cancer research and treatment.

Sincerely,

Qingyu S. Zhou

Qingyu S. Zhou, Ph.D.
Associate Professor of Pharmaceutical Sciences
Taneja College of Pharmacy, University of South Florida
Tampa, Florida, USA

Contents

Foreword

It is a privilege to introduce *Vitamin C and Cancer: Mechanisms and Therapeutic Synergies,* a timely and thoughtful contribution to the field of oncology research. For decades, vitamin C has been known to be an essential nutrient for human health, from its historical role in preventing scurvy to its more recent use in strengthening the immune system. Historically, the potential of vitamin C as a therapeutic agent in cancer has been a subject of both great promise and spirited debate. The Nobel Laureate Linus Pauling was a profound proponent of the use of high doses of vitamin C in disease prevention, although he was met with substantial opposition.

In this book, Dr. Lunawati Bennett provides historical perspective on the use of vitamin C in the study of various types of cancer as well as her own experimental findings. She examines how pharmacological doses of vitamin C can induce oxidative stress selectively in cancer cells, impair signaling pathways, and enhance the efficacy of several anticancer drugs.

What makes this book particularly valuable is its dual appeal. For scientists and clinicians, it provides a foundation that may inspire new approaches in combining vitamin C with existing chemotherapeutics. For healthcare providers, it offers a deeper understanding of how a familiar vitamin can act in complex ways within cancer biology.

I commend Dr. Bennett for her commitment to advancing this important area of research. I trust readers will find *Vitamin C and Cancer: Mechanisms and Therapeutic Synergies,* both informative and thought-provoking, and I hope it sparks further innovation in the ongoing fight against cancer.

E. Blake Watkins, PhD
Professor and Chair, Department of Pharmaceutical Sciences
Union University College of Pharmacy
Jackson, TN 38305 USA

Preface

Interest in the anticancer properties of vitamin C has re-emerged in recent years, supported by new evidence that high (pharmacological) concentrations can act as a pro-oxidant in cancer cells and enhance the effects of certain antineoplastic agents. *Vitamin C and Cancer: Mechanisms and Therapeutic Synergies,"* presents a systematic, laboratory-based investigation into these mechanisms across multiple cancer models and chemotherapeutic drugs. The goal of this book is to provide a comprehensive understanding of vitamin C's role in cancer treatment and its potential for safe and effective integration into modern oncology.

This volume is composed of eighteen chapters. Chapter 1 introduces key concepts in cancer biology, while Chapter 2 focuses on vitamin C - its biological roles, pharmacology, and high-dose effects as an adjunctive therapy. Chapter 3 details the materials and experimental methods used throughout the studies, ensuring transparency and reproducibility. Chapter 4 presents data on the effect of vitamin C on non-cancerous models, including rat spleen, kidney, and fibroblast cells. Beginning with Chapter 5, the book transitions into detailed discussions examining how vitamin C interacts with different antineoplastic agents across distinct cancer cell models, from liver cancer, osteosarcoma, breast cancer, prostate cancer, pancreatic cancer, chronic myelogenous and chronic lymphocytic leukemia, non–small cell lung cancer, malignant pleural mesothelioma, renal, to neuroblastoma cancers, each revealing unique mechanistic and therapeutic responses. Each model was treated with vitamin C alone and in combination with selected antineoplastic agents, including doxorubicin, etoposide, sorafenib, paclitaxel, afatinib, temsirolimus, and bortezomib - tested at their lowest effective concentrations to evaluate additive or synergistic effects. Functional assays such as Hoechst, Rhodamine 123, and H2DCFDA were employed to assess apoptosis, mitochondrial membrane potential, and reactive oxygen species generation, while scratch assays were used to evaluate cell migration and wound healing. Western blot analysis was employed to identify different cell signaling involved in cancer.

Throughout these studies, vitamin C demonstrated variable yet often synergistic effects when combined with antineoplastic. In several cancer models, the combination treatments enhanced cytotoxicity and apoptosis, frequently associated with increased reactive oxygen species production and mitochondrial disruption - findings that support a pro-oxidant, mitochondria-mediated mechanism of action. In other models, responses were neutral or modest, suggesting that vitamin C's synergy depends on cell type, redox status, and signaling context. The inclusion of non-cancerous cells provided a crucial safety perspective, underscoring the importance of dose control and selective cytotoxicity. When unexpected results arose - such as reduced caspase activity or signs of epithelial–mesenchymal transition - possible mechanisms were explained to guide future studies.

The final chapter integrates these findings through comprehensive summary tables - including Chou–Talalay combination-index data, mechanistic insights, and translational outcomes - to provide a comparative overview of vitamin C interactions across systems. It also discusses the limitations of current data and outlines essential next steps: *in vivo* validation, mechanistic exploration of caspase-independent cell-death pathways, pharmacokinetic and dose-response optimization, and rigorously designed clinical trials prioritizing patient safety and monitoring. While the cumulative results underscore promising synergistic potentials between vitamin C and several anticancer drugs, they equally emphasize the need for cautious translation from bench to bedside, guided by mechanistic understanding and clinical prudence.

While promising, these results also revealed an important truth: *vitamin C's effects are not universal, nor uniformly synergistic.* In certain models - such as renal (A-498) and prostate (LNCaP) cancer - early or concurrent treatment produced *less-than-additive responses* or was moderated by *compensatory survival signaling pathways*, highlighting the dynamic interplay between redox modulation and intracellular feedback networks. In these cases, synergy emerged *only under specific timing conditions*, such as extended exposure or adjusted sequencing with targeted therapies. These findings emphasize that vitamin C is not merely an "add-on" treatment, but a *biologically active signaling modulator* whose therapeutic potential depends on dosage, cellular context, and treatment schedule.

This book is intended for a broad readership of scientists, physicians, oncologists, pharmacists, and other health professionals interested in the evolving science of vitamin C in oncology. Researchers will find detailed experimental data and mechanistic insights that may inspire new studies. Clinicians may gain a clearer understanding of preclinical evidence supporting cautious exploration of high-dose intravenous vitamin C in cancer therapy. Pharmacists and healthcare providers will benefit from learning how vitamin C can shift from antioxidant to pro-oxidant behavior at pharmacological doses, influencing its therapeutic potential.

This work represents years of independent experimental effort, motivated by the desire to clarify the scientific basis of vitamin C's role in cancer therapy. It is my hope that *Vitamin C and Cancer*: *Mechanisms and Therapeutic Synergies* will serve as both a reference and an inspiration - encouraging continued research, collaboration, and thoughtful application of vitamin C in the fight against cancer.

Respectively yours,
November 2025

Lunawati Bennett MS, MRE, PhD, PharmD, FACN, CNS
Professor of Pharmaceutical Sciences
Union University
College of Pharmacy
Jackson, Tennessee 38305, USA

Chapter 1

An Introduction to Cancer Biology

Lunawati L. Bennett*, PhD, PharmD,
Ola Boateng, MBA
and Xinyue Shen, PharmD
Union University, College of Pharmacy, Jackson, Tennessee, USA

Abstract

Cancer is a leading cause of death worldwide, accounting for nearly 10 million deaths in 2020. The most common cancer is lung, breast, colorectal, prostate, skin (non-melanoma), stomach, and liver. Cancer arises from the transformation of normal cells into tumor cells in a multi-stage process from a pre-cancerous lesion to a malignant tumor.

Several causes of cancer include genetic and external agents. External agents can be categorized into biological carcinogens such as infection from certain viruses, bacteria, or parasites, physical carcinogens such as ultraviolet and ionizing radiation, and chemical carcinogens such as asbestos, tobacco, alcohol, aflatoxin/food contaminant, and arsenic/drinking water contaminant. Treatment of cancer usually includes surgery, radiotherapy, and/or systemic therapy (chemotherapy, hormonal treatments, targeted biological therapies). Treatment of cancer is inherently challenging due to the heterogeneity of cancer, genetic mutations, and drug resistance among others.

This chapter covers diverse cancers ranging from the most common liver cancer known as hepatocellular carcinoma, to more difficult to treat breast cancer known as triple negative breast cancer, as well as non-solid cancers such as chronic lymphocytic leukemia and chronic myelogenous leukemia. The role of ascorbic acid or vitamin C will be discussed briefly with each cancer being discussed.

Keywords: cancer, aberrant signaling pathway, malignancy, hepatic cancer, breast cancer, triple negative breast cancer, chronic lymphocytic leukemia, chronic myelogenous leukemia, malignant pleural mesothelioma, osteosarcoma, lung cancer, neuroblastoma, renal cancer, prostate cancer, pancreatic cancer, and colorectal cancer

* Corresponding Author's Email: llbennett@uu.edu

Abbreviations

HCC	hepatocellular carcinoma;
EGFR	epidermal growth factor receptor;
VC	vitamin C;
PDL1	programmed death ligand;
CML	chronic myelogenous leukemia;
CLL	chronic lymphocytic leukemia;
TKI	tyrosine kinase inhibitor;
GI	gastrointestinal;
CRC	colorectal cancer;
PCa	prostate cancer;
MDR	multi drug resistant;
SF	Sorafenib;
DX	doxorubicin;
ET	Etoposide;
mTOR	mammalian target of rapamycin;
OS	osteosarcoma,
TNBC	Triple negative breast cancer;
CRPC	castration resistant prostate cancer;
MAPK	mitogen activated protein kinase;
MEK	mitogen activated protein kinase kinase;
FDA	Food and Drug Administration;
ERK	epidermal growth factor.

Introduction[1]

Within the realm of oncology, the ceaseless pursuit of unraveling the complexities inherent to diverse cancer types has become a scientific imperative. This chapter stands as a dedicated exploration into the intricate molecular landscapes and clinical peculiarities of hepatic cancer, breast cancer, malignant pleural mesothelioma, osteosarcoma, neuroblastoma, non-small cell lung cancer, renal cancer, pancreatic cancer, prostate cancer, chronic myelogenous leukemia, chronic lymphocytic leukemia, and colorectal cancers.

A meticulous examination of the epidemiological trends, risk factors, and diagnostic modalities unique to the respective cancer, providing a comprehensive foundation for clinicians, researchers, and students dedicated to the pursuit of understanding cancer biology.

The treatment of cancer is inherently challenging due to several complex factors. Cancer is not a single disease but a group of diseases with diverse characteristics (heterogeneity). Cancer cells can vary widely, even within the same type of cancer,

---

[1] Portions of this chapter (Neuroblastoma and Breast Cancer) were written by students under the editorial supervision of the primary author.

making it challenging to develop universal treatment strategies. Cancer often arises from genetic mutations which are unique to each patient. In addition, cancer cells can spread to different parts of the body, a process known as metastasis. Detecting and treating cancer in its advanced stages, when metastasis has occurred, can be more difficult and less effective.

Cancer cells have adaptability to resist treatment over time, while certain types of cancer still lack effective targeted therapies, making treatment options limited. Cancer can create an immunosuppressive environment, allowing cancerous cells to evade the body's natural defense mechanisms.

The intricate web of carcinogenesis and the heterogeneity exhibited by different cancers present formidable challenges to researchers and clinicians alike. Understanding the unique genetic aberrations, signaling pathways, and microenvironmental factors characterizing each malignancy is crucial for the development of targeted therapies.

Liver Cancer

Liver cancer is a significant global health concern representing the seventh most common and the second leading cause of cancer-related deaths [1-2]. There were 906,000 new cases and 830,000 patients who died of liver cancer throughout the world in 2020. The number of new cases and deaths from liver cancer could rise to greater than 55% by 2040 [3]. It is the top three cause of cancer related death in 46 countries. The countries with the highest incidence of liver cancer are typically show lower level of economic development and geographically include North and West Africa (Gambia, Egypt, and Guinea) and East and Southeast Asia (Cambodia, Mongolia, and Vietnam) [4].

Liver cancer is a heterogenous group of malignances ranging from hepatocellular carcinoma (HCC) (75 to 85%), intrahepatic cholangiocarcinoma (ICC) (10 to 15%), to several rare subtypes, such as hepatoblastoma (HB), the most common pediatric liver cancer [5-8].

The common risk factors of liver cancer include genetic aberrations, chronic hepatitis B virus (HBV) or chronic hepatitis V virus (HCV) infection, non-alcoholic fatty liver disease (NAFLD), aflatoxin contamination in foods, alcohol consumption, obesity, and diabetes [1]. Other risk factors include older age and male [3, 5].

HCC usually arises from interaction between activated proto-oncogenes and inactivated tumor suppressors. *CTNNB1* (coding for β-catenin with 22% mutation rate) and *TP53* (29% mutation rate) are the most frequently altered proto-oncogenes and tumor suppressor genes [5]. *CTNNB1* mutation is also identified in more than 10% hepatocellular adenoma (HCA), which is a benign liver neoplasm with higher risk to become malignant [5]. Mutations of exon 3 had been identified as the most common alterations of β-catenin in liver cancer [9]. Exon 3 protects β-catenin protein from degradation and in return constitutively turns on β-catenin signaling cascade [10-11]. Phosphorylation of serine/threonine encoded by exon 3 of *CTNNB1* leads to ubiquitination-mediated degradation of β-catenin. Since mutated β-catenin contributes to hepatocarcinogenesis, inhibition of β-catenin as novel targets for the treatment of liver cancer may be viable options in decreasing downstream events such as aberrant metabolism and signaling transduction pathway [5, 7].

Altered pathways in HCC are also involved growth factor receptors such as vascular endothelial growth factor receptor (VEGFR), epidermal growth factor receptor (EGFR), and/or its cytoplasmic intermediates such as PI3K/AKT/mTOR and RAF/ERK/MAPK, and key pathways in cell differentiation Hippo, Hedgehog, Notch Wnt/β-catenin, JAK/STAT [8]. Moreover, coactivation of Wnt/β-catenin/ROCK and Akt/mTOR pathways was found in 14.4% of patients with liver cancer. These patients showed poorer survival than those with either Wnt/ROCK/β-catenin or AKT/p13K/mTOR pathway activation alone [12-13].

There are many different methods for the staging of liver cancer in clinical practice, including Okuda, Barcelona Clinic Liver Cancer (BCLC), Cancer of the Liver Italian Program (CLIP), Chinese University Prognostic Index (CUPI), Japan Integrated Staging (JIS), and tumor–node–metastasis (TNM). Most methodologies are based on the size of the cancer and its metastasis status [14-15]. Clinically, these different staging methods are highly correlated with treatment strategies for liver [16]. Evaluation should also consider tumor status, performance status and liver function (Child–Pugh score).

For patients with early-stage (0-A), liver resection or ablation (radiofrequency or microwave) the accepted treatment option. For patients with intermediate stage (B), liver transplantation, trans arterial chemoembolization and systemic drug therapy using targeted drugs and immunotherapy are available treatment options. For patients with advanced stage (C), these patients usually receive systemic drug treatment first, followed by other options. Patients with end-stage liver cancer (D) can only receive supportive therapy since therapies are no longer effective [17].

Among solid tumor, liver cancer has elevated level of inter- and intra-tumor heterogeneity which greatly hampered the effectiveness of drugs [17-18]. Given the cause and genetics of liver cancer among patients vary widely, there are only a handful targeted agents such as Sorafenib or Lenvatinib being approved for the treatment.

Sorafenib was the first targeted liver cancer drug to pass Phase III clinical trials and receive approval by Food and Drug Administration (FDA) for the treatment of unresectable HCC and advanced renal cell carcinoma. Sorafenib is an oral multiple tyrosine kinase inhibitor (TKI) that inhibits angiogenesis, cell proliferation, and cell differentiation by targeting both the RAF/MEK/ERK pathway and receptor tyrosine kinases [19]. The specific targets of this small-molecule inhibitor are VEGFR, platelet-derived growth factor (PDGFR), stem cell factor receptor (c-KIT), and Fms-like tyrosine-kinase receptor (FLT-3), among others [20-21]. By interfering with these signaling pathways, sorafenib has the potential to interrupt cellular processes in cancer cells, leading to apoptosis, cell death, and decreased in cell proliferation [22]. However, modest clinical benefits with severe side effects and frequent development of drug resistance cause limitation of Sorafenib usage [23-25].

Recently, the systemic management of HCC has been revolutionized by the combination therapy using atezolizumab, a programmed death ligand (PDL1) inhibitor plus bevacizumab, a VEGF antibody [23]. This combination significantly extended the median overall survival by six months to 19.2 months versus sorafenib at 13.6 months [26-27]. This treatment has been recommended and approved by many societies and countries as the first-line treatment for unresectable malignant liver cancer. Other drugs that have been explored or in the clinical trials include tremelimumab (anticytotoxic T lymphocyte-associated antigen 4/anti-CTLA-4), durvalumab (anti-PD-L1), nivolumab and ipilimumab (anti-CTLA-4 monoclonal antibody), and ramucirumab (anit-VEGFR-2) [28-30]. Other anti-cancer drugs that have been explored to treat HCC include cisplatin, fluorouracil, and doxorubicin [16, 31-32].

Considering the limited efficacy of traditional treatments in addressing advanced liver cancer, the imperative for continuous exploration and innovation in therapeutic approaches becomes evident. Currently, there have been no reported investigations of using vitamin C as an adjuvant in the literature regarding its role in HCC. Through sustained exploration, we can pave the way for groundbreaking solutions that hold the promise for improving outcomes in patients with HCC.

Malignant Pleural Mesothelioma

Malignant pleural mesothelioma (MPM) is a rare, lethal, and aggressive cancer that affects the pleural cavity, the outer lining of the lung [33-34]. It is primarily caused by exposure to asbestos; a mineral naturally found in the environment. Asbestos, when broken up during mining, produces dust that may accumulate in the lungs, stomach, or heart. Although asbestos has been used in commercial buildings for centuries, it contains carcinogenic fibers that can lead to cancer [34]. While the use of asbestos is currently forbidden in Western countries, the incidence of MPM is still expected to rise in regions where asbestos remain legal or prevalent, such as in rural areas or industrialized countries that still use asbestos for building renovations [35-36]. Furthermore, environmental exposure continues to be widespread as human activities disturb natural deposits [37].

The incidence of MPM varies globally. Between 1990 and 2017, the worldwide incidence of MPM decreased from 0.52 to 0.44 per 100,000 people [38]. Using the Bayesian APC model, a study projected that the incidence rates of MPM in China would rise from 1.4 per one million persons in 2016 to 1.9 per one million persons in 2030. The estimated number of new incident cases is expected to increase to about 2,775 in 2030 [39]. According to the World Health Organization, between 2018 and 2040, there is a predicted gradual increase in the trend of MPM, shifting from 3,060 to 4,699 cases [40].

MPM predominantly affects males, with approximately 80% of cases attributed to occupational or environmental asbestos exposures with a median survival of 6 to 18 months and a 5-year survival rate of less than 5% [37, 41-43]. This poor prognosis can be attributed to several factors, such as the absence of reliable tools for screening and identifying specific biomarkers and lack of effective systemic therapies. Patients are often being diagnosed at advanced stages [44-45]. In the U.S, a significant milestone was achieved on March 19, 2024, as the United States Environmental Protection Agency (EPA) issued a landmark ruling to ban chrysotile asbestos [46-47].

MPM manifests in three histological subtypes: epithelioid (associated with the best outcomes), sarcomatoid (linked to the worst outcomes), and biphasic. Carcinogenesis in MPM is a multistep process driven by the deep penetration of asbestos fibers into the lung epithelium and pleural space. This process induces mutations through a repeated cycle of pleural irritation, damage, and repair, resulting in the release of pro-oncogenic proteins and growth factors [48-50]. Notably, there is a long latency period of 30 to 50 years between the first asbestos exposure and the diagnosis of MPM [44-45]. Clinical symptoms of MPM are typically insidious and nonspecific, including dyspnea, cough, and/or chest pain [43-45].

The diagnostic algorithm for MPM initiates with a morphological assessment of cytology or histological specimens. Several biomarkers such as pan cytokeratin, Calretinin, CK5/6, Thrombomodulin (CD141), HBME-1, WT-1, D2-40, EMA, CEA, B72.3 (TAG-72), BG8, CD15, TTF-1, MOC31, claudin-4, and BerEP4 (HEA), are then utilized through immunohistochemistry (IHC) on formalin-fixed, paraffin-embedded, or cell block samples to differentiate mesothelial from epithelial lineage [48-51].

The current standard care for MPM involves surgery with the intent to cure if the disease is diagnosed at an early stage, or palliative care utilizing combination chemotherapy with platinum agents such as carboplatin or cisplatin, along with anti-folates like pemetrexed [52-54]. The use of neoadjuvant or subsequent-line agents in treating MPM has not been clearly established.

To date, there is no documented information about utilization of VC as an adjuvant in treating MPM. Therefore, any effort to enhance treatment options for this aggressive and lethal cancer is a welcome addition. By persistently delving into this unexplored territory, uncovering innovative solutions may have the potential to enhance outcomes in the treatment of MPM.

Osteosarcoma

Osteosarcoma (OS) is a primary malignant bone tumor derived from bone-forming mesenchymal system cells that primarily affect children and adolescents. This cancer presents a significant challenge due to their high rates of local invasion and metastasis. Local invasion occurs in 85% of OS patients while distant metastasis to the lungs occurs in 74% of the cases [55].

The incidence of OS occurs in 0.2-3 cases per 100,000 annually in children and 0.8-11 cases per 100,000 annually in adolescents [56-58]. Around 4% of all childhood malignancies are due to OS [59]. In the United States, there are an estimated 3,600 new cases of OS each year, with approximately 1,720 deaths [60]. Worldwide, the incidence of OS is about 3.4 per million per year [61]. In Europe, the incidence is particularly higher in patients aged 15 to 19 years, with an incidence of 8-11 per million per year. Below 15 years of age, the incidence is higher in females, while after 15 years the incidence is higher in males [62-63].

The rapid bone cell turnover and growth typical of childhood or pubertal growth spurts are likely linked to the risk of developing OS. It primarily localizes long bones of the extremities near the most proliferative growth plates, such as the distal femur, proximal tibia, and proximal humerus. The most common symptoms, depending on the location and growth rate of cancer, include reduced joint movement, local pain, and swelling around the cancer mass. Pain and swelling may be more intense with physical activity, during the night, and become more persistent over time [59].

Most OS cases appear to be sporadic, occurring in patients without a family history [64]. The initiation of tumorigenesis involves the malignant transformation of cells and functional alterations in the tumor microenvironment, including osteoblasts, osteoblasts, osteoclasts, endothelial cells, blood vessels, tumor-associated fibroblasts, and malignant mesenchymal stem cells [65-66]. Extracellular vehicles play a significant role in tumor progression by acting as mediators regulating communication among cells. EVs mediate intracellular communication by delivering bioactive molecules such as DNA, mRNAs, non-coding RNAs, proteins, lipids, and metabolites to regulate interactions among tumor cells, the tumor microenvironment, and distant organs and tissues [67-68].

Molecular abnormalities with wide genetic instability, including deletions or losses of genes on chromosomes 3q, 6q, 10, 13, 17p, 18q, and gains and amplifications on chromosomes 1p, 1q, 6p, 8q, and 17p, have been identified [69-70]. There is growing evidence that OS is associated with the activation of numerous oncogenes such as cyclin D1, mouse double minute 2 homolog (MDM2), and c-Myc [64]. Other signaling pathways involved in the tumorigenesis of OS include PI3K/Akt with Wnt/β-catenin pathways have been identified as important regulators of OS [59, 71].

Treatment for OS includes surgical amputation, radiation, and chemotherapy. Radiation treatment is controversial due to its questionable effectiveness and increased risk of infection [72]. Surgery combined with new chemotherapies using cisplatin, adriamycin, methotrexate, and cyclophosphamide has significantly improved overall survival and quality of life and is recognized as the standard treatment. The combination therapy of doxorubicin, cisplatin, and high doses of methotrexate (referred to as MAP) is used as the first-line therapy alongside limb-sparing surgery to remove the primary cancer. However, changes in genetic and epigenetic characteristics of OS can cause drug resistance through increased drug metabolism, evasion of apoptosis, or reduced drug uptake [55].

Clinical trials in Phase I or I/II are being conducted to treat metastatic OS, with almost half trials use immunotherapies such as interleukin-2 (IL-2), programmed cell death (PD-1) inhibitors, or tyrosine kinase (TK) inhibitors. They have shown promising results [73-75]. In addition, bisphosphonates have shown promising preclinical activity by inhibiting farnesyl pyrophosphate synthase, which plays important role in inhibiting osteoclast activity [76].

Treatment strategy for using high dose of VC only has not been reported. However, the combined effect of VC and cisplatin treatment showed that the chemo sensitizing effect of VC is linked to reactive oxygen species (ROS) production, due to alterations in the cellular redox state and modification of glycolysis and mitochondrial function.

Therefore, there is a significant rationale to combine cisplatin with VC as a therapeutic strategy against OS [77].

Clinical trials incorporating predictive biomarker assays that improve outcomes such as mammalian target of rapamycin (mTOR), programmed cell death ligand 1 (PD-L1), or understanding detailed physiological, cellular, and biochemical factors, may allow our understanding of personalized drug treatment. Current treatment strategies, including surgery and chemotherapy, have improved survival rates, but the complexity of the disease, marked by genetic and molecular abnormalities, poses ongoing challenges, particularly with drug resistance.

Emerging therapies, such as immunotherapies or combinations of antineoplastic and VC, offer promising avenues for improving patient outcomes. Continued research and clinical trials remain vital to developing more effective and personalized strategies against this devastating cancer. As our understanding of redox biology and tumor microenvironment deepens, integrating VC into multimodal treatment regimens may not only enhance therapeutic efficacy but also restore hope for patients facing one of the most challenging malignancies of our time.

Brain Cancer

Brain cancer accounted for approximately 23,890 new cases and 18,020 new deaths in the U.S. in 2020. Brain cancers are extremely heterogenous with more than one hundred classified types with potentially different risk factors with the five-year relative survival is estimated at 35.8% [78-80]. On average, individuals diagnosed with brain cancer may experience a reduction in life expectancy by around 20 years. Brain cancer is ranked third leading cause of solid cancer-related deaths between the ages of 20 and 39 [81-82].

According to the WHO, they are classified as primary (originating from brain cells) or secondary or metastatic brain cancer which are more prevalent. All secondary brain cancers are malignant, while primary brain cancer can be benign or malignant [79]. The most common malignant brain cancers originate from glial cells with the most malignant is glioblastoma multiforme (GBM) shows the highest malignancy and invasiveness [83-84].

Neuroblastoma is the most common extracranial cancer in children that originates from the embryonic neural crest cell derivatives in the sympathetic nervous system. About 700 children are diagnosed each year in the United States, which represents 8% of pediatric cancers. It has an insidious onset and rapid progression, accounting for 15% of childhood cancer deaths. The most common age of presentation is between 18 and 22 months with most cases being diagnosed before the age of 5. Older children are more likely to have aggressive cancers that are resistant to multimodal and cytotoxic therapies while infants less than 18 months can be successfully treated with surgery alone [85].

About 50% of neuroblastoma have severe clinical course, marked by widespread metastases to the bone and bone marrow. For these cases, despite intensive therapeutic measures such as induction chemotherapy, surgery, myeloablative therapy with stem cell rescue, local radiation therapy, and the use of retinoids and/or immunotherapy for biological response modification, the survival rate remains below 35% [86-87].

Approximately 1-2% of neuroblastoma patients have familial forms of the disease. Among these, about 75% of hereditary neuroblastoma cases are linked to *ALK* gene, while another 5% are due to mutations in the *PHOX2B* gene. These genetic factors highlight the complex and multifaceted etiology of neuroblastoma [88].

The treatment regimen for high-risk neuroblastomas consists of three distinct phases: induction of remission, consolidation of remission, and maintenance phase that focus on eradicating minimal residual disease. The induction phase typically revolves around a regimen developed at the Memorial Sloan-Kettering Cancer Center, involving dose-intensive cycles of cisplatin and etoposide, alternating with vincristine, doxorubicin, cyclophosphamide, and topotecan [89].

Although most high-risk neuroblastomas exhibit an initial response to therapy, eventual relapses due to drug resistance or formation of rare resistant clones within a heterogeneous tumor environment. Isotretinoin was introduced to reduce relapse risk in high-risk neuroblastoma patients, but uncertainties remain about its optimal dosing, pharmacokinetics, and long-term toxicity. Despite progress, many high-risk patients still relapse [89].

There is limited information about use of VC in neuroblastoma. One study showed VC affects the expression of intercellular adhesion molecule-1 (ICAM-1) induced by tumor necrosis factor-α (TNF-α) in human neuroblastoma cells (SK-N-SH). TNF-α activates the NF-kB signaling pathway, leading to increased ICAM-1 expression. The findings reveal that VC reduces both the surface expression and mRNA levels of ICAM-1 in a concentration-dependent manner. Additionally, VC inhibits NF-kB activation and the degradation of IkBα, which is induced by TNF-α. Therefore, VC appears to downregulate ICAM-1 expression by inhibiting the NF-kB pathway [90].

VC has been shown to be highly effective in killing neuroblastoma cells at lower concentrations compared to other tumor cell lines. This effect is believed to result from disruptions in intracellular iron levels, caused by the downregulation of the tumor flare reaction (TfR). This leads to VC-induced apoptosis and oxidative stress, which can damage DNA and impair glycolysis in cancer cells, while sparing normal cells. However, the exact mechanism behind VC's selective cytotoxicity, particularly regarding ATP depletion, is still being studied [91-92].

Continued exploration of these pathways may not only clarify the molecular determinants of vitamin C's selectivity but also open new avenues for integrating redox modulation into the management of pediatric and refractory neuroblastoma.

Gastrointestinal Cancer

Gastrointestinal (GI) cancer significantly contributes to global cancer-related fatalities, affecting various segments of the digestive system such as pancreatic, liver, colorectal, esophageal, and gastric. In 2020, the US recorded 1,806,590 new cancer cases and 606,520 deaths, with GI cancer being a leading cause. The distribution of specific GI cancer types reveals notable regional variations. In Asia, there is a higher prevalence of esophageal, gastric, and liver cancers, while in Europe and North America, colorectal and pancreatic cancers are more common. This geographical diversity extends to gender-based disparities, with GI cancers affecting men twice the rate of women. Notably, 8 in 100 men and 4 in 100 women develop GI cancer before the age of 75 [93].

This insight prompts a closer exploration of the interplay between lifestyle factors and the development of GI cancers, highlighting modifiable risk factors that demand thorough consideration. Among these factors, high-fat diets (HFD), obesity, alcohol, tobacco, and infections emerge as pivotal contributors, adding layers of complexity to GI cancer. The influence of HFD and obesity transcends mere inflammation, delving into the realms of metabolic reprogramming and alterations of various carcinogenic molecules [94]. A global rise in obesity rates to 18% for men and 21% for women by 2025 intensify concerns about an imminent increase in the prevalence of GI cancers. This apprehension is grounded by the understanding that alterations in insulin signaling and inflammation from fat tissues significantly contribute to the escalating burden of GI malignancies [94-95].

Despite modifying risk factors, the prognosis of GI cancers frequently remains unfavorable due to late-stage diagnoses - a trend reflected in mortality rates across different sites. Colorectal cancer, however, distinguishes itself as an exception, benefiting from advances in early detection and treatment, leading to a generally more favorable prognosis [93].

Colorectal cancer (CRC) holds a significant place among the ‘big four’ cancer types in the United States, standing alongside breast, lung, and prostate cancer. Globally, it ranks as the third most common cancer in men and the second most common in women. While CRC incidence is relatively low before the age of 50, a significant increase is observed with advancing age. In developed countries, the median age at diagnosis hovers around 70 years [96-97].

Beyond demographics, additional risk factors of CRC include family history, inflammatory bowel disease, smoking, excessive alcohol consumption, high intake of red and processed meat, obesity, and diabetes. Recent studies have also introduced the potential role of infectious agents, such as *Helicobacter pylori*, *Fusobacterium*, and others, which are currently under investigation [98].

Colorectal cancer has a significant global impact, affecting over 1.85 million individuals annually and resulting in more than 850,000 deaths. Survival rates for individuals diagnosed with metastatic CRC show approximately 70% to 75% survive within one year, 30% to 35% beyond three years, and fewer than 20% beyond five years from diagnosis [99]. However, it’s important to note that the five-year relative survival rate is more favorable in high-income countries such as Australia, Canada, the US, and various European nations. The stage at which the cancer is diagnosed is identified as the most crucial prognostic factor, significantly influencing survival outcomes [98].

Research has extensively focused on key tumor suppressor genes like p53 and recurrent cytogenetic aberrations. Common mutations in CRC are *APC*, *CTNNB1*, *KRAS, BRAF*, *SMAD4*, *TGFBR2*, and *PIK3CA*, influencing key signaling pathways like *Wnt*, *β-catenin, EGFR, MAPK,* and *p85,* as well as genes regulating critical cellular behaviors such as DNA repair and proliferation. Detecting these mutations provides insights into CRC progression, enabling early diagnosis and facilitating early treatment [100].

For over 50 years, fluoropyrimidines, administered by IV as 5-fluorouracil (5-FU) or orally as capecitabine, have served as conventional first-line chemotherapy treatment. These pyrimidine antagonists disrupt DNA synthesis, and their combination with leucovorin, a folic acid derivative, enhances cytotoxic inhibitory effects [99]. Although 5-FU-based chemotherapy remains a major treatment for CRC, it presents disadvantages due to systemic toxicity, lack of effectiveness and selectivity, and the development of resistance [101].

For patients with wild-type *RAS* colorectal cancer, the primary treatment goals are life extension and achieving secondary resection, typically through anti-EGFR therapy combined with bevacizumab. In *RAS*-mutant tumors, a chemotherapy doublet with bevacizumab remains a standard option. For *BRAF*-mutant cases, treatment decisions are less straightforward; however, a triplet regimen consisting of 5-fluorouracil (5-FU), folinic acid, oxaliplatin, and irinotecan in combination with bevacizumab may be appropriate for well-tolerant patients. Overall, combination chemotherapy and targeted regimens are increasingly utilized to overcome multi-drug resistance and improve therapeutic outcomes [102].

High-dose intravenous VC (IVC) therapy has been shown to suppress cancer growth as a potential Warburg effect inhibitor in a concentration-dependent manner, reversing the glucose-induced oncogenic effect in HCT116, a CRC model [103].

Due to its redox potential and involvement in several cellular processes, VC is being investigated in clinical trials as a treatment modality for various types of GI cancers. Cells harboring *KRAS* and *BRAF* mutations overexpress Glucose Transporter 1 (GLUT1) and sodium-dependent vitamin C transporter 2 (SVCT2). This leads to increased intracellular vitamin C transport, resulting in ROS generation and ultimately cell death [104]. Therefore, high-dose VC is proposed to overcome resistance to *EGFR*-targeted therapy in *BRAF/KRAS* mutated CRC. Furthermore, VC exerts its anti-neoplastic effect through various mechanisms by interfering with anaerobic glycolysis and hindering angiogenesis [105-106].

Other studies show that high-dose VC modulates the tumor microenvironment by promoting immune cell infiltration and delaying cancer growth in a T cell–dependent manner. VC not only enhances the cytotoxic activity of adoptively transferred $CD8^+$ T cells but also cooperates with immune checkpoint therapy (ICT). The combination of VC and ICT can even be curative in models of mismatch repair–deficient gastrointestinal cancer [107].

These findings underscore vitamin C's emerging role as an immunometabolism modulator, offering a promising avenue for integrating redox regulation with immunotherapeutic strategies in cancer treatment.

Pancreatic Cancer

Pancreatic cancer is a leading cause of cancer-related death worldwide, and its global burden has more than doubled over the past 25 years. In 2018, there were 458,918 new cases of pancreatic cancer documented globally, accounting for 2.5% of all cancers. Pancreatic cancer is more prevalent in men than in women and is rarely diagnosed before the age of 55. It predominantly affects elderly populations, with the highest incidence observed in individuals over 70 years old [108-109].

Approximately 90% of pancreatic cancers are pancreatic ductal adenocarcinoma (PDAC) with the 5-year survival rate of 11%. The highest incidence rates of PDAC are observed in Black individuals, followed by White, Hispanic, and Asian populations [110-112]. Common symptoms of pancreatic cancer include: 1) abdominal pain that may be persistent, dull, or aching and can be exacerbated by eating or lying down. It is often due to tumor invasion of adjacent structures or local inflammation, 2) jaundice, or yellowing of the skin and sclera, occurs when the tumor obstructs the bile duct, leading to the accumulation of bilirubin in the bloodstream, 3) significant weight loss despite a normal or increased appetite. This is due to metabolic changes associated with cancer, such as increased energy expenditure and reduced nutrient absorption, 4) nausea and vomiting due to gastric outlet destruction, and 5) steatorrhea due to impaired digestion and absorption of fats [113-114].

Pancreatic cancer is characterized by a series of genetic mutations and epigenetic alterations. The most frequent genetic mutations include: *KRAS, TP53, CDKN2A, SMAD4*. Mutations in the KRAS gene are present in approximately 90% of PDAC cases. *KRAS* is an oncogene that encodes a GTPase involved in cell signaling pathways regulating growth and survival. Mutations in KRAS lead to constitutive activation of downstream signaling pathways, promoting uncontrolled cell proliferation and survival [115]. The *TP53* gene, which encodes the p53 tumor suppressor protein, is mutated in about 50-75% of PDAC cases. p53 plays a crucial role in DNA repair, cell cycle regulation, and apoptosis. Loss of functional p53 impairs the cell's ability to respond to DNA damage and promotes tumor progression. The *CDKN2A* gene encodes proteins that inhibit cyclin-dependent kinases, which are essential for cell cycle progression. Mutations in *CDKN2A* result in the loss of cell cycle control and contribute to cancer development. *SMAD4*, a key player in the TGF-β signaling pathway, is frequently mutated or deleted in pancreatic cancer. This disruption affects cell growth and differentiation, further driving cancer progression [115].

The potential for curing pancreatic cancer lies in a combination of thorough resection and systemic multi-agent chemotherapy. Despite this approach, the overall recurrence rate remains high, ranging from 70-80%. For patients diagnosed with locally advanced or metastatic PDAC, the condition is generally deemed non-curative, and the focus shifts to palliative management. Numerous trials have demonstrated that systemic chemotherapy, often utilizing a combination of 5-FU, folinic acid, irinotecan, and oxaliplatin (FOLFIRINOX) can enhance overall survival in advanced PDAC cases. Adjuvant radiation is also employed, but it is essential to acknowledge the potential toxicity of chemotherapy drugs in the treatment process [116-117]. Combination regimens such as FOLFIRINOX or gemcitabine plus nab-paclitaxel have prolonged the median overall survival to 8.5–13 months, but with a significant toxic burden. Numerous attempts have been made to improve systemic therapies, but they have either failed to improve efficacy or have added significant toxic side effects [118].

Addition of IVC to antineoplastic showed synergistic effect. A phase I/IIa study investigating the pharmacokinetic interaction between IVC, and gemcitabine showed that pharmacological IV induced cell death in pancreatic cancer cells with diverse mutational backgrounds by depleting cellular NAD+ of cancer cells but not normal cells, leading to ATP depletion. While ATP depletion led to cell death, over-acetylated tubulin inhibited motility and mitosis. Collagen was increased, and cancer cell epithelial-mesenchymal transition (EMT) was inhibited, accompanied by a reduction in metastasis. EMT is a process where epithelial cells acquire mesenchymal properties, increasing their migratory and invasive capabilities. This transition is crucial for tumor metastasis. In pancreatic cancer, EMT is driven by various signaling pathways, including TGF-β and Wnt/β-catenin [119].

Collectively, these findings suggest that IVC represents a safe and promising adjunct in the management of advanced pancreatic cancer. By enhancing oxidative stress selectively within tumor cells, modulating redox sensitive signaling pathways, and potentially improving chemosensitivity to gemcitabine, IVC provides a multifaceted therapeutic approach with minimal systemic toxicity. The dual capacity of VC to promote metabolic vulnerability in cancer cells while preserving normal cellular integrity underscores its translational potential. Continued clinical evaluation through well-designed, randomized studies will be essential to define optimal dosing, combination strategies, and patient selection criteria. Ultimately, integrating IVC into standard chemotherapeutic regimens may help transform the treatment landscape for this highly lethal malignancy, offering renewed hope for improved survival and quality of life.

Breast Cancer

Breast cancer is the most common cancer among women worldwide and can be classified into various subtypes based on the presence or absence of specific receptors. Treatment plans vary according to these subtypes. Common treatments for breast cancer include surgery, radiation, chemotherapy, hormone therapy, immunotherapy, and targeted drug therapy. The current 5-year relative survival rate for women in the United States with non-metastatic invasive breast cancer is 91%. This increasing survival rate is attributed to widespread annual mammograms and early biomarker detection tests [120]. While breast cancer predominantly affects women, men can also develop the disease [121].

In the U.S., 1 in 8 women will experience invasive breast cancer in their lifetime, whereas approximately 1 in 1,000 men will have breast cancer [122]. The incidence of breast cancer increases with age, primarily occurring in those over 50. According to the

American Cancer Society, breast cancer rates are highest among non-Hispanic white women.

Breast cancer is a highly heterogeneous neoplasm. Gene expression analysis has facilitated the identification and classification of distinct molecular subtypes. These subtypes are categorized based on the immunohistochemical presence of hormone receptors into four groups: estrogen receptor-positive (ER+), progesterone receptor-positive (PR+), human epidermal growth factor receptor-positive (HER2+), and triple-negative breast cancer (TNBC) [123].

The four major breast cancer subtypes are luminal A (LumA), luminal B (LumB), HER2+, and TNBC. LumA is characterized by being ER+ and/or PR+ and HER2-negative (HER2-). LumB, which has a more aggressive phenotype than LumA, is further divided into LumB HER2- (ER+ and/or PR+ and HER2-) and LumB HER2+ (ER+ and/or PR+ and HER2+) [124]. Cancers that do not fall into the LumA or LumB categories are considered hormone negative. TNBC is identified by the absence of ER, PR, and HER2 expressions and typically has the worst prognosis among the subgroups [125-126].

The 5-year relative survival rate for women in the US with non-metastatic invasive breast cancer is 91%, and the 10-year survival rate is 85%. Early detection significantly improves the likelihood of curing and surviving breast cancer. Mammograms are commonly used for early diagnosis, but their efficacy and accuracy can be limited, particularly in younger women with dense breast tissue [127].

Treatment modalities vary based on the cancer's stage and characteristics. For early, localized, and operable breast cancer, the general approach includes surgery, radiation, chemotherapy, targeted therapy, hormone therapy, and immunotherapy [128].

Hormone therapy is used for hormone receptor-positive cancers. It blocks hormone production or interferes with hormone behavior to slow or stop tumor growth. Hormonal therapy can cause hot flashes, vaginal dryness, mood swings, and joint pain. Long-term use, particularly of aromatase inhibitors, can lead to osteoporosis and increased fracture risk.

Targeted therapy drugs target specific abnormalities in cancer cells that allow them to grow and spread. Examples include trastuzumab (Herceptin ®) and pertuzumab (Perjeta ®), which target the HER2 protein. Immunotherapy helps the body's immune system recognize and attack cancer cells. Although not yet as common for breast cancer, it is being studied in clinical trials for its potential [129].

Common pharmacological agents for breast cancer, including trastuzumab, capecitabine, paclitaxel, doxorubicin, and cisplatin, have significant side effects. Cardiotoxicity and marrow neoplasia are notable concerns. Cardiotoxicity, associated with anthracyclines and trastuzumab, results from free radical production and impaired heart function. Dexrazoxane can reduce the risk of doxorubicin-induced cardiotoxicity, and continuous intravenous infusion of doxorubicin is less cardiotoxic than bolus administration [130-131].

Drug resistance is a growing issue in cancer treatment. Mechanisms of drug resistance include multi-drug resistance (MDR), suppression of apoptosis, changes in drug metabolism, epigenetic alterations, improved DNA repair, and gene amplification

[132]. MDR arises when cancer cells expel drugs more effectively, reducing drug absorption. DNA repair mechanisms, such as nucleotide excision repair and homologous recombination repair, contribute to resistance against drugs like cisplatin and doxorubicin. Gene amplification, seen in about 10% of cancer cases, increases the number of target genes, leading to resistance to drugs like methotrexate.

Studies have shown that high doses of VC can induce changes in the LumA cell line, affecting sphingomyelin metabolism, reducing cell viability, modulating cell cycle-related genes, and downregulating estrogen receptors in MCF-7 cells [126]. These alterations reflect the pleiotropic nature of pharmacologic VC, which targets multiple metabolic and signaling axes simultaneously. The disruption of sphingomyelin metabolism can impair membrane integrity and receptor clustering, contributing to altered hormone responsiveness and apoptosis induction. Moreover, modulation of genes involved in the cell cycle underscores VC's ability to suppress proliferation through G1/S checkpoint control, while the downregulation of estrogen receptors further attenuates hormonal signaling that drives MCF-7 cell survival and growth. Collectively, these findings reinforce the concept that high-dose VC not only acts as a pro-oxidant but also functions as a regulator of lipid metabolism, transcriptional activity, and hormonal pathways in hormone-sensitive breast cancer models.

Prostate Cancer

Prostate cancer (PCa) is a significant malignancy affecting men and is a major contributor to global mortality rates [133]. It is especially prevalent among men over the age of 65, with approximately six out of ten cases occurring in this age group. PCa is more common in Caribbean men of African ancestry and African American men compared to men of other races, though the reasons for this disparity remain unclear. Due to its high prevalence, PCa is the second most diagnosed solid-organ cancer in men, after lung cancer [134-135]. In 2018, PCa resulted in 358,989 deaths worldwide and approximately 1.3 million new diagnoses [136]. Currently, about 10 million men globally live with PCa, with roughly 700,000 having metastatic forms of the disease [137-138].

Prostate is divided into central, transitional, and peripheral regions. More than 95% of PCa cases are adenocarcinomas, primarily of acinar origin, with a few being of ductal origin [139]. If diagnosed at an early stage, the survival rate for men with localized PCa can be as high as 99% for over ten years [140]. However, managing a customized treatment plan is often necessary for those with slow-growing or indolent cancers. Conversely, some cases of relapsed PCa, following definitive treatment, may become aggressive and resistant to standard care. Approximately 5% of men with PCa are diagnosed with distant metastases, often in multiple sites, while 15% are diagnosed with locoregional metastases [138]. Men with late-stage PCa (distant metastases) have a poor five-year survival rate of only 30%. Metastatic PCa is responsible for over 400,000 deaths annually, and this mortality rate is expected to double by 2040 [137].

Treatment options for PCa include active surveillance, chemotherapy, radiation therapy, hormonal therapy, surgery, and cryotherapy, depending on the cancer's characteristics, such as prostate-specific antigen levels, grade, stage, and potential recurrence [141]. Active surveillance is used for low-grade, slow-growing localized PCa until treatment becomes necessary. Radical prostatectomy (RP) is the most common surgical approach, accounting for up to 90% of procedures. Radiotherapy is curative in 60% of localized PCa cases [141-143]. The proliferation and differentiation of PCa are largely driven by androgen receptors. Localized PCa usually responds to androgen deprivation therapy but most patients eventually develop castration-resistant PCa (CRPC) or metastatic CRPC (mCRPC) eventually become end-stage disease with no further effective solutions available [144].

Docetaxel (Taxotere ®) is a common chemotherapy drug for PCa [145]. This antimicrotubular agent inhibits microtubule depolymerization, suppressing mitotic cell division and causing apoptosis [146] However, resistance and relapse due to multidrug resistance (MDR1) gene encoding P-glycoprotein highlight the importance of combination therapy [147]. Combination therapy has proven effective for treating castration-resistant PCa, though no drugs currently cure CRPC. Approved and ongoing clinical trials include androgen deprivation therapy combined with radiation therapy, and other agents such as Sipuleucel T, docetaxel, abiraterone, and apalutamide. Despite these options, mCRPC remains incurable, with ongoing research focused on understanding the disease's growth, metastasis, tumorigenesis, tumor microenvironment, and interactions that promote progression [148].

Despite these limitations, integrating *VC* with current antineoplastic therapies may represent a promising adjunctive strategy. Evidence from both preclinical and early translational studies suggests that VC can enhance oxidative stress within tumor cells, sensitize resistant clones to therapy, and modulate pathways involved in apoptosis, DNA repair, and cellular metabolism. While metastatic castration-resistant prostate cancer (mCRPC) remains incurable, the redox-modulating potential of VC offers a unique avenue for overcoming therapeutic resistance and improving patient outcomes. Continued investigation into optimal dosing, delivery routes, and mechanistic synergies between VC and established drugs could pave the way for its inclusion as a supportive or combination treatment in advanced prostate cancer.

Chronic Myelogenous Leukemia

Chronic myelogenous leukemia (CML) is cancer that primarily affects adults between 45 to 65 years old. CML rarely occurs in younger individuals or in children. This cancer represents about 15-20% of adult leukemias in Western countries, with an estimated incidence of 1-2 cases per 100,000 people annually in the US. CML affect males more than females with ratio approximately 1.5:1 [149-150].

While CML can arise sporadically, certain risk factors are associated with an increased likelihood of developing the disease such as previous exposure to ionizing radiation, as demonstrated in survivors of the atomic bombings in Japan, who exhibited an increased incidence of CML. Family history of CML, or other genetic predispositions do not significantly elevate the risk of CML [151].

About 95% of CML cases are due to genetic abnormality known as the Philadelphia (Ph) chromosome, which arises from a reciprocal translocation between chromosomes 9 and 22 that result in the fusion of the BCR (breakpoint cluster region) gene on chromosome 22 and the ABL1 (Abelson murine leukemia) gene on chromosome 9 [152]. This BCR-ABL fusion gene produces a constitutively active tyrosine kinase that drives uncontrolled cellular proliferation, reduced apoptosis, and impaired cell differentiation in hematopoietic cells [153]. The BCR-ABL tyrosine kinase signaling pathway plays a central role in the development and progression of CML, making it a prime target for therapeutic interventions [154].

Treatment Options include tyrosine kinase inhibitors (TKIs), hematopoietic stem cell transplantation, Interferon-alpha, and chemotherapy. TKIs are now the mainstay of CML treatment. Imatinib, the first TKI approved for CML, revolutionized CML therapy by targeting the BCR-ABL tyrosine kinase. Subsequent TKIs, such as dasatinib, nilotinib, bosutinib, and ponatinib, provide options for patients with imatinib resistance or intolerance [155]. TKIs have transformed CML from a fatal disease to a manageable chronic condition for most patients [156].

Vitamin C has been identified to enhance the activity of the ten-eleven translocation (TET) family of enzymes, which are involved in DNA demethylation. This process plays a role in the regulation of cancer stem cells, particularly in leukemias. In CML, the activity of TET enzymes is often reduced, leading to aberrant DNA methylation that can promote cancer cell proliferation. Vitamin C's role in enhancing TET activity can, therefore, potentially help restore normal gene expression patterns and reduce the leukemia stem cell population [157]. In addition, VC may enhance the efficacy of TKIs by promoting oxidative stress in CML cells while also acting on pathways that support leukemia cell death [158]. VC may also promote differentiation in leukemia stem cells, potentially making them more susceptible to standard therapies and reducing the risk of relapse [159]. Future preclinical and clinical studies are warranted to define optimal dosing, administration routes, and combinational strategies integrating VC with existing targeted therapies.

Chronic Lymphocytic Leukemia

Chronic lymphocytic leukemia (CLL) is cancer that primarily affects older adults, characterized by the accumulation of impaired but mature B-lymphocytes in the blood, bone marrow, and lymphoid tissues. CLL is most common form of leukemia in adults in Western countries, but it is rare in Asian populations [160]. In the United States, CLL accounts for approximately 25-30% of all leukemia cases, with an estimated incidence of 4-6 cases per 100,000 people annually [161]. CLL is rare in people under 40 years old, with a median age at diagnosis 70 years old. It is more common in men than in women, with a male-to-female ratio of approximately 1.7:1 [162].

CLL is due to the clonal expansion of $CD5^+$ B cells that are arrested at an intermediate stage of differentiation. The leukemic cells evade apoptosis process due to genetic mutations and alterations in the B-cell receptor (BCR) signaling pathway which plays a critical role in the survival and proliferation of CLL cells. Overactivity of this pathway promotes cancer growth and progression [163]. Additionally, CLL cells create an immunosuppressive microenvironment that can impair T-cell function, allowing the leukemia cells to evade immune surveillance [164].

This cancer has a highly variable clinical course, with survival ranging from months to decades, depending on the risk factors and genetic profile of the patient. While some patients may never require treatment, others experience rapid disease progression and require early intervention. The median overall survival for CLL varies significantly, with early-stage patients having a life expectancy close to that of the general population, while those with high-risk features, such as 17p deletions, have shorter survival [160].

The management of CLL depends on disease stage, symptoms, and genetic factors. Treatment is generally not initiated in asymptomatic patients but is considered in those with disease progression or significant symptoms using chemotherapy/immunotherapy, targeted therapy, or monoclonal antibodies.

Chemoimmunotherapy with fludarabine, cyclophosphamide, and rituximab (FCR) was historically the standard of care for younger, fit patients without TP53 mutations, while bendamustine combined with rituximab (BR) has also been used in older or less fit patients [165]. The development of targeted therapies has transformed the treatment landscape for CLL, particularly for high-risk patients. Ibrutinib, a Bruton's tyrosine kinase (BTK) inhibitor, is highly effective in treating CLL by inhibiting the BCR signaling pathway, essential for CLL cell survival. Ibrutinib is approved as a first-line treatment and for relapsed or refractory CLL [166]. Another targeted therapy is phosphoinositide 3-kinase (P13K) and BCL-2 Inhibitors. Idelalisib, a PI3K inhibitor, is often used in combination with rituximab for relapsed or refractory CLL who cannot tolerate chemotherapy [167]. Venetoclax, targets the anti-apoptotic protein BCL-2, induces cell death in CLL cells and is effective in patients with 17p deletions or TP53 mutations. It can be used as monotherapy or in combination with other agents [168].

Vitamin C has been studied for its potential role in CLL, primarily due to its properties as an antioxidant and its ability to influence cellular processes such as apoptosis and immune function. High-dose VC has been shown to exert pro-oxidative effects that may selectively target cancer cells while sparing normal cells, making it an attractive candidate for cancer therapy [169]. However, clinical studies specifically evaluating vitamin C as a monotherapy for CLL are limited and inconclusive.

As an adjunctive therapy in CLL treatment to enhance the effects of chemotherapy or targeted therapies, VC can improve the cytotoxicity of certain chemotherapeutic agents leading to better outcomes [170-171]. Preclinical research has indicated that VC can sensitize CLL cells to the effects of fludarabine and rituximab, making it a candidate for combination therapy strategies [172]. Overall, the adjunctive use of vitamin C (VC) in chronic lymphocytic leukemia (CLL) therapy holds significant translational potential. By enhancing the cytotoxic effects of established agents such as fludarabine and rituximab, VC may help overcome chemoresistance and augment apoptosis through redox modulation and mitochondrial stress pathways. Furthermore, VC's ability to alter cellular antioxidant balance and promote pro-oxidant signaling can sensitize malignant B cells to immune-mediated cytotoxicity. Future studies should focus on optimizing dosing regimens, administration routes, and pharmacologic combinations to harness VC's synergistic potential while maintaining selectivity for leukemic cells over normal lymphocytes.

Non-Small Cell Lung Cancer

Non-small cell lung cancer (NSCLC) accounts for approximately 85% of all lung cancer cases, making it the most common type of lung cancer worldwide. It is especially prevalent among smokers, former smokers, and non-smokers. NSCLC incidence rates vary geographically, with the highest rates found in North America, Europe, and parts of Asia. This variation reflects differences in smoking prevalence and exposure to environmental carcinogens [173]. It is more common in men over 65 years [174]. This cancer has the highest incidence and mortality rates, with over 1.8 million new cases and 1.6 million deaths annually. Lung cancer remains the leading cause of cancer-related mortality worldwide, with NSCLC contributing significantly to this statistic [175]. With a steady decline in smoking rates, the incidence of mortality also has been decreased [173].

Histological subtypes include adenocarcinoma, squamous cell carcinoma, and large cell carcinoma. The pathogenesis of NSCLC often involves a series of genetic and molecular alterations that lead to uncontrolled cell proliferation, resistance to cell death, and eventually cancer progression. Common genetic mutations include *EGFR*, *KRAS*, and anaplastic lymphoma kinase (*ALK*) genes, and environmental factors like tobacco smoking. contribute to the mutational burden seen in lung cancer, promoting genomic instability and increased mutation rates in lung epithelial cells [176-177].

The prognosis for NSCLC varies widely depending on the stage at diagnosis, histological subtype, and molecular characteristics. Early-stage NSCLC, where the tumor is localized, has a five-year survival rate of 60-80% with surgical resection and appropriate adjuvant therapy. However, the five-year survival rate for advanced-stage NSCLC remains poor, ranging from 6-20% [178]. The advent of targeted therapies and immune checkpoint inhibitors has improved survival rates for certain NSCLC subtypes, but overall, late-stage NSCLC is associated with a high mortality rate [179].

Several biomarkers play a critical role in NSCLC diagnosis, prognosis, and treatment selection. These include genetic mutations in EGFR (common in non-smokers), KRAS (more prevalent in smokers), and ALK rearrangements. Other biomarkers include programmed death- ligand 1(PD-L1) expression, which can help predict responses to immunotherapy, and mesenchymal epithelial transition factor receptor (MET) amplifications, seen in an advanced NSCLC case [180]. Biomarker testing is essential for determining eligibility for targeted therapies, such as EGFR inhibitors erlotinib, osimertinib or ALK inhibitors alectinib, crizotinib, and can significantly improve outcomes in patients with these mutations [181]. Immune checkpoint inhibitors, such as pembrolizumab and nivolumab, have shown promise in treating advanced NSCLC in patients with high PD-L1 expression. By targeting the PD-1/PD-L1 pathway, these therapies enhance immune system activity against the cancer cells [182].

Vitamin C has been explored as a complementary therapy in cancer treatment due to its antioxidant properties and potential pro-oxidative effects at high concentrations. While its role in cancer therapy remains controversial, there is growing evidence suggesting that high-dose VC may enhance the efficacy of standard treatments in NSCLC [183]. Preclinical studies have shown that high-dose VC can induce oxidative stress, disrupt cancer cell metabolism, and enhance the efficacy of chemotherapy and radiation therapy [184].

Combining VC with cisplatin may increase cytotoxicity in NSCLC cells and improving treatment outcomes [185]. VC can sensitize cancer cells to chemotherapy by increasing oxidative stress within the tumor microenvironment, leading to higher rates of cancer cell death [186]. A phase I trial demonstrated that high-dose VC was well-tolerated and showed signs of tumor regression in combination with chemotherapy, although the overall survival benefit remains uncertain due to limited sample sizes and study duration [187]. Another clinical trial showed improvement in quality of life in NSCLC patients treated with VC and chemotherapy, though the effect on overall survival was not conclusive [188].

Collectively, these studies highlight the potential of vitamin C (VC) as a valuable adjuvant to standard chemotherapy regimens in non–small cell lung cancer (NSCLC). By enhancing oxidative stress within the tumor microenvironment, VC can potentiate the cytotoxic activity of agents like cisplatin, leading to increased cancer cell apoptosis and improved treatment response. Clinical evidence indicates that high-dose intravenous VC is generally well-tolerated and may contribute to tumor regression and better quality of life in NSCLC patients, even though definitive survival benefits remain to be proven. Continued investigation through larger, controlled trials is essential to establish optimal dosing schedules, patient selection criteria, and mechanistic insights that could transform VC from an experimental adjunct to a clinically integrated component of NSCLC therapy.

Renal Cancer

Renal cancer is relatively rare compared to other cancers but has been on the rise in recent decades. According to the Global Cancer Observatory, renal cancer was estimated to cause approximately 431,288 new cases and 179,368 deaths worldwide in the next decade, emphasizing the urgency of addressing this significant global health trend [189-190]. The highest incidence rates are observed in North America and Europe, while lower rates are reported in Asia and Africa. Risk factors for developing renal cancer include smoking, obesity, hypertension, and genetic syndromes, such as von Hippel-Lindau (VHL) disease and hereditary papillary renal cell carcinoma.

The most common subtype of kidney cancer is renal cell carcinoma (RCC) that account for 90% of cases. RCC are further divided into clear cell (ccRCC) account for 70% of the cases, papillary (pRCC-type 1 and 2) account for 10–15%, and chromophobe (chRCC) account for 5% [191]. Each has distinct genetic alterations and clinical manifestations. Histological subtypes are linked to overall survival and cancer specific survival, with a better prognosis is usually with chRCC subtype [192].

The pathophysiology of kidney cancer is complex and often involves multiple pathways such as *mTOR, MAPK/ERK*, and the *PI3K/AKT* signaling pathway implicated in cancer progression and metastasis. In advanced stages, this cancer can metastasize to various organs, including the lungs, liver, bones and adrenal gland [193-194].

Treatment of renal cancer varies based on the stage of the disease and individual patient factors. The treatment modalities include chemotherapy, surgical, radiofrequency ablation (RFA), targeted therapy and immunotherapy. Chemotherapy is generally not effective for RCC and is rarely used, except in specific cases of advanced or metastatic disease [195].

Tyrosine kinase inhibitors (TKIs) such as sunitinib, pazopanib, cabozantinib, axitinib, sorafenib have been approved to treat advanced RCC. These agents target specific pathways involved in cancer growth and angiogenesis [196-197]. Besides TKIs, another targeted therapy such as immune checkpoint inhibitors (ICIs), such as nivolumab and pembrolizumab, have also revolutionized the treatment landscape for RCC and metastatic RCC by enhancing the body's immune response against cancer cells. In addition, various combinations of TKIs and ICIs have been assessed and are currently considered the preferred regimen for all metastatic RCC patients [196-198].

Vitamin C has been explored as both a monotherapy and adjunctive treatment in renal cancer, primarily due to its potential to enhance the efficacy of conventional treatments, to reduce oxidative stress, and to promote apoptosis in renal cancer cells. However, its use in clinical practice remains largely experimental, with most studies focusing on its role as an adjunctive therapy. The use of high-dose vitamin C as a monotherapy for kidney cancer is not well-established. While preclinical studies have shown that VC can induce oxidative stress, interfere with cancer cell metabolism, induce apoptosis in renal cancer cells, clinical trials focusing on VC as monotherapy are limited [199].

Renal cancer management continues to evolve with advances in targeted therapies, immunotherapy, and personalized medicine. Research is ongoing to identify new biomarkers for early detection and prognosis, as well as to develop more effective treatment strategies.

Conclusion

The exploration of various cancers ranging from hepatocellular carcinoma (HCC) and malignant pleural mesothelioma (MPM) to breast cancer and chronic leukemias, reveals the complexity and heterogeneity inherent to oncological diseases. Each type of cancer is defined by its unique etiology, pathophysiological mechanisms, diagnostic markers, and prognosis. The diversity in cancer biology underscores the need for personalized and multifaceted treatment approaches.

In HCC, a condition primarily associated with chronic liver disease and cirrhosis, advances in biomarkers and imaging techniques have enabled earlier detection. Treatment modalities, including surgical resection, liver transplantation, and targeted therapies like sorafenib, highlight the evolving landscape of HCC management. In MPM, a cancer strongly linked to asbestos exposure, the pathophysiological profile marked by aggressive pleural thickening requires a combination of chemotherapy, surgery, and emerging immunotherapeutic agents.

The osteosarcoma and neuroblastoma information elucidate the challenges faced in pediatric oncology. While osteosarcoma is often addressed with surgical intervention and multi-agent chemotherapy, neuroblastoma treatment is more varied, involving immunotherapy, differentiation agents, and molecular-targeted strategies. Biomarkers amplification in neuroblastoma provides critical prognostic information that shapes therapeutic decisions.

CRC and pancreatic cancer both present substantial treatment challenges due to late-stage diagnoses and metastatic potential. In CRC, advancements in the understanding of molecular pathways, such as Wnt/β-catenin and microsatellite instability, have informed the use of targeted agents like bevacizumab and cetuximab. Pancreatic cancer, notorious for its dismal prognosis, has seen incremental improvements with the advent of FOLFIRINOX and gemcitabine-based regimens.

Breast cancer and prostate cancer are often typified by their hormonal dependencies. The roles of estrogen and androgen receptors have paved the way for targeted endocrine therapies, including tamoxifen and enzalutamide. The integration of precision medicine approaches, including gene expression profiling and PARP inhibitors, has expanded the therapeutic against these prevalent malignancies.

In CML and CLL, breakthroughs in targeted therapy, TKIs such as imatinib, have transformed the treatment landscape, turning these once-fatal diseases into manageable chronic conditions. In NSCLC, a leading cause of lung cancer mortality, there has been significant progress with the introduction of immune checkpoint inhibitors and targeted therapies aimed at mutations like *EGFR* and *ALK*.

Renal carcinoma, with its complex pathophysiological mechanisms involving VHL gene mutations, has benefited from targeted treatment approaches like VEGF inhibitors and immune-based therapies. These developments have improved survival rates and provided new hope for patients.

The role of VC has been discussed as an adjunctive therapy, exploring its pro-oxidant and antioxidant properties and its ability to modulate various cellular pathways. The use of VC at pharmacological concentrations has demonstrated potential in enhancing the efficacy of traditional chemotherapeutic agents and in selectively inducing cytotoxicity in cancer cells while sparing normal tissues. This dual role of VC, as both a complementary agent and a potential standalone treatment, offers an intriguing prospect for future cancer therapy.

The cumulative understanding of these cancers underscores that while significant strides have been made, the fight against cancer remains formidable. The interplay between genetics, environmental factors, and cellular biology continues to shape the development of novel therapies. Integrative approaches that combine conventional treatments with adjunctive agents like VC represent a promising frontier in oncology. Future research should prioritize clinical trials that substantiate these findings, refining our knowledge and enhancing outcomes for patients worldwide.

References

[1] Choi S., Kim B.K., Yon D.K., Lee S.W., Chang H.H., Park S., et al., Global burden of primary liver cancer and its association with underlying etiologies, sociodemographic status, and sex differences from 1990-2019: A DALY-based analysis of the Global Burden of Disease 2019 study. *Clin Mol Hepatology* 2023; 29 :433-452.

[2] Bray F., Ferlay J., Soerjomataram I., Siegel R.L., Torre L.A., Jemal A. Global cancer statistic 2018: GLOBOCAN estimates of incidence and mortality worldwide for 36 cancers in 185 countries. CA *Cancer J Clin* 2020 ; 70 :313.

[3] Rumgay H., Arnold M., Ferlay J., Vignat J., McGlynn K.A., Soerjomataram I. Global burden of primary liver cancer in 2020 and predictions to 2040. *J Hepatol* 2022 ; 77 : 1598-1606.

[4] Yu S., Wang H., Hu T., Chen X. Disease burden of liver cancer attributable to specific etiologies in China from 1990 to 2019: An age-period cohort analysis. *Sci Prog* 2021 ; 104 :368504211018081.

[5] Liu F., Gai X., Wu Y., Zhang B., Wu X., Cheng R., et al., Oncogenic β-catenin stimulation of AKT2-CAD-mediated pyrimidine synthesis is targetable vulnerability in liver cancer. PNAS. 2022 ; 119(39) : e2202157119.

[6] Sia D., Villanueva A., Friedman S.L., Llovet J.M. Liver cancer cell of origin, molecular class, and effects on patient prognosis. *Gastroenterology* 2017 ;152 : 745–761.

[7] Bioulac-Sage P., Laumonier H., Laurent C., Zucman-Rossi J., Balabaud C. Hepatocellular adenoma: What is new in 2008. *Hepatol. Int.* 2008 ; 2 : 316–321.

[8] Monga S.P. β-catenin signaling and roles in liver homeostasis, injury, and tumorigenesis. *Gastroenterology* 2015 ; 148 : 1294–1310.

[9] Garcia-Lezana T., Lopez-Canovas J.L., Villanueva A. Signaling pathways in hepatocellular carcinoma. *Adv Cancer Res*. 2021 ; 149 : 63-101.

[10] Harada N., Tamai Y., Ishikawa T., Taketo M.M. Intestinal polyposis in mice with a dominant stable mutation of the beta catenin gene. *EMBO.J* 1999 ; 18 : 5931-5942.

[11] Harada N., Miyoshi H., Murai N., Tamai Y., Oshima M., Taketo M.M. Lack of tumorigenesis in the mouse liver after adenovirus-mediated expression of a dominant stable mutant of beta-catenin. *Cancer Res* 2002 ; 62 : 1971-1977.

[12] Toh T.B., Lim J.J., Hooi L., Rashid M.B.M.A., Chow E.K. Targeting Jak/stat pathway as a therapeutic strategy against SP/CD44+ tumorigenic cells in Akt/β catenin-driven hepatocellular carcinoma. *J Hepatol* 2020 ; 72 : 104-118.

[13] Hoxhaj G., Manning B. The p13K-AKT network at the interface of oncogenic signaling and cancer metabolism. *Nat Rev Cancer* 2020 ; 20 : 74-88.

[14] Chen Z.H., Hong Y.F., Lin J., Li X., Wu D.H., Wen J.Y., et al., Validation and ranking of seven staging systems of hepatocellular carcinoma. *Oncol Lett* 2017 ;14 : 705–714.

[15] Zhang J.F., Shu Z.J., Xie C.Y., Jin X.H., Gu W., Jiang F.J., et al., Prognosis of unresectable hepatocellular carcinoma: Comparison of seven staging systems (TNM, Okuda, BCLC, CLIP, CUPI, JIS, CIS) in a Chinese cohort. *PLoS ONE* 2014 ; 9 : e88182.

[16] Huang P.S., Wang L.Y., Tsai M.M., Lin T.K., Yeh C.T., Lin K.H. Evaluation and application of drug resistance by biomarkers in the clinical treatment of liver cancer. *Cells* 2023; 12: 869.

[17] Reig M., Forner A., Rimola J., Ferrer-Fabrega J., Galle P.R., Mazzaferro V., et al., BCLC strategy for prognosis prediction and treatment recommendation: The 2022 update. *J. Hepatol.* 2022 ; 76 : 681–693.

[18] Jiang S.H., Li S., Dong F.Y., Yang J.Y., Liu D.J., Wang J.H., et al., Increased serotonin signaling contributes to the Warburg effect in pancreatic tumor cells under metabolic stress and promotes growth of pancreatic tumors in mice. *Gastroenterology* 2017 ; 153 : 277-291.

[19] Abdelgalil A.A., Alkahtani H.M., Al-Jenoobi F.I. Sorafenib. *Profile Drug Subst* Excip Relat *Methodol* 2019 ; 44 : 239–266.

[20] Olten M.A., Matuz R., Sitar-Taut A., Rednic N., Minciuna I.A., Orasan O., et al., Renal Cell Carcinoma with Extensive Tumor Thrombus Into the Inferior Vena Cava and Right Atrium in a 70-Year-Old Man. *Am. J. Men's Health* 2019 ; 13 : 1557988319846404.

[21] Pearson H., Marshall L.V., Carceller F. Sorafenib in pediatric hepatocellular carcinoma from a clinician perspective. *Pediatr Hematol Oncol* 2020 ; 37 :412–423.

[22] Li Z.J., Dai H.Q., Huang X.W., Feng J., Wang Z.X., Liu Y.J., et al., Artesunate synergizes with sorafenib to induce ferroptosis in hepatocellular carcinoma. *Acta Pharmacol Sin* 2021 ; 42 : 301–310.

[23] Zhang X., Zhu X.J., Zhong Z., Du J.C., Cui X.L., Hu Y.H, et al., Small molecule-induced differentiation as a potential therapy for liver cancer. *Adv Sci* 2022 ; 9 : 2103619.

[24] Mousa A.B. Sorafenib in the treatment of advanced hepatocellular carcinoma. Saudi J. *Gastroenterol.* 2008 ; 14 : 40-42.

[25] Zhu Y.J., Zheng B., Wang H.Y., Chen L. New knowledge of the mechanisms of sorafenib resistance in liver cancer. *Acta Pharmacol Sin* 2017 ; 38 : 614–622.

[26] Jain A., Chitturi S., Peters G., Yip D. Atezolizumab and bevacizumab as first line therapy in advanced hepatocellular carcinoma: Practical considerations in routine clinical practice. *World J Hepatol* 2021 ; 13, 1132–1142.

[27] Qin S., Ren Z., Feng Y.H., Yau T., Zhao H., Gu S., et al., Atezolizumab plus Bevacizumab versus Sorafenib in the Chinese Subpopulation with Unresectable Hepatocellular Carcinoma: Phase 3 Randomized, Open-Label IMbrave150 Study. *Liver Cancer 2021* ; 10 : 296–308.

[28] Llovet J.M., Castet F., Heikenwalder M., Mazzaferro V., Pikarsky E., Zhu A.X., et al., Immunotherapies for hepatocellular carcinoma. *Nat Rev Clin Oncol* 2022 ; 19 : 151–161.

[29] Yau T., Kang Y.K., Kim T.Y., El-Khoueiry A.B., Sangro B., Kudo M., et al., Efficacy and Safety of Nivolumab Plus Ipilimumab in Patients with Advanced Hepatocellular Carcinoma Previously Treated with Sorafenib: The Checkmate 040 Randomized Clinical Trial. *JAMA Oncol* 2020 ; 6: e204564.

[30] De Luca E., Marino D., Di Maio M. Ramucirumab, A Second-Line Option for Patients with Hepatocellular Carcinoma: A Review of The Evidence. *Cancer Manag Res* 2020 ; 12 : 3721–3729.

[31] Tan C., Cao J., Chen L., Xi X., Zhu Y., Ma L., et al., Noncoding RNAs Serve as Diagnosis and Prognosis Biomarkers for Hepatocellular Carcinoma. *Clin Chem* 2019 ; 65 : 905–915.

[32] Tomimaru Y., Eguchi H., Nagano H., Wada H., Kobayashi S., Takeda Y, et al., MicroRNA-21 induces resistance to the anti-tumor effect of interferon-alpha/5-fluorouracil in hepatocellular carcinoma cells. *Br. J. Cancer* 2010 ; 103 : 1617–1626.

[33] Karunakaran K.B., Yanamala N., Boyce G., Ganapathi Raju M.K. Malignant pleural mesothelioma interactions with 364 novel protein-protein interactions. *Cancer* 2021 ;13 : 1660.

[34] Mutti L., Peikert L., Robinson B.W.S., Carbone M., Thomas A., Hassan R. Scientific advances, and new frontiers in mesothelioma therapeutics. *J Thorac Oncol* 2018 ; 13 : 1269-1283.

[35] Carbone M., Baris Y.I., Bertino P., Way S., Yang H., Miller A. Erionite exposure in North Dakota and Turkish villages with mesothelioma. *PNAS* 2011 ; 108 : 13618–13623.

[36] Baumann F., Buck B.J., Metcalf R.V., Merkler D.J., Carbone M. The presence of asbestos in the natural environment is likely related to mesothelioma in young individuals and women from Southern Nevada. *J Thorac Oncol* 2015 ; 10 : 731–737.

[37] Gray S.G. Emerging avenues in immunotherapy for the management of malignant pleural mesothelioma. *BMC Pulmonary Med* 2021 ; 21 : 148.

[38] Hemminki K., Forsti A., Chen T., Hemminki A. Incidence, mortality, and survival in malignant pleural mesothelioma before and after asbestos in Denmark, Finland, Norway and Sweden. *BMC cancer* 2021 ; 21 : 1189.

[39] Zhai Y., Hui Z., Chen W., Ying J., Li J., Gao S. The epidemic of malignant mesothelioma in China: a prediction of incidence during 2016-2030. *Trans Lung Cancer Res* 2022 ; 11 : 2403-2411.

[40] WHO. Cancer tomorrow -A tool that predicts the future cancer incidence and mortality burden worldwide from the current estimates in 2018 up until 2040. Available online : *https://gco.iarc.fr/tomorrow/home.*

[41] Roe O.D., Stella G.M. Malignant pleural mesothelioma: history, controversy and future of a man-made epidemic. *Eur Respira Rev* 2015; 24, 115–131.

[42] Peto J., Decarli A., La Vecchia C. The European mesotelioma epidemic. *Br J Cancer* 1999; 79: 666–672.

[43] Fennell D.A., Gaudino G., O'Byrne K.J., van Meerbeeck J. Advances in the systemic therapy of malignant pleural mesothelioma. *Nat Clin Pract Oncol* 2008 ; 5 : 136–147.

[44] Schrepel A., Astoul P., Baas P. Guidelines of the European Respiratory Society and the European Society of Thoracic Surgeons for the management of malignant pleural mesothelioma. *Eur Respir J* 2010 ; 35 : 479–495.

[45] Creaney J., Robinson B.W. Malignant mesothelioma biomarkers - from discovery to use in clinical practice for diagnosis, monitoring, screening, and treatment. *Chest* 2017 ; 152 : 143–149.

[46] Callis Leo. EPA makes 'historic' ruling to ban hazardous material: "a symbol of how then law can and must be used. *http://www.msn.com*. Retrieved April 13, 2024.

[47] Schaerbeek E., van Meerbeeck J.P., Lamote K. Clinical utility of diagnostic biomarkers in malignant pleural mesothelioma: a systematic review and meta-analysis. *Eur Respir Rev* 2021 ; 30: 210057.

[48] Scherpereel A., Opitz I., Bergmans T., Glatzer M., Fennell D., Hoda M.A., et al., ERS/ESTS/EACTS/ESTRO guidelines for the management of malignant pleural mesothelioma. *Eur Respir J* 2020 ; 55 : 1900953.

[49] Arnold D.T., Maskell N.A. Biomarkers in mesothelioma. *Ann Clin Biochem* 2018 ; 55 : 49–58.

[50] Lamote K., Nackaerts K., van Meer Beeck J.P. Strengths, weaknesses, and opportunities of diagnostic breath omics in pleural mesothelioma-a hypothesis. *Cancer Epidemiol Biomarkers Prev* 2014 ; 23 : 898–908.

[51] Robinson B.W.S., Creaney J., Lake R. Soluble mesothelin-related protein - a blood test for mesothelioma. *Lung Cancer* 2005; 49: S109–S111.

[52] Ceresoli G., Zucali P.A., Favaretto A.G., Morenghi E., Cavina R., Parra H.J., et al., Phase II study of pemetrexed plus carboplatin in malignant pleural mesothelioma. *J Clin Oncol* 2006 ; 24 : 1443–1448.

[53] Schulte J.J., Husain A.N. Update on the pathologic diagnosis of malignant mesothelioma. *Transl Lung Cancer Res* 2020 ; 9 : 917-923.

[54] Kindler H.L., Ismalia N., Armato III S.G., Jahan T., Jones C.M., Pass H., et al., Treatment of malignant pleural mesothelioma: American Society of Clinical Oncology Clinical Practice Guideline. *J Clin Oncol* 2018 ; 36 : 1343-1373.

[55] Xiang Y., Yang Y., Liu J., Yang X. Functional role of MicroRNA/p13K/AKT axis in osteosarcoma. *Frontiers Oncology* 2023 ; 10.3389/fonc.2023.1219211.

[56] Roth R.E., Ho X.D., Xu J., Wood D., Martson A., Maasalu K. Alternative splicing of leptin receptor overlapping transcript in osteosarcoma. *Exp Biol Med* (Maywood) 2020 ; 245 :1437–1443.

[57] Xu R., Feng F., Yu X., Liu Z., Lao L. LncRNA SNHG4 promotes tumor growth by sponging miR-224-3p and predicts poor survival and recurrence in human osteosarcoma. *Cell Proliferation* 2018 ; 51 : e12515.

[58] Isakoff M.S., Bielack S.S., Meltzer P., Gorlick R. Osteosarcoma: current treatment and a collaborative pathway to success. *J Clin Oncol* 2015 ; 33 :3029–35.

[59] Martins-Neves S.R., Sampaio-Ribeiro G., Gomes C.M.F. Self-renewal and pluripotency in osteosarcoma stem cells' chemoresistance: Notch, Hedgehog, and Wnt/β-catenin interplay with embryonic markers. *Int J Mol Sci* 2023; 24: 8401.

[60] *https://seer.cancer.gov/statfacts/html/bones.html*. Access May 20, 2024.

[61] Mirabello L., Troisi R.J., Aavage S.A. International osteosarcoma incidence patterns in children and adolescent, Middle Ages, and elderly persons. *Int J Cancer* 2009; 125: 229-234.

[62] Ritter J., Bielak S.S. Osteosarcoma. *Ann Oncol* 2010; 21: vii320-vii325.

[63] Cole S., Gianferante D.M., Zhu B., Mirabello L. Osteosarcoma: A surveillance, Epidemiology, and end results program-based analysis from 1975 to 2017. *Cancer* 2022 ; 128 : 2107-2118.

[64] Angulo P., Kaushik G., Subramaniam D., Dandawate P., Neville K., Chastain K., et al., Natural compounds targeting major cell signaling pathways: a novel paradigm for osteosarcoma therapy. *J Hematol & Oncol* 2017 ; 10 :10.

[65] Liao Y., He J., Huang D., Xiong J., Sun W., Sun W. Extracellular vesicles in tumorigenesis, metastasis, chemotherapy resistance and intercellular communication in osteosarcoma. *Bioengineered* 2023 ; 14 : 113-128.

[66] Kok V.C., Yu C.C. Cancer-derived exosomes; their role in cancer biology and biomarker development. *Int J Nanomedicine* 2020 ; 15 : 8019-8036.

[67] Jeppesen D.K., Fenix A.M., Franklin J.L. Reassessment of exosome composition. *Cell* 2019 ; 177 : 428-445.

[68] Sil S., Dagur R.S., Liao K. Strategies for the use of extracellular vesicles for the delivery of therapeutics. *J Neuroimmune Pharmacol* 2020 ; 15 : 422-442.

[69] Martin J.W., Squire J.A., Zielenska M. The genetics of osteosarcoma. *Sarcoma* 2012 ; 627254.

[70] Czarnecka A.M., Firley W., Sobzuk P., Fiedorowicz M., Grieb P., Rutkowski P. Molecular biology of osteosarcoma. *Cancers* 2020 ; 12 : 2130.

[71] Zhang J., Yu X.H., Yan Y.G., Wang C., Wang WJ. P13/Akt signaling in osteosarcoma. *Clin Chim Acta* 2015 ; 444 : 182-192.

[72] Amirhossein A., Goldin M., Kulidjian A.A.W Osteosarcoma: a comprehensive review. *SICOT J* 2018 ; 4 : 1-12.

[73] Harris M.A., Hawkins C.J. Recent and ongoing research into metastatic osteosarcoma treatments. *Int J Mol Sci* 2022 ; 23 : 3817.

[74] Duffaud F., Mir O., Boudou-Rouquette P., Panel N., Italiano A., Collard O. Efficacy and safety of regorafenib in adult patients with metastatic osteosarcoma: a non-comparative randomized, double blind, placebo-controlled, phase 2. *Lancet Oncol* 2019 ; 20 : 120-133.

[75] Le Cessna A., Berard P., Blay J.Y., Gaspar N, Penel N, Cousin S, et al., Programmed cell death 1 (PD-1) targeting in patients with advanced osteosarcoma: Results from the PEMBROSARC study. *Eur J Cancer* 2019 ; 119 : 151-157.

[76] Goldsby R.E., Fan T.M., Wagner L.M., Isakoff M.S., Randall R.L., Lee S., et al., Feasibility, and dose discovery analysis of zoledronic acid with concurrent chemotherapy in the treatment of newly diagnosed metastatic osteosarcoma: A report from the Children's Oncology Group. *Eur J Cancer* 2013 ; 49 : 2384-2391.

[77] Oka N., Komuro A., Amano H., Honda M., Nishimura S., Akagi M, et al., Ascorbate sensitizes human osteosarcoma cells to the cytostatic effects of cisplatin. *Pharmacol Res Perspect* 2020 ; e00632.

[78] Williamson M.R., Klug M.G., Schwartz G.G. Brain cancer incidence rates and the presence of nuclear reactors in US States: a hypothesis-generating study. *Environ Geochem Health* 2021 ; 43 : 3967-3975.

[79] Louis D.N., Perry A., Reifenberger G., von Deimling A., Figarella B.D., Cavence WK. The 2016 World Health Organization classification of tumors of the central nervous system: A summary. *Acta Neuropathologica* 2016 ; 131 : 803-820.

[80] Ahmad F., Varghese R., Panda S., Areeshi M.Y., Fagoonee S., Haque S. Smart Nano formulations for brain cancer theragnostic: challenges and promises. *Cancers* 2022 ; 14 : 5389.

[81] Mercaldo F., Brunese L., Martinelli F., Santone A., Cesarelli M. Explainable convolutional neural networks for brain cancer detection and localization. *Sensors* 2023 ; 23 : 7614.

[82] *National Cancer Institute. Neuroblastoma Treatment (PDQ).* 2020. https://www.cancer.gov/types/neuroblastoma/hp/neuroblastoma-treatment-pdq on April 9, 2021.

[83] Rushing E.J. WHO classification of tumors of the nervous system: preview of the upcoming 5th edition. *Memo Mag Euro Med Oncol* 2021 ; 14 : 188-191.

[84] Polivka J., Holubec L., Kubikova T., Priban V., Hes O., Treskova I. Advances in experimental targeted therapy and immunotherapy for patients with glioblastoma multiforme. *Anticancer Res* 2017 ; 37 : 21-33.

[85] Newman E.A., Abdessalam S., Aldrink J.H., Austin M., Heaton T.E., Bruny J., et al., APSA Cancer committee. Update on neuroblastoma. *J Pediatric Surg* 2019 ; 54(3) :383-389.

[86] Capasso M., Devoto M., Hou C., Glessner J.T., Attiyeh E.F., Mosse Y.P., et al., Common variations in BARD1 influence susceptibility to high-risk neuroblastoma. *Nat Genet* 2009 ;41(6) :718-723.

[87] Maris J.M., Hogarty M.D., Bagatell R., Cohn S.L. Neuroblastoma. *Lancet* 2007 ; 23 ;2106-2120.

[88] Brodeur G.M., Bagatell R. Mechanisms of neuroblastoma regression. *Nature Rev Clin Oncol* 2014 ; 11(12) :704-713.

[89] Maris J.M. Recent advances in neuroblastoma. *N Engl J Med* 2010 ; 362(23) :2202-2211.

[90] Tolbert V.P., Matthey K.K. Neuroblastoma: clinical and biological approach to risk stratification and treatment. *Cell Tissue Res* 2018 ;372(2) :195-209.

[91] Carosio R., Zuccari G., Orienti I., Mangraviti S., Montaldo P.G. Sodium ascorbate induces apoptosis in neuroblastoma cell lines by interfering with iron uptake. *Mol Cancer* 2007 ; 6 :55.

[92] Ma E., Chen P., Wilkins H.M., Wang T., Swerdlow R.H., Chen Q. Pharmacologic ascorbate induces neuroblastoma cell death by hydrogen peroxide mediated DNA damage and reduction in cancer cell glycolysis. *Free Radic Biol Med* 2017 ; 113 :36-47.

[93] Arnold M., Abnet C.C., Neale R.E., Vignat J., Giovannucci E.L., McGlynn K.A., et al., Global Burden of 5 Major Types of Gastrointestinal Cancer. *Gastroenterology* 2020 ; 159(1) :335-349.e15.

[94] Murphy N., Jenab M., Gunter M.J. Adiposity and gastrointestinal cancers: epidemiology, mechanisms and future directions. *Nat Rev Gastroenterol Hepatol* 2018 ; 15(11) :659-670.

[95] Tong Y., Gao H., Qi Q., Liu X., Li J., Gao J., et al., High fat diet, gut microbiome and gastrointestinal cancer. *Theragnostic* 2021 ; 11(12) :5889-5910.

[96] Ferlay J., Soerjomataram I., Dikshit R., Eser S., Mathers C., Rebelo M., et al., Cancer incidence and mortality worldwide: sources, methods and major patterns in GLOBOCAN 2012. *Int J Cancer* 2015 ; 136(5) : E359-386.

[97] Rahib L., Smith B.D., Aizenberg R., Rosenzweig A.B., Fleshman J.M., Metrician L.M. Projecting cancer incidence and deaths to 2030: the unexpected burden of thyroid, liver, and pancreas cancers in the United States. *Cancer Res* 2014 ; 74(11) :2913-2921.

[98] Biller L.H., Schrag D. Diagnosis and Treatment of Metastatic Colorectal Cancer: A Review. *JAMA* 2021 ; 325(7) :669-685.

[99] Brenner H., Kloor M., Pox C.P. Colorectal cancer. *Lancet* 2014 ;383(9927) :1490-1502.

[100] Wu Z., Li Y., Zhang Y., Hu H., Wu T., Liu S., et al., Colorectal Screening Methods and Molecular Markers for Early Detection. *Technol Cancer Res Treat* 2020 ; 19 :1533033820980426.

[101] Modest D.P., Pant S., Sartore-Bianchi A. Treatment sequencing metastatic colorectal cancer. *Eur J Cancer* 2019; 109:70-83.

[102] Alzahrani S.M., Al Doghaither H.A., Al-Ghafari A.B., Pushparaj P.N. 5-Fluorouracil and capecitabine therapies for the treatment of colorectal cancer (Review). *Oncol Rep* 2023 ;50(4) :175.

[103] Yu C., Min S., Lev F. Vitamin C inhibits the growth of colorectal cancer cell HCT116 and reverses the glucose-induced oncogenic effect by downregulating the Warburg effect. *Med Oncol* 2023 ; 40, 297.

[104] Machmouchi A., Chehade L., Temraz S., Shamseddine A. Overcoming EGFR resistance in metastatic colorectal cancer using vitamin C: A review. *Biomedicine* 2023 ; *11*(3) : 678.

[105] El Halabi I., Bejjany R., Nasr R., Mukherji D., Temraz S, Nassar F.J., et al., Ascorbic Acid in Colon Cancer: From the Basic to the Clinical Applications. Int J Mol Sci 2018 ; 19, 2752.

[106] Dachs G.U., Gandhi J., Wohlrab C., Carr A.C., Morrin H.R., Pullar J.M., et al., Vitamin C Administration by Intravenous Infusion Increases Tumor Ascorbate Content in Patients with Colon Cancer : A Clinical Intervention Study. Front Oncol 2021 ; 10, 600715.

[107] Magri A., Germano G., Lorenzato A., Lamba S., Amodio V., Arena S., et al., High-dose vitamin C enhances cancer immunotherapy. *Sci Trans Med* 2020 ; 12 (532) : eaay8707.

[108] Siegel R., Miller K.D., Jemal A. Cancer statistics, 2023. *Cancer J Clinicians* 2023 ; 73(1) : 17-48.

[109] Rawla P., Sunkara T., Gaduputi V. Epidemiology of Pancreatic Cancer: Global Trends, Etiology and Risk Factors. *World J Oncol* 2019 ; 10(1) :10-27.

[110] Stoffel E.M., Brand R.E., Goggins M. Pancreatic cancer: changing epidemiology and new approaches to risk assessment, early detection, and prevention. *Gastroenterology* 2023 ; 164 (5) : 752-765.

[111] National Cancer Institute. Surveillance, Epidemiology and End Results Program. *www.seer.cancer.gov*. Accessed February 10, 2023.

[112] Klein A.P. Pancreatic cancer epidemiology: understanding the role of lifestyle and inherited risk factors. *Nat Rev Gastroenterol Hepatol* 2021 ; 18 :493–502.

[113] Kisiel J.B., Taylor W.R. Diagnostic approaches in pancreatic cancer: From imaging to biomarkers. *J Gastrointestinal Oncology* 2024 ; 15(4) : 1012-1023.

[114] Yoshida K., Nakamura Y. Advances in biomarker discovery and imaging techniques for pancreatic cancer. *J Translational Medicine* 2023 ; 21(1), 298.

[115] Wang H., Zhang Y. Recent advances in understanding the molecular mechanisms of pancreatic cancer. *Cancer Biology & Medicine* 2024 ; 21(2): 243-259.

[116] Kolbeinsson H.M., Chandana S., Wright G.P., Chung M. Pancreatic Cancer: A Review of Current Treatment and Novel Therapies. *J Invest Surg* 2023 ; '36(1) :2129884.

[117] Tzeng C.W.D., Erdek M.A. Treatment of locally advanced and metastatic pancreatic cancer: Current strategies and future directions. *Oncology Reviews* 2024 ; 18(1): 46-61.

[118] Hochster C.M.R., Ko M.A.M.Z., Ross H.A.M., Jones D.G.S., Williams T.L., Tempero W.S., et al., Erlotinib plus gemcitabine compared with gemcitabine alone in patients with advanced pancreatic cancer : A phase III trial of the National Cancer Institute of Canada Clinical Trials Group. *J Clin Oncol* 2007 ; 25 :1960–1966.

[119] Polireddy K., Dong R., Reed G., Chen P., Williamson S., Pessetto Z., et al., High dose parenteral ascorbate inhibited pancreatic cancer growth and metastasis: mechanisms and a phase I/IIa study. *Sci Rep* 2017 ; 7 : 17188.

[120] Cameron E., Pauling L. Supplemental ascorbate in the supportive treatment of cancer: Prolongation of survival times in terminal human cancer. *PNAS* 1976 ; 73(10) :3685-3689.

[121] Gucalp A., Traina T.A., Eisner J.R., Parker J.S., Selitsky S.R., Park B.H., et al., Male breast cancer: A disease distinct from female breast cancer. *Breast Cancer Res Treat* 2019; 173(1):37-48.

[122] Alkabban F.M., Ferguson T. Breast Cancer. In: *Stat Pearls* [Internet]. Treasure Island (FL): Stat Pearls Publishing; 2023 Jan-. Available from: https://www.ncbi.nlm.nih.gov/books/NBK482286/.

[123] Orrantia-Borunda E., Nuñez P.A., Acuña-Aguilar L.E., Gómez-Valles F.O., Ramírez-Valdespino CA. Chapter 3 *Subtypes of Breast Cancer.* In: Mayrovitz HN, editor. Exon Publications 2022.

[124] Yin L., Duan J.J., Bian X.W., Yu S.C. Triple negative breast cancer molecular subtyping and treatment progress. *Breast Cancer Res* 2020 ; 22 :61.
[125] Wolff A.C., Hammond H., Hicks D.G., Dowsett M., McShane L.M., Allison K.H., et al., Recommendations for human epidermal growth factor receptor 2 testing in breast cancer: American Society of Clinical Oncology/College of American Pathologists clinical practice guideline update. *J Clin Oncol* 2013; 31:3997–4013.
[126] Codini M., Fiorani F., Mandarano M., Cataldi S., Arcuri C., Mirarchi A., et al., Sphingomyelin Metabolism Modifies Luminal A Breast Cancer Cell Line under a High Dose of Vitamin C. *Int J Mol Sci* 2023;24(24), 17263.
[127] Li J., Guan X., Fan Z., Ching L.M., Li Y., Wang X., et al., Non-Invasive Biomarkers for Early Detection of Breast Cancer. *Cancers (Basel)* 2020 ; 12(10) : 2767.
[128] PDQ Adult Treatment Editorial Board. Breast Cancer Treatment (PDQ®): Health Professional Version. 2023 Nov 13. In: *PDQ Cancer Information Summaries* [Internet]. Bethesda (MD): National Cancer Institute (US); 2002-. Available from: https://www.ncbi.nlm.nih.gov/books/NBK65744/. Accessed Feb 10, 2024.
[129] Ben-Dror J., Shalamov M., Sonnenblick A. The history of early breast cancer treatment. *Genes* 2022 ; 13 (6) : 960.
[130] Marty M., Espié M., Llombart A., Monnier A., Rapoport B.L., Stahalova V. Dexrazoxane Study Group. Multicenter randomized phase III study of the cardioprotective effect of dexrazoxane (Cardioxane) in advanced/metastatic breast cancer patients treated with anthracycline-based chemotherapy. *Ann Oncol* 2006 ; (4) :614-622.
[131] Hortobagyi G.N., Frye D., Buzdar A.U., Ewer M.S., Fraschini G., Hug V., et al., Decreased cardiac toxicity of doxorubicin administered by continuous intravenous infusion in combination chemotherapy for metastatic breast carcinoma. *Cancer.* 1989 ; 63(1) :37-45.
[132] Mansoori B., Mohammadi A., Davudian S., Shirjang S., Baradaran B. The Different Mechanisms of Cancer Drug Resistance: A Brief Review. *Adv Pharm Bull* 2017 ; 7(3) :339-348.
[133] Wasim S., Lee S.Y., Kim J. Complexities of prostate cancer. *Int J Mol Sci* 2022 ; 23 : 14257.
[134] Ferlay J., Soerjomataram I., Dikshit R., Eser S., Mathers C., Rebelo M., et al., Cancer incidence and mortality worldwide: Sources, methods and major patterns in GLOBOCAN 2012. *Int J Cancer* 2015, 136 : E359–E386.
[135] *American Cancer Society. Global Cancer Statistics,* 4/4/2024. https://pressroom.concer.org/.
[136] Rawla P. Epidemiology of Prostate Cancer. *World J Oncol* 2019, 10, 63–89.
[137] Sandhu S., Moore C.M., Chiong E., Beltran H., Bristow R.G., Williams S.G. Prostate cancer. *Lancet* 2021; 398: 1075–1090.
[138] Siegel R.L., Miller K.D., Jemal A. Cancer statistics, 2018. *CA Cancer J Clin* 2018; 68: 7–30.
[139] Virgo K.S., Basch E., Loblaw D.A., Oliver T.K., Rumble R.B., Carducci M.A, et al., Second-Line Hormonal Therapy for Men with Chemotherapy-Naive, Castration-Resistant Prostate Cancer: American Society of Clinical Oncology Provisional Clinical Opinion. *J Clin Oncol* 2017 ; 35 : 1952–1964.
[140] Crew B.A. Closer look at a revered robot. *Nature* 2020 ; 580 : S5–S7.
[141] Sekhoacha M., Riet K., Motloung P., Gumenku L., Adegoke A., Mashele S. Prostate cancer review: genetics, diagnosis, treatment options, and alternative approaches. *Molecules* 2022 ; 27 : 5730.
[142] Jamaspishvili T., Berman D.M., Ross A.E., Scher H.I., De Marzo A.M., Squire J.A., et al., Clinical implications of PTEN loss in prostate cancer. *Nat Rev Urol* 2018 ; 15 : 222–234.
[143] Harmenberg U., Hamdy F.C., Widmark A., Lanners B., Nilsson S. Curative radiation therapy in prostate cancer. *Acta Oncol* 2011 ; 50 (Suppl.1) : 98–103.
[144] Ritch C.R., Cookson M.S. Advances in the management of castration resistant prostate cancer. *BMJ* 2016 ; 355 : i4405.

[145] Jain K.K. Personalized medicine for cancer: From drug development into clinical practice. *Expert Opin Pharmacotherapy* 2005 ; 6 : 1463–1476.

[146] Zhu Y., Liu C., Nadiminty N., Lou W., Tummala R., Evans C.P., et al., Inhibition of ABCB1 Expression Overcomes Acquired Docetaxel Resistance in Prostate Cancer. *Mol Cancer Ther* 2013 ; 12 : 1829–1836.

[147] Abidi A. Cabazitaxel: A novel taxane for metastatic castration-resistant prostate cancer-current implications and future prospects. *J. Pharmacol. Pharmacotherapy* 2013 ; 4 : 230–237.

[148] Braga-Basaria M., Muller D.C., Carducci M.A., Dobs A.S., Basaria S. Lipoprotein profile in men with prostate cancer undergoing androgen deprivation therapy. *Int J Impot Res* 2006 ; 18 : 494–498.

[149] Kantarjian H., O'Brien S., Shan J., Huang X. Cytogenetic and molecular responses and outcome in chronic myelogenous leukemia: need for new response definitions? *Cancer* 2008.

[150] Sampaio M.M., Santos M.L.C., Marques H.S., de Sa Santos L.K., Santos M.N., Souza C.L., et al., Chronic myeloid leukemia-from the Philadelphia chromosome to specific target drugs : A literature review. *World J of Clin Oncol* 2021 ; 12 : 69-94.

[151] von Bubnoff N., Duyster J. Chronic Myelogenous Leukemia: Treatment and Monitoring. *Dtsch Arztebl Int* 2010 ; 107 : 114–122.

[152] Ross T.S., Mgbemena V.E. Re-evaluating the role of BCR/ABL in chronic myelogenous leukemia. *Mol Cell Oncol* 2014 ; 1(3) : e963450.

[153] Rowley J.D. A new consistent chromosomal abnormality in chronic myelogenous leukemia identified by quinacrine fluorescence and Giemsa staining. *Nature* 1973 ; 243(5405) : 290-293.

[154] Flis S., Chojnacki T. Chronic myelogenous leukemia, a still unsolved problem: pitfalls and new therapeutic possibilities. *Drug Des Devel Ther* 2019 ; 13 : 825–843.

[155] Hochhaus A., Breccia M., G Saglio G., V García-Gutiérrez V Expert opinion management of chronic myeloid leukemia after resistance to second-generation tyrosine kinase inhibitors. *Leukemia* 2020 ; 34 : 1495-1502.

[156] Bhatia R. Novel approaches to therapy in CML. *Hematology Am Soc Hematol Educ Program* 2017; (1): 115–120.

[157] Agathocleous M. Vitamin C promotes stem cell function and reduces blast crisis in CML. *Nature* 2017; 549(7673): 476-479.

[158] Pires D.A., Brandão-Rangel M.A.R., Silva-Reis A., Olímpio F.R.S., Oliveira C.R., Silva J.R., et al., Vitamin C inhibits lipopolysaccharide-induced hyperinflammatory state of chronic myeloid leukemia cells through purinergic signaling and autophagy. *Nutrients* 2024 ; 16, 383.

[159] Isola S., Gammeri, Furci F., Gangemi S., Pioggia G., Allegra A. Vitamin C Supplementation in the Treatment of Autoimmune and Onco-Hematological Diseases: From Prophylaxis to Adjuvant Therapy. *Int J Mol Sci* 2024, 25, 7284.

[160] Shanafelt T.D., Rabe K.G., Kay N.E., Bowen D.A., Slager S.L., Hanson C.A., et al., Age at diagnosis and the utility of prognostic testing in patients with chronic lymphocytic leukemia. *Cancer* 2010; 116 (20): 4777-4787.

[161] Siegel R.L., Miller K.D., Jemal A. Cancer statistics 2020. *Cancer J Clin* 2020 ; 70(1) : 7-30.

[162] Howlader N., Noone A.M., Krapcho M. SEER Cancer Statistics Review, 1975–2017. *National Cancer Institute* 2020. https://seer.cancer.gov/archive/csr/1975_2017/browse_csr.php.

[163] Burger J.A., Chiorazzi N. B cell receptor signaling in chronic lymphocytic leukemia. *Blood* 2014 ; 114(2): 3635-3644.

[164] Svanberg R., Janum S., Patten P.E.M., Ramsay A.G., Niemann C.U. Targeting the microenvironment in chronic lymphocytic leukemia. *Haematologica* 2021 ; 106 : 2312-2324.

[165] Eichhorst B., Fink A.M., Bahlo J., Kovacs G., Lange E., Kiehl M., et al., First-line chemoimmunotherapy with bendamustine and rituximab versus fludarabine, cyclophosphamide, and rituximab in patients with previously untreated chronic lymphocytic

leukemia: A randomized, open-label, phase 3, non-inferiority trial. *Lancet Oncology* 2016 ; 17(7) : 928-942.

[166] Byrd J.C., Furman R.R., Coutre S.E., Flinn I.W., Burger J.A., Blum K.A., et al., Targeting BTK with ibrutinib in relapsed chronic lymphocytic leukemia. *N Engl J Med* 2013 ; 369 (1) : 32-42.

[167] Furman R.R., Sharman J.P., Coutre S.E., O'Brien S. Idelalisib and rituximab in relapsed chronic lymphocytic leukemia. *N Engl J Med* 2014 ; 370 : 997-1007.

[168] Roberts A.W., Davids M.S., Pagel J.M., Kipps T.J., Seymour J.F. Targeting BCL2 with venetoclax in relapsed chronic lymphocytic leukemia. *N Engl J Med* 2016; 374: 311-322.

[169] Mastrangelo D., Massai L., Fioritoni G., Lo Coco F., Noguera N., Testa U. High dose of vitamin C and leukemia: in vitro update. *Myeloid Leukemia* 2018; 10.5772/intechopen.71484.

[170] Mussa A., Idris R.A.M., Ahmed N., Ahmad C., Lazim N.M., Uskoković V., et al., High-dose vitamin C for cancer therapy. *Pharmaceuticals (Basel)* 2022;15(6):711.

[171] Darwiche W., Gomila C., Ouled-Haddou H., Marolleau J.P., Ghamlouch H. Ascorbic acid synergistically enhances the therapeutic effect of targeted therapy in chronic lymphocytic leukemia. *J Exp Clin Cancer Res* 2020; 39.

[172] Carr A.C., Lykkesfeldt J. Vitamin C: From bench to bedside. *Nutrients* 2021 ; 13(4) : 1102.

[173] National Cancer Institute. *Cancer Statistics. International Agency for Research on Cancer* https://www.cancer.gov/policies/linking.

[174] Bray F., Ferlay J., Soerjomataram I. Global cancer statistics. *CA Cancer J Clin* 2018 ; 68(6) : 394-424.

[175] World Health Organization. *Cancer fact sheet*. Geneva : WHO. 2021.

[176] Herbst R.S., Morgensztern D., Boshoff C. The biology and management of NSCLC. *Nature* 2018 ; 553 (7689) : 446-454.

[177] Cheng T.Y.D., Cramb S.M., Baade P.D., Youden D.R., Reid M.E. The International Epidemiology of Lung Cancer: latest trends, disparities, and tumor characteristics. *J Thorac Oncol* 2016 ; 11(10) :1653-71.

[178] National Cancer Institute. *Non-Small Cell Lung Cancer Treatment (*PDQ®)–Health Professional Version 2022.

[179] Hirsch F.R., Scagliotti G.V., Mulshine J.L., Kwon R., Curran W.J., Wu Y.L., et al., Lung cancer: current therapies and new targeted treatments. *Lancet* 2017 ; 389 (10066) : 299-311.

[180] Reck M., Rodríguez-Abreu D., Robinson A.G., Hui R., Csőszi T., Fülöp A., et al., Pembrolizumab versus chemotherapy for PD-L1–positive NSCLC. *N Engl J Med* 2016 ; 375(19) :1823-1833.

[181] Cooper A.J., Sequist L.V., Lin J.J. Third-generation EGFR and ALK inhibitors: mechanisms of resistance and management. *Nat Rev Clin Oncol* 2022 ;19(8) :499-514.

[182] Borghaei H., Gettinger S., Vokes E.E., Burgio M.A., Pluzanski A., Frontera O.A., et al., Five-year outcomes from the randomized, phase III trials Checkmate 017 and 057 : Nivolumab versus docetaxel in previously treated NSCLC. *J Clin Oncol* 2021 ; 39(7) :723-733.

[183] Doskey C.M., Buranasudja V., Wagner B.A., Wilkes J.G., Du J., Cullen J.J., et al., Tumor cells have decreased ability to metabolize hydrogen peroxide : implications for pharmacologic ascorbate in cancer therapy. *Redox Biology* 2016 ; 10 :274-284.

[184] Ngo B., Van Riper J.M., Cantley L.C., Yun J. Targeting cancer vulnerabilities with high-dose Vitamin C. *Nat Rev Cancer* 2019 ; 19(5) : 271-282.

[185] Gillberg L., Ørskov A.D., Jones P.A., Gronbaek K. Vitamin C - a novel player in regulation of the cancer epigenome. *Seminars in Cancer Biology* 2018 ; 51 : 59-67.

[186] Nowak A.Z., Nowak P.J., Rysz A.C. High-Dose vitamin C in advanced-stage cancer patients. *Nutrients* 2021 ; 13 : 735.

[187] Guo D., Liao Y., Na J., Wu L., Yin Y., Mi Z., et al., The involvement of ascorbic acid in cancer treatment. *Molecules* 2024 ; 29(10) : 2295.

[188] Lamas D.J., Inés Tasat D.R., Cabral P. Impact of high-dose Vitamin C on quality of life of cancer patients undergoing chemotherapy. *J Cancer Res and Clin Oncol* 2020 ; 146(8) : 1945-1954.

[189] Cirillo L., Innocenti S., Becherucci F. Global epidemiology of kidney cancer. *Nephrol Dial Transplant* 2024 ; 39 :920-928.

[190] Sung H., Ferlay J., Siegel R.L., Laversanne M., Soerjomataram I., Jemal A., et al., Global Cancer Statistics 2020: GLOBOCAN Estimates of Incidence and Mortality Worldwide for 36 Cancers in 185 Countries. CA : A *Cancer J Clin* 2021 ; 71(3) : 209-249.

[191] Mancini M., Righetto M., Baggio G .Gender-related approach to kidney cancer management: Moving forward. *Int J Mol Sci* 2020 ; 21(9) :3378.

[192] Patard J.J., Leray E., Rioux-Leclercq N., Cindolo L., Ficarra V., Zisman A., et al., Prognostic Value of Histologic Subtypes in Renal Cell Carcinoma: A Multicenter Experience. *J Clin Oncol* 2005; 23:2763–2771.

[193] Capitanio U., Montorsi F. Renal cancer. *Lancet* 2016; 387: 894-906.

[194] Bianchi M, Sun M, Jedres C. Distribution of metastatic sites in renal cell carcinoma: a population-based analysis. Ann Oncol 2012 ; 23 :973-980.

[195] Wolf M.M., Rathmell W.K., Beckermann K.E. Modeling clear cell renal cell carcinoma and therapeutic implications. *Oncogene* 2020; 39 (17): 3413-3426.

[196] Catalano M., Procopio G., Sepe P., Santoni M., Sessa F., Villari D., et al., Tyrosine kinase and immune checkpoints. Tyrosine kinase and immune checkpoints inhibitors in favorable risk metastatic renal cell carcinoma: trick or treat? *Pharmacol Ther* 2023 ; 249 :108499.

[197] Aparicio L.M.A., Fernandez I.P., Cassinello J. Tyrosine kinase inhibitors reprogramming immunity in renal cell carcinoma: rethinking cancer immunotherapy. *Clin Transl Oncol* 2017 ; 19(10) :1175-1182.

[198] Robert J., Motzer R.J., Konstantin P.K., Haanen J., Rini B., Albiges L., et al., Avelumab plus Axitinib versus Sunitinib for Advanced Renal-Cell Carcinoma. *N Eng J Med* 2019 ; 380 : 1103-1115.

[199] Böttger F., Vallés-Martí A., Cahn L., Jimenez C.R. High-dose intravenous vitamin C, a promising multi-targeting agent in the treatment of cancer. *J Exp Clin Cancer Res* 2021 ; 40 (1) : 343.

Chapter 2

The Background of Vitamin C

Lunawati L. Bennett*, PhD, PharmD

Union University, College of Pharmacy, Jackson, Tennessee, USA

Abstract

Vitamin C has been known for decades to treat scurvy, manifests as lethargy and weakness due to lacking consumption of fresh fruits and vegetables. Vitamin C or ascorbate is also useful to treat and to prevent many illnesses such as common cold and heart diseases since this water-soluble vitamin plays essential multifunctional micronutrient in many enzymatic reactions. In 1972, Ewan Cameron, a Scottish surgeon hypothesized that vitamin C could suppress cancer development by inhibiting hyaluronidase preventing cancer cells to metastasize. Together with Linus Pauling, a renowned chemist and two-time Nobel Prize Laureate, they treated terminally ill cancer patients with high doses or also known as pharmacological concentration of vitamin C. Their studies showed patients improved quality of life and there was a four-fold increase in mean survival time. However, clinical trials conducted by Mayo Clinic around the same time failed to show any positive outcomes in treating cancer patients, which dampened early enthusiasm about the role of vitamin C in cancer treatment.

In recent times, several newer studies have shown that VC can kill cancer cells which rekindled current interest in studying this vitamin's effects on cancers. This chapter covers the background of vitamin C from its discovery, its absorption, transport and biological properties, its role in health, in various diseases and cancers, its prooxidant and antioxidant properties, and its use as adjuvant medication.

Keywords: pharmacological concentration of vitamin C, high dose of vitamin C, ascorbic acid, cancer, hydrogen peroxide, free radicals, reactive oxygen species, anti-neoplastic

* Corresponding Author's Email: llbennett@uu.edu

Abbreviations

VC	Vitamin C;
PVC	Pharmacological concentration of vitamin C;
ASc	Ascorbate;
AA	Ascorbic acid;
H_2O_2	Hydrogen peroxide;
GSH	glutathione;
ROS	Reactive oxygen species;
RNS	Reactive nitrogen species;
GLUT	Glucose transporter;
IV	intravenous;
SVCT1	sodium-dependent transporter-1;
DHA	dehydroascorbic acid.

Introduction

Isolated in 1928, vitamin C (VC) also known as ascorbic acid (AA) or ascorbate (Asc) - is essential for human health. These terms will be used interchangeably throughout this chapter. VC plays a crucial role in several metabolic functions, including the activation of vitamin B and folic acid; the conversion of cholesterol to bile acids; and the transformation of certain amino acids such as tyrosine, tryptophan, glycine, proline, and lysine. It also protects the body from free radical damage and helps maintain connective tissue integrity [1].

Most plant and animal species can synthesize VC from glucose and galactose through the uronic acid pathway. However, humans and other primates cannot synthesize VC due to the lack of enzyme gluconolactone oxidase [2]. As an antioxidant, VC protects the body from the harmful effects of free radicals, including reactive oxygen species (ROS), reactive nitrogen species (RNS), pollutants, and toxins [1].

Linus Pauling and Ewan Cameron were pioneers in advocating high doses of VC for treating various conditions, ranging from common cold to cancer [3]. Since then, megadose of VC has been widely used in the treatment and prevention of numerous disorders, including diabetes mellitus, atherosclerosis, cataracts, glaucoma, stroke, heart disease, and cancer.

History

During the 16th to 19th centuries, scurvy was a severe disease primarily affecting sailors who spent months at sea without access to fresh fruits and vegetables [4]. In 1747, James Lind, a surgeon with the British Royal Navy, conducted the first human clinical trial to treat scurvy. He administered various potential remedies, including cider, vinegar, and citrus fruits (oranges and lemons), to a group of 12 scurvy-stricken sailors. The only individuals who recovered were those who received lemons and oranges [5]. Subsequently, citrus juice was adopted by British sailors as a preventive measure against scurvy [3-5].

It took nearly 200 years before Albert Szent-Györgyi, a Hungarian biochemist, isolated VC, and Norman Haworth synthesized the compound. Initially, it was identified as hexuronic acid, which was later named L-ascorbic acid (ascorbate) [6]. For their contributions, Haworth and Szent-Györgyi were awarded the Nobel Prize in 1937 [6-8].

Vitamin C is a water-soluble organic compound with the IUPAC name (5R)-5-[(1S)-1,2-Dihydroxyethyl]-3,4-dihydroxyfuran-2(5H)-one. Its oxidized form, dehydroascorbic acid (DHA), is also referred to as vitamin C. Among the four stereoisomers, only L (+)-ascorbic acid exhibits biological activity [4].

Many of the known functions of VC are attributed to its action as an electron donor. VC has two ionizable hydroxyl groups with pKa values of 4.2 and 11.6, meaning at physiological pH, it is present as the ascorbate monoanion, as illustrated in Figure1 [5, 9]. VC is an excellent antioxidant, both thermodynamically and kinetically, and can neutralize many highly ROS species [10].

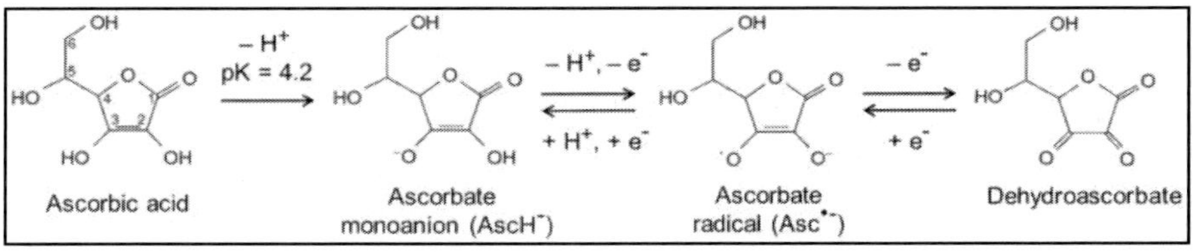

Figure 1. Chemical structure of ascorbate and its oxidation products. At physiological pH, ascorbate exists as the ascorbate monoanion and can undergo two consecutive, reversible, one-electron oxidations to produce the ascorbate radical and dehydroascorbate (DHA) [9].

Health Impact

Vitamin C plays a crucial role as a multifunctional micronutrient in various enzymatic reactions, including collagen synthesis, iron absorption, immune function maintenance, and antioxidant. Most plants and animals can synthesize VC from glucose and galactose, but humans cannot produce VC due to the absence of the enzyme L-gulono-γ-lactone oxidase [11]. Under physiological pH conditions, VC predominantly exists as the ascorbate anion, resulting from the dissociation of the 3-hydroxyl group [12].

Dietary sources of VC include citrus fruits such as oranges, grapefruits, lemons, and limes, as well as berries and tropical fruits like kiwi, pineapple, mango, papaya, and guava [4, 13-15]. Vegetables, particularly tomatoes, leafy greens, and cruciferous vegetables, are also good sources, with the highest amounts per serving found in red and yellow bell peppers. Plant-based sources of VC range from 14 mg to 190 mg per cup [13-15]. VC supplements are widely available in various forms, including tablets, capsules, chewable, and powders, typically providing doses ranging from 100 mg to 1000 mg or more.

In the plasma of healthy individuals, the reduced form of VC is dominant, while the oxidized form, dehydroascorbic acid (DHA), is present at very low levels, approximately 1-2% of total VC concentrations [12, 16]. In certain organs, such as brain, adrenals, liver, and white blood cells, high intracellular levels of VC are found to meet its role as an essential enzyme cofactor [15-17].

Vitamin C deficiency can lead to symptoms such as fatigue, gum disease, skin hemorrhages, respiratory infections, weakness, poor wound healing, ecchymoses, xerosis, edema, and musculoskeletal pain [14, 18].

The Recommended Dietary Allowances (RDA) for VC vary by age, sex, and life stage. For most adults, the RDA is 90 mg/day for men and 75 mg/day for women. For optimal plasma concentration, a typical target is about 70 µmol/L [19]. The RDA for infants to adolescents ranges from 15 mg/day to 75 mg/day. These recommendations are designed to maintain health, prevent deficiency, and provide antioxidant protection. Higher intakes are advised for smokers and individuals experiencing increased oxidative stress due to stress, illness, or chronic disease [14]. Pregnant and lactating women require RDAs of 85 mg and 120 mg/day, respectively, to support fetal development and milk production.

During periods of illness or increased physical stress, VC supplementation can be beneficial. Dosage for supplementation ranges from 100 mg to 2000 mg/day. About 50% of healthy adults can have hypovitaminosis C due to plasma concentration less than 23 umol/L despite taking diet recommended daily doses of VC [19]. Severe VC deficiency shown as plasma concentration of 11umol/L can cause scurvy [20]. Doses of 200-1000 mg per day are commonly used to support the immune system, but it is important to avoid excessive doses of the tolerable upper intake level (UL). The UL for VC is set at 2,000 mg/day for adults, while for ages 1 to 18 years, it ranges from 400 mg/day to 1800 mg/day. Excessive intake can lead to gastrointestinal disturbances such as diarrhea, nausea, and abdominal cramps. Adverse effects above the UL can include diarrhea, bloating, abdominal pain, increased risk of kidney stone formation in predisposed individuals, such as hemolysis in people with glucose-6-phosphate dehydrogenase (G6PD) deficiency [21].

Absorption, Transport, Metabolism, and Drug-Interaction

The absorption and metabolism of VC involve complex processes influenced by dosage, dietary factors, health status, and individual variability. VC is absorbed primarily in jejunum and ileum. Human cells can store and reabsorb VC sufficiently for 2-6 weeks. In the blood, approximately 24% of VC is bound to proteins [4].

Vitamin C absorption occurs through both active transport and passive diffusion. Passive diffusion is less efficient and contributes minimally compared to active transport. At physiological doses, VC uptake into cells is mediated by sodium-dependent vitamin C transporters SVCT1 and SVCT2 [22-24]. SVCT1 is a high-capacity transporter with low affinity, while SVCT2 has high affinity but lower capacity [25-26].

The primary excretion of VC occurs via kidneys through urine, predominantly through SVCT1. Studies have shown that approximately 70% of VC is excreted through urinary elimination [27]. SVCT2 plays a crucial role in supplying VC to the brain and supporting vascular development [28]. Although VC can also be absorbed through passive diffusion at high doses, this mechanism is less effective compared to active transport [29]. The body tightly regulates plasma VC levels; any excess beyond tissue saturation is filtered by the kidneys and excreted in the urine. The renal threshold for VC is around 1.4 mg/dL (80 μmol/L), before it begins to be excreted.

The oxidized form of VC, dehydroascorbate (DHA), is transported from the intestine to the blood by glucose transporters (GLUT) GLUT-2 and GLUT-8, and from the blood to tissues by GLUT-1, GLUT-3, and GLUT-4, as intestinal cells do not express these transporters [23, 30]. Excess glucose can competitively inhibit DHA uptake. Within cells, VC is rapidly regenerated from DHA by glutathione (GSH) and NADPH [31]. Excess DHA can be further degraded into oxalate and other metabolites, which are then excreted in the urine [32-34]. Figure 2 describes the location of VC transporters [29].

Several factors influence VC absorption. Efficiency decreases with higher doses; at low dietary intakes (30-180 mg/day), about 70-90% of VC is absorbed, but when intake exceeds 1 g/day, absorption drops to less than 50%. The bioavailability of VC from natural food sources and supplements is generally similar. Some supplements, such as ester-C or liposomal vitamin C, are marketed as having enhanced absorption [29, 34]. Certain substances can enhance VC absorption, such as flavonoids found in fruits and vegetables, while high doses of iron supplements can decrease absorption. Conditions like Crohn's or celiac disease can impair VC absorption.

Vitamin C is distributed widely throughout the body, with the highest concentrations in the adrenal glands, pituitary gland, thymus, retina, brain, and leukocytes. Plasma VC concentration is tightly regulated, typically ranging from 50 to 70 μmol/L in healthy individuals [4, 34]. It interacts with various nutrients and compounds, influencing their absorption, metabolism, and effectiveness. VC enhances the absorption of non-heme iron (from plant-based sources) by reducing ferric iron (Fe^{3+}) to ferrous iron (Fe^{2+}), which is more readily absorbed. Consuming VC-rich foods or supplements with iron-rich meals can improve iron bioavailability, especially for individuals at risk of iron deficiency. VC regenerates oxidized vitamin E (α-tocopherol) to its active antioxidant form, boosting vitamin E's capacity to protect cell membranes from oxidative damage. VC also works synergistically with other antioxidants, such as glutathione, and beta-carotene, to neutralize free radicals and reduce oxidative stress. This synergy enhances overall antioxidant defense and cellular protection. High doses of VC may interfere with vitamin B12 absorption and utilization, potentially leading to decreased serum levels of vitamin B12 in vulnerable populations. VC may also enhance the bioavailability and cellular uptake of vitamin D, supporting bone health, immune function, and overall well-being. Adequate levels of both vitamins are essential for optimal health outcomes [35-39].

The Impact of High-Dose on Diseases

High-dose VC or pharmacological concentration of VC (PVC) has been extensively researched for its potential therapeutic effects beyond basic nutritional needs. This interest is due to its antioxidant properties and its roles in collagen synthesis, immune function, and cellular health.

Collagen provides structural support to bones and joints. A deficiency in VC can impair collagen synthesis, potentially leading to weakened bones and an increased risk of joint disorders. PVC is crucial for wound healing by promoting collagen formation at the wound site, enhancing tissue repair, and supporting the formation of scar tissue necessary for tissue regeneration [32, 40-41].

Pharmacological concentration of vitamin C is thought to reduce inflammation, oxidative stress, and endothelial dysfunction in septic patients. Evidence from the VICTAS (Vitamin C, Thiamine, and Steroids in Sepsis) trial suggests that high-dose intravenous (IV) Vitamin C, often combined with hydrocortisone and thiamine, may reduce mortality and improve recovery times in septic patients [42]. However, larger randomized controlled trials (RCTs) have produced mixed results, and further research is needed to establish definitive benefits and protocols. PVC, which can only be achieved by IV, can improve endothelial function and reduce arterial stiffness by enhancing nitric oxide production and reducing oxidative stress. Some studies have shown that PVC can lower blood pressure and improve vascular function in hypertensive and diabetic patients, although results are variable and not yet sufficient to recommend it as a standalone therapy [38].

The antioxidant properties of VC may protect against neurodegeneration by reducing oxidative stress and inflammation. Some observational studies suggest a link between higher VC intake and a reduced risk of cognitive decline, but clinical trials have not conclusively demonstrated that HVC supplementation can prevent or treat Alzheimer's or Parkinson's disease.

Vitamin C may also support mitochondrial function and reduce oxidative stress. Some small trials have indicated that PVC can alleviate symptoms in patients with chronic fatigue syndrome and fibromyalgia, though more robust evidence is required [32].

High-dose VC, both oral and topical, has been shown to improve wound healing and reduce the appearance of wrinkles and fine lines. A study found that HVC reduced healing time and improved cosmetic outcomes in patients undergoing surgical procedures. VC acts as a cofactor for enzymes involved in the hydroxylation of proline and lysine residues within procollagen molecules. Hydroxylation is essential for the proper formation of collagen's triple helix structure, which enhances its stability and functionality. By facilitating collagen hydroxylation, VC helps stabilize the triple helix structure of collagen fibers, which is crucial for the strength and resilience of connective tissues throughout the body. PVC may also be beneficial for severe burns and surgical recovery [43].

The Impact of High-Dose on Cancers

The potential anti-cancer properties of VC have been recognized since the 1960s, when it was demonstrated to be highly toxic to *in vitro* Ehrlich ascites carcinoma cells, while remaining nontoxic to normal body tissues [44]. In the 1970s, Scottish surgeon Ewan Cameron and his colleague Allan Campbell began investigating the use of both oral and intravenous (IV) VC for cancer treatment. Their work, further supported by Linus Pauling, suggested that IVC or PVC could improve survival in patients with advanced cancer [45-47]. This collaboration highlighted the potential of VC therapy in cancer management.

However, this promising outlook faced setbacks when two double-blinded, randomized clinical trials conducted by the Mayo Clinic using high-dose oral VC did not demonstrate significant benefits [48-49]. Consequently, the use of VC for cancer treatment was deemed ineffective and dismissed by the research and medical communities [50].

The discrepancy in results between these studies is largely attributed to differences in administration methods. While Pauling's group administered VC both orally and intravenously, the Mayo Clinic trials relied solely on oral administration without realizing that maintaining high plasma levels of VC through oral administration is challenging [50].

Oral VC plasma levels are regulated by intestinal absorption (bioavailability), tissue accumulation, and renal elimination [51]. Consequently, plasma concentrations cannot exceed 100 μM with oral intake and with supplements. At an oral dose of 100 mg, 200 mg, 1000 mg or 2500 mg, the steady-state plasma concentration is approximately 50-60, 80, and 80-90 μM, respectively [52-53]. Oral doses of 3 g six times daily can only achieve plasma concentrations of 220 μM. Bioavailability after a single 200 mg dose is 100% but declines to 33% after a 1250 mg dose. Plasma VC levels are tightly regulated by SVCTs, which limit absorption and reabsorption in the intestine and kidneys, usually not exceeding ~100 μM.

In contrast, IV administration can achieve PVC in plasma at millimolar concentrations [50]. For example, infusing 10 g of VC in cancer patients results in plasma concentrations ranging from 1 to 5 mM [54-55]. IV administration bypasses these controls by transporters, kidney and others; therefore, PVC can achieve plasma levels up to 100-fold higher than oral, with maximum levels reaching up to 15 mM [43]. IV administration bypasses the regulation of intestinal uptake, resulting in plasma concentrations about 6.5 times higher than the oral route [43]. Pharmacokinetic modeling predicts plasma levels of 220 μM for a maximum tolerated oral dose of 3 g every 4 hours, compared to 13,350 μM and 15,380 μM for 50 g and 100 g IV doses, respectively [56]. IV administration can increase VC plasma levels 30 to 70 times higher than the highest tolerated oral dose [56]. In cancer patients, whether they undergo chemotherapy or not, IVC doses ranging from 0.1 to 3 g/kg body weight result in maximum concentrations ranging from 2 to 37 mM [57-63].

In animal studies, PVC given at 0.1-0.8 g/kg body weight for 2-4 weeks not only inhibited cancer growth but also reduced cell invasiveness and increased survival [56,

64-68]. Xenograft experiments showed that PVC at 4 g/kg body weight once or twice daily increased blood and tissue concentrations to greater than 30 mM, significantly reducing cancer growth rates in glioblastoma, ovarian, and pancreatic carcinoma cells in mice [69].

In addition, PVC may protect against cancer by enhancing collagen synthesis [70]. VC can potentiate the intrinsic production of serum hyaluronidase inhibitor (PIH), which protects against cancer cell spread [71]. Additionally, VC supports natural resistance to malignant growth by potentiating oxidative stress in cancer cells, which enhances their susceptibility to apoptosis [72]. In fibrosis, VC increases the effectiveness of malignant cell encapsulation in fibrous tissue, extends lymphocytic infiltration, and protects the adeno-pituitary axis against depletion caused by cancer-related stress [29].

Vitamin C content of cancer cells has been measured and yielded variable results. Brain and colorectal cancers were found to have significantly less VC compared to normal tissues, while breast, oral, skin, and lung cancers contained more VC than their normal counterparts [73-74].

To assess whether VC at physiological (0.1 mM) and pharmacological (0.3-20 mM) concentrations can selectively kill cancer cells, normal and cancer cell types were incubated in media containing VC ranging from 0 to 20 mM. The results indicated that normal cells were unaffected by 1 to 2 hours of incubation in 20 mM VC, while five cancer cell lines had effective concentration (EC) values of < 4 mM and EC50 values of < 10 mM for 75% of the cancer cells tested [69, 75]. Furthermore, cancer cell death was associated with extracellular rather than intracellular VC, dependent on extracellular hydrogen peroxide (H_2O_2) formation upon VC oxidation, which displayed a linear relationship with the formation of ascorbyl radical (Asc*). VC generated detectable levels of H_2O_2 in extracellular media in the presence of serum, but not in whole blood, suggesting that PVC achievable through IV administration may act as a prodrug for delivery H_2O_2 to tissues [75]. In pancreatic tumor cell lines, elevated levels of H_2O_2 from PVC have been shown to decrease tumor growth [69, 75].

Emerging data suggest that the oxidized form of VC, dehydroascorbate (DHA), might be pharmacologically active. High doses of VC can act as a prooxidant, generating H_2O_2, which can be toxic to cancer cells while sparing normal cells [69, 75-77].

Laboratory investigations have reported that IV Vitamin C exhibits redox properties and inhibits cell proliferation in various cancer cell lines, including those from the prostate, pancreas, liver, colon, mesothelioma, and neuroblastoma. Pharmacokinetic studies have highlighted significant differences in blood concentrations of VC depending on the route of administration, with IV administration bypassing the tight control mechanisms observed with oral intake, resulting in substantially higher plasma concentrations. Therefore, it is crucial to distinguish between the 'pharmacological' concentration of VC, which can only be achieved through IV administration, and the 'physiological' levels attained through oral intake. Only the pharmacological doses administered via IV have the potential to act as a drug.

Antioxidant vs. Prooxidant Profile

Vitamin C is known for its potent antioxidant properties, including the donation of electrons, scavenging of ROS and reactive nitrogen species (RNS), and protection against free-radical damage to various tissues. Additionally, VC can regenerate other antioxidants such as glutathione and vitamin E back to their active states [78]. However, VC also exhibits pro-oxidant activity by reducing catalytic metals like Fe^{3+} to Fe^{2+}, which enhances the pro-oxidant chemistry of these metals and facilitates the generation of ROS [12].

The cytotoxic mechanism of VC can be linked to the intracellular generation of H_2O_2 produced upon VC oxidation. This occurs because cancer cells selectively take up more VC compared to normal cells through facilitated transport via glucose transporters (GLUTs) due to their increased metabolic need for glucose [77-79]. H_2O_2 is catalyzed by the enzyme catalase to produce oxygen and water. Since catalase activity in cancer cells is 10-100 times lower than in normal cells, cancer cells are more sensitive to VC [44].

PVC-related cancer cell death is thought to be mediated by H_2O_2 formation, which, in the presence of reduced transition metal catalysts, can produce highly reactive hydroxyl radical (OH•) species. In the extracellular fluid, ascorbic acid loses one electron to form an ascorbate radical, which then reduces ferric iron to ferrous iron [17].

$$AscH^{-} + Fe^{3+} \rightarrow Fe^{2+} + Asc^{\bullet -} + H^{+}$$

An electron was donated to molecular oxygen, forming a superoxide anion ($O_2^{\bullet -}$) which reacts with hydrogen to produce H_2O_2.

$$2O_2 \rightarrow 2O_2^{\bullet -} + 2H^{+} \rightarrow H_2O_2 + O_2$$

Then in the classic Fenton reaction, ferrous iron is oxidized by H_2O_2 to generate ferric iron and a highly reactive hydroxyl radical ($OH^{\bullet}$)

$$Fe^{2+} + H_2O_2 \rightarrow Fe^{3+} + OH^{\bullet} + OH^{-}$$

It is also likely that reduced metal centers (Fe^{2}) can donate their electron to molecular oxygen to produce superoxide radical anions ($O_2^{\bullet -}$).

$$Fe^{2+} + O_2 \rightarrow Fe^{3+} + O_2^{\bullet -}$$

Vitamin C as a pro-oxidant converts Fe^{3+} back to Fe^{2+} to continue the cyclic oxidation/reduction of Fe^{2+} coupled to the generation of superoxide radical anions [17]. Mobilization of intracellular iron storage by VC followed by the Fenton reaction giving highly reactive hydroxyl radicals [79].

Vitamin C is oxidized to DHA with a half-life of about 70 minutes [79-80]. The ability of VC or DHA to kill cancer cells while sparing normal cells is explained by the fact that DHA, which is taken up by the GLUT1 glucose transporter, is reduced by GSH, NADH, and NADH-dependent enzymes. This reduction leads to the depletion of glutathione, thioredoxin, and NADPH, thereby increasing intracellular oxidative stress [17]. The accumulation of ROS inside cells inactivates glyceraldehyde 3-phosphate dehydrogenase (GAPDH), leading to decreased formation of glycolytic adenosine 5-triphosphate (ATP) and pyruvate. This results in an energetic crisis that triggers cell death [80-82].

Cancer cells are typically under higher oxidative stress than normal cells, and an additional increase in pro-oxidant levels can trigger cell death [82-85]. Persistent redox adaptation in cancers contributes to the development of aggressive traits and resistance to cancer therapies [82]. The majority of ROS/RNS include H_2O_2, hydroxyl radicals (OH•), superoxide radicals (O_2•), nitric oxide (NO•), and peroxynitrite ($ONOO^-$). ROS have both physiological functions and pathological effects within cells [86]. When the balance between pro-oxidants and antioxidants shifts, oxidative stress occurs, leading to adaptive responses that result in mutations and genomic instability [82]. Metastatic abilities of various cancers, such as prostate and breast cancer, correlate with the cellular redox state [87]. Redox imbalance can lead to activation of the mitogen-activated protein kinases (MAPK) signaling cascade and cancer cell migration [88].

The need for VC increases during anti-cancer therapy and treatment of related complications [89-91]. As the disease progresses, VC plasma levels decline compared to earlier stages [92-93]. Studies have shown that severe VC deficiency was found in 30% of hospice residents with advanced cancer and 50% in terminal cancer patients [93].

Although animal model studies have demonstrated significant tumor growth reductions with PVC, results as a single anti-cancer agent have been inconsistent. For instance, a study using PVC dosing from 30 to 110 g/m^2 for 4 consecutive days a week for 4 weeks showed no response in 17 participants. Another study with 24 participants using 0.4 to 1.5 g/kg body weight three times weekly for 10 weeks also did not observe objective tumor-related responses [58-60]. On the other hand, sole IVC administration of 15-65 g twice a week in two patients with metastatic renal cell carcinoma and non-Hodgkin's lymphoma showed complete remission [94-95].

In addition to direct ROS neutralization, VC is crucial for regenerating other antioxidants, such as vitamin E, making VC an important redox node alongside glutathione [96]. Furthermore, VC influences critical intracellular signal transduction pathways. It acts as a cofactor for enzymes that regulate the activity of transcription factors like hypoxia-inducible factor-1α (HIF-1α) and nuclear factor kappa-light-chain-enhancer of activated B cells (NF-κB) during oxygen deprivation or inflammation [97].

The Effects of Combination Cancer Therapy

Although high-dose VC or PVC alone has demonstrated the ability to reduce cancer growth in various mouse models, its clinical potential as an anticancer therapy may be enhanced when used in combination with other cancer treatments. Numerous preclinical and clinical studies suggest that PVC does not interfere with chemotherapy or radiotherapy and may even act synergistically [50, 98].

For example, a study comparing standard paclitaxel/carboplatin therapy over six months with the same regimen plus concurrent VC for twelve months showed that the combination improved overall survival by 8.75 months. However, this difference did not reach statistical significance [62]. In two non-randomized phases I studied, IVC combined with gemcitabine or erlotinib in patients with metastatic pancreatic cancer resulted in reduced tumor size, improved performance status, and median overall survival of 13 months and 182 days [61, 63].

In phase II clinical trials, groups of 20 patients receiving a combination of arsenic trioxide, dexamethasone, and 1 g IVC demonstrated median overall survival of 962 days and 11 months, and progression-free survival of 316 days and 4 months, respectively [99-100]. Another study with 22 participants who received arsenic trioxide, bortezomib, and VC reported a median progression-free survival of 5 months, with 12-month progression-free survival and overall survival rates of 34% and 74%, respectively [101-102].

The addition of VC to chemotherapy regimens has also been associated with pain relief. Pain, a common symptom in cancer patients, can be related to the primary tumor, disease progression, metastasis, and side effects of treatment [103]. Initial reports in 1974 noted significant pain relief, including complete relief from bone pain and headaches, following administration of 10 g of VC for up to 10 days [71]. Subsequent studies have shown that IVC, ranging from 25 to 100 g over four weeks, can alleviate pain associated with cancer metastases and other symptoms [43].

Moreover, in vitro studies have shown that VC treatment leads to a dose- and time-dependent decrease in prostate cancer cell viability and thymidine incorporation into DNA. While the addition of catalase, an enzyme that degrades H_2O_2, did not affect cell viability, superoxide dismutase, which generates H_2O_2, did not prevent the decrease in cell viability, indicating that the cytotoxic effects of VC are related to H_2O_2 production [17].

Additionally, the combination of VC with chemotherapeutic agents like etoposide, cisplatin, doxorubicin, and gemcitabine has shown synergistic effects, resulting in decreased tumor size and increased survival [17, 56]. PVC has been observed to induce cell death in pancreatic cancer cells with diverse mutational backgrounds by depleting cellular NAD+ and ATP, increasing α-tubulin acetylation, and inhibiting epithelial-mesenchymal transition and metastasis [102].

In a study involving 1000 patients, those who received 10 g of intravenous VC daily for 10 days followed by oral VC had survival times more than four times longer than those who did not receive VC [103]. High-dose VC treatment appears to be safe in advanced cancer patients, with manageable side effects such as transient headache, dizziness, nausea, flu-like symptoms, and minor laboratory abnormalities (e.g., anemia, hypernatremia, hypercalcemia) when appropriate precautions are taken. As the mechanisms of action of VC become better understood, its combination with other therapies appears increasingly rational and hypothesis driven [98].

Conclusion

Early research, including the pioneering work of Linus Pauling, suggested potential benefits of high-dose VC in cancer treatment. However, subsequent controlled trial by Mayo Clinic did not support these initial findings. More recent studies have yielded mixed results, with some patients reporting improvements in quality of life and slower cancer progression, particularly when IVC is used alongside conventional therapies.

The National Cancer Institute continues to explore the role of high-dose VC in integrative cancer care, investigating its safety, efficacy, and underlying mechanisms. Due to its low toxicity and relatively low cost, VC holds promise as a valuable addition to cancer treatment regimens, either as a standalone therapy or in combination with other treatments. While definitive clinical benefits remain to be established, preclinical studies and early-phase clinical trials suggest that high-dose VC could be a beneficial adjunct in the fight against cancer.

References

[1] Chambial S., Dwivedi S., Shukla K.K., John P.J., Sharma P. Vitamin C in disease prevention and cure: An overview. *Ind J Clin Biochem* 2013 ; 28 (4) : 314-328.

[2] Nishikimi M., Fukuyama R., Minoshima S., Shimizu N., Yagi K. Cloning and chromosomal mapping of the human nonfunctional gene for L-gulono-gamma-lactone oxidase, the enzyme for L-ascorbic acid biosynthesis missing in man. *J Biol Chem* 1994 ; 269 : 13685-13688.

[3] Dunitz JD. Linus Carl Pauling. 28 February 1901-19 August 1994. *Biographical memoirs of fellows of the Royal Society* 1996; 42: 316-318.

[4] Kietzmann T. Vitamin C: from nutrition to oxygen sensing and epigenetics. *Redox Biology* 2023 ; 63 : 102753.

[5] Kuiper C., Vissers M.C.M. Ascorbate as a co-factor for Fe- and 2-oxoglutarate dependent dioxygenases: physiological activity in tumor growth and progression. *Frontiers in Oncology* 2014 ; 4, 359.

[6] Niki E. Historical perspective: Albert Szent-Györgyi and the discovery of vitamin C. *Nutrition Reviews* 1991; 49(2): 65-67.

[7] Szent-Gyorgyi A. Observation on the function of peroxidase systems and the chemistry of the adrenal cortex: description of a new carbohydrate derivative. *Biochem J* 1928 ; 22 : 1387-1409.

[8] Carpenter K.J. The discovery of vitamin C. *Annals of Nutrition and Metabolism* 1986; 30(2): 89-96.

[9] Kall M.A. Ascorbic acid: properties and determination. In: Caballero B, ed. *Encyclopedia of Food Sciences and Nutrition*. Oxford: Academic Press 2003; 316-324.

[10] *Buettner G.R., Jurkiewicx B.A. Catalytic metals, ascorbate and free radicals: combinations to avoid. Radiat Res* 1996 ; 145 : 532 – 541.

[11] Meschi′ M., Gazivoda K. Therapeutic Perspective of Vitamin C and Its Derivatives. *Antioxidants* 2019 ; 8 : 247.

[12] Roa F.J., Pena E., Gatica M., Escobar-Acuna K., Saavedra P., Maldon D.O., et al., Therapeutic use of vitamin C in cancer : physiological considerations. *Frontiers in Pharmacology* 2020 ; 11 : 211.

[13] Golde D.W. Vitamin C in cancer. *Integrative Cancer Therapies* 2003 ; 2: 158–159.

[14] National Institutes of Health (NIH), *Office of Dietary Supplements*. (2020). Vitamin C. https://ods.od.nih.gov/factsheets/VitaminC-HealthProfessional. Access August 31, 2024.

[15] *USDA National Nutrient Database for Standard Reference.* https://fdc.nal.usda.gov/. Access August 31, 2024.

[16] May J.M., Qu Z., Neel D.R., Li X. Recycling vitamin C from its oxidized forms by human endothelial cells. *Biochim. Biophys. Acta Mol. Cell Res* 2003 ; 1640 : 153–216.

[17] Vissers M.C.M., Das A.B. Potential Mechanisms of Action for Vitamin C in Cancer: Reviewing the Evidence. *Front. Physiol* 2018 ; 9 : 1–13.

[18] Prokop D.J., Kivirikko K.I. Collagens: Molecular biology, diseases, and potential for therapy. *Ann Rev Biochem* 1995 ; 64 : 403-434.

[19] Carr A.C., Rowe S. Factors Affecting Vitamin C Status and Prevalence of Deficiency: A Global Health Perspective. *Nutrients* 2020 ; 12, 1963.

[20] Rowe S., Carr A.C. Global vitamin c status and prevalence of deficiency: A cause for concern? *Nutrients* 2020 ; 12, 2008.

[21] Michels A.J., Frei B., Myzak M.C. Vitamin C. In Ross R, Caballero B, Cousins R, Tucker KL, Ziegler T. Eds. *Modern Nutrition in Health and Disease* 11th ed. Lippincott Williams & Wilkins 2012; 289-304.

[22] Liang W.J., Johnson D., Jarvis S.M. Vitamin C transport systems of mammalian cells. *Mol Member Biol* 2001 ; 18 : 87–95.

[23] Rumsey S.C., Kwon O., Xu G.W., Burant C.F., Simpson I., Levine M. Glucose transporter isoforms GLUT1 and GLUT3 transport dehydroascorbic acid. *J. Biol Chem* 1997 ; 272 : 18982-18989.

[24] Wang H., Dutta B., Huang H., Devoe L.D., Leibach F.H., Ganapathy V., et al., Human Na+-dependent vitamin C transporter 1 (hSVCT1): primary structure, functional characteristics and evidence for a non-functional splice variant. *Biochim Biophys Acta Biomed* 1999 ; 1461 : 1-9.

[25] Tsukaguchi H., Tokui T., Mackenzie B., Berger U.V., Chen X.Z., Wang Y., et al., A family of mammalian Na+-dependent L-ascorbic acid transporters. *Nature* 1999 ; 399 :70-75.

[26] Daruwala R., Song J., Koh W.S., Rumsey S.C., Levine M. Cloning and functional characterization of the human sodium-dependent vitamin C transporters hSVCT1 and hSVCT2. *FEBS Lett* 1999 ; 460 : 480-484.

[27] Corpe C.P., Tu H., Eck P., Wang J., Walter F. Vitamin C transporter Slc23a1 links renal reabsorption, vitamin C tissue accumulation, and perinatal survival in mice. *J Clin Invest* 2010 ; 120 : 1069-1083.

[28] Sotiriou S., Gispert S., Cheng J., Wang Y., Chen A., Hoogstraten-Miller S, et al., Ascorbic-acid transporter Slc23a1 is essential for vitamin C transport into the brain and for perinatal survival. *Nat Med* 2002 ; 8 : 514-517.

[29] Padayatty S.J., Levine M. Vitamin C: The known and the unknown and Goldilocks. *Oral Diseases* 2016 ; 22(6) : 463-493.

[30] Corpe C.P., Eck P., Wang J., Al-Hasani H., Levine M. Intestinal dehydroascorbic acid (DHA) transport mediated by the facilitative sugar transporters, GLUT2 and GLUT8. *J Biol Chem* 2013; 288: 9092-9101.

[31] Linster C.L., Van Scheveningen E. Vitamin. *FEBS J* 2007 ; 274 : 1-22.

[32] Carr A.C., Maggini S. Vitamin C and Immune Function. *Nutrients* 2017 ; 9(11), 1211.

[33] Combs G.F., McClung J.P. *The Vitamins: Fundamental Aspects in Nutrition and Health* 5th ed. Academic Press. 2017.

[34] Lykkesfeldt J. Ascorbate and dehydroascorbic acid as biomarkers of oxidative stress: Validity of clinical studies. *J Clin Nutr and Metab* 2012 ; 27(1) :1-8.

[35] Hunt J.R. Bioavailability of iron, zinc, and other trace minerals from vegetarian diets. *Amer J of Clin Nutrition* 2003 ; 78(3) : 633S-639S.

[36] Traber M.G., Stevens J.F. Vitamin C and E: Beneficial effects from a mechanistic perspective. *Free Radical Biology and Medicine* 2011 ; 51(5) : 1000-1013.

[37] Schleicher R.L., Carroll M.D., Ford E.S., Lacher D.A. Serum vitamin C and the prevalence of vitamin C deficiency in the United States: 2003-2004 National Health and Nutrition Examination Survey (NHANES). *Amer J Clin Nutrition* 2009 ; 90(5): 1252-1263.

[38] *Institute of Medicine (US) Panel on Dietary Antioxidants and Related Compounds.* Dietary Reference Intakes for Vitamin C, Vitamin E, Selenium, and Carotenoids. National Academies Press (US). 2000.

[39] Nair R., Maseeh A. Vitamin D: The "sunshine" vitamin. *J Pharmacol & Pharmacotherapy* 2012 ; 3(2) : 118-126.

[40] Pullar J.M., Carr A.C., Vissers M.C. The roles of vitamin C in skin health. *Nutrients* 2017 ; 9(8): 866.

[41] Murad S., Grove D., Lindberg K.A., Reynolds G., Sivarajah A., Pinnell S.R. Regulation of collagen synthesis by ascorbic acid. *PNAS* 1981 ; 78(5) : 2879-2882.

[42] Marik P.E, Khangoora V, Rivera R, Hooper MH, Catravas J. Hydrocortisone, vitamin C, and thiamine for the treatment of severe sepsis and septic shock: a retrospective before-after study. Chest 2017 ; 151 (6) :1229-1238.

[43] Padayatty J, Sun H, Wang Y. Vitamin C pharmacokinetics: implications for oral and intravenous use. Ann. Intern. Med. 2004 ;140 : 533–537.

[44] Benade L, Howard T, Burk D. Synergistic Killing of Ehrlich Ascites Carcinoma Cells by Ascorbate and 3-Amino-1,2,4, -triazole. Oncology 1969 ; 23 : 33–43.

[45] Pauling L. Vitamin C therapy of advanced cancer. *New Engl J Med* 1980 *; 302* : 694–695.

[46] Pauling L., Anderson R., Banic S. Workshop on vitamin C in immunology and cancer. *Inter J Vit and Nutr Res* 1981 ; 23 : 209–219.

[47] Pauling L., Moertel C. A proposition: Megadose of vitamin C is valuable in the treatment of cancer. *Nutrition Reviews 1986 ;* 44 : 28-29.

[48] Casciari J., Riordan N.H., Schmidt T.L. Cytotoxicity of ascorbate, lipoic acid, and other antioxidants in hollow fiber in vitro tumors. *Br J Cancer* 2002 ; 84 : 1544–1550.

[49] Moertel G., Fleming T.R., Creagan E.T. High-dose vitamin C versus placebo in the treatment of patients with advanced cancer who have had no prior chemotherapy. A randomized double-blind comparison. *N Engl J Med* 1985 *;* 312 : 137–141.

[50] Du J., Cullen J.J., Buettner G.R. Ascorbic acid: chemistry, biology and the treatment of cancer. *Biochim Biophys Acta* 2012 ; 1826 : 443-457.

[51] Levine M., Padayatty S.J., Espey M.G. Vitamin C: A Concentration-Function Approach Yields Pharmacology and Therapeutic Discoveries. *Adv Nutr* 2011 ; 2 : 78–88.

[52] Graumlich J.F., Ludden T.M., Conry-Cantilena C. Pharmacokinetic model of ascorbic acid in healthy male volunteers during depletion and repletion. *Pharm Res* 1997 ; 14 : 1133–1139.

[53] Levine M., Conry-Cantilena C., Wang Y., Welch R.W., Washko P.W., Dhariwal K.R., et al., Vitamin C pharmacokinetics in healthy volunteers: Evidence for a recommended dietary allowance. *PNAS* 1996 ; 93 : 3704–3709.

[54] Drisko A., Chapman J., Hunter V.J. The use of antioxidants with first-line chemotherapy in two cases of ovarian cancer. *J Am Coll Nutr* 2003 ; 22 : 118–123.

[55] Riordan D., Casciari J.J., Gonzalez M.J., Jackson J.A. A pilot clinical study of continuous intravenous ascorbate in terminal cancers patients. *P R Health Sci J* 2005 ; 24 : 269–276.

[56] Carr A.C., Cook J. Intravenous Vitamin C for Cancer Therapy - Identifying the Current Gaps in Our Knowledge. *Front Physiol* 2018 ; 9.

[57] Hoffer L.J., Robitaille L., Zakarian R., Melnychuk D., Kavan P., Agulnik J., et al., High-Dose Intravenous Vitamin C Combined with Cytotoxic Chemotherapy in Patients with Advanced Cancer : A Phase I-II Clinical Trial. *PLoS ONE* 2015 ; 10, e0120228.

[58] Nielsen T.K., Højgaard M., Andersen J.T., Jørgensen N.R., Zerahn B., Kristensen B., et al., Weekly ascorbic acid infusion in castration-resistant prostate cancer patients : A single-arm phase II trial. *Transl Androl Urol* 2017 ; 6 : 517–528.

[59] Stephenson C.M., Levin R.D., Spector T., Lis C.G. Phase I clinical trial to evaluate the safety, tolerability, and pharmacokinetics of high-dose intravenous ascorbic acid in patients with advanced cancer. *Cancer Chemother Pharmacol.* 2013 ; 72 : 139–146.

[60] Hoffer L.J., Levine M., Assouline S., Melnychuk D., Padayatty S.J., Rosadiuk K., et al., Phase I clinical trial of i.v. ascorbic acid in advanced malignancy. *Ann Oncol* 2008 ; 19 : 1969–1974.

[61] Welsh J.L., Wagner B.A., van Erve T.J., Zehr P.S., Berg D.J., Halfdanarson T.R., et al., Pharmacological ascorbate with gemcitabine for the control of metastatic and node-positive pancreatic cancer (PACMAN) : Results from a clinical trial. *Cancer Chemother Pharmacol* 2013 ; 71 : 765–775.

[62] Ma Y., Chapman J., Levine M., Polireddy K., Drisko J., Chen Q. High-Dose Parenteral Ascorbate Enhanced Chemosensitivity of Ovarian Cancer and Reduced Toxicity of Chemotherapy. *Sci Transl Med.* 2014 ; 6 : 222ra18.

[63] Monti D.A., Mitchell E., Bazzan A.J., Littman S., Zabrecky G., Yeo C.J., et al., Phase I Evaluation of Intravenous Ascorbic Acid in Combination with Gemcitabine and Erlotinib in Patients with Metastatic Pancreatic Cancer. *PLoS ONE* 2012 ; 7, e29794.

[64] Casciari J.J., Riordan H.D., Miranda-Massari J.R., Gonzalez M.J. Effects of high dose ascorbate administration on L-10 tumor growth in guinea pigs. *PR Health Sci J* 2005 ; 24 : 145–150.

[65] Yang G., Yan Y., Ma Y., Yang Y. Vitamin C at high concentrations induces cytotoxicity in malignant melanoma but promotes tumor growth at low concentrations. *Mol Carcinog* 2017 ; 56 : 1965–1976.

[66] Verrax J., Calderon P.B. Pharmacologic concentrations of ascorbate are achieved by parenteral administration and exhibit antitumoral effects. *Free Radic Biol Med* 2009 ; 47 : 32–40.

[67] Yeom C.H., Lee G., Park J.H., Yu J., Park S., Yi S.Y., et al., High dose concentration administration of ascorbic acid inhibits tumor growth in BALB/C mice implanted with sarcoma 180 cancer cells via the restriction of angiogenesis. *J. Transl. Med.* 2009 ; 7, 70.

[68] Du J., Martin S.M., Levine M., Wagner B.A., Buettner G.R., Wang S.H., et al., Mechanisms of Ascorbate-Induced Cytotoxicity in Pancreatic Cancer. *Clin Cancer Res* 2010 ; 16 : 509–520.

[69] Chen Q., Espey M.G., Sun A.Y. Pharmacologic doses of ascorbate act as a prooxidant and decrease growth of aggressive tumor xenografts in mice. *PNAS* 2008 ; 105 : 11105–11109.

[70] Cameron E., Campbell A. The ortho molecular treatment of cancer. II. Clinical trial of high-dose ascorbic acid supplements in advanced human cancer. *Chem Biol Interact* 1974 ; 9 : 285–315.

[71] van der Reest J., Gottlieb E. Anti-cancer effects of vitamin C revisited. Cell Research. *2*016 ; 26 : 269–270.

[72] Szydlowski E, Stankiewicz A. Antioxidant status and lipid peroxidation in colorectal cancer. *J Toxicol Env Heal* 2001 ; 64 :213–222.

[73] Langemann H., Torhorst J., Kabiersch A., Krenger W., Honegger C.G. Quantitative determination of water- and lipid-soluble antioxidants in neoplastic and non-neoplastic human breast tissue. *Int J Cancer* 1989 ; 43 :1169–1173.

[74] Anthony H.M., Schorah C.J. Severe hypovitaminosis C in lung-cancer patients: the utilization of vitamin C in surgical repair and lymphocyte-related host resistance. *Br J Cancer* 1982 ; 46 :354–67.

[75] Chen Q., Espey M.G., Krishna M.C. Pharmacologic ascorbic acid concentrations selectively kill cancer cells: Action as a pro-drug to deliver hydrogen peroxide to tissues. *PNAS* 2005 ; 102 : 13604–13609.

[76] Valenti M.T., Zanatta M., Donatelli L. Ascorbic acid induces either differentiation or apoptosis in MG-63 osteosarcoma lineage. *Anticancer Res* 2014 ; 34 :1617-1627.

[77] Fritz H., Flower G., Weeks L., Cooley K., Callachan M., McGowan J., et al., Intravenous Vitamin C and Cancer. *Integr Cancer Ther* 2014 ; 13 : 280–300.

[78] Rivière J., Ravanat J.L., Wagner J.R. Ascorbate and H2O2 induced oxidative DNA damage in Jurkat cells. *Free Radic Biol Med* 2006 ; 40 : 2071–2079.

[79] Pawlowska E., Szczepanska J., Blasiak J. Pro- and antioxidant effects of vitamin C in cancer in correspondence to its dietary and pharmacological concentrations. *Oxidative Medicine and Cellular Longevity* 2019 ; 7286737.

[80] Wang W., Knovich M.A., Coffman L.G., Torti F.M., Torti S.V. Serum ferritin : past, present and future. *Bio Chim Biophys Acta Gen Subj* 2010 ; 1800 : 760-769.

[81] Richardson D.R., Ponka P. The molecular mechanisms of metabolism and transport of iron in normal and neoplastic cells. *Biochim Biophys Acta Rev Bimembral* 1997 ; 1331 : 1-40.

[82] Chaiswing L., St. Clair W.H., St. Clair D.K. Redox paradox: A novel approach to therapeutics-resistant cancer. *Antioxidants & Redox Signaling* 2018 ; 29 : 1237-1272.

[83] Aykin-Burns N., Ahmad I.M., Zhu Y., Oberley L.W., and Spitz D.R. Increased levels of superoxide and H_2O_2 mediate the differential susceptibility of cancer cells versus normal cells to glucose deprivation. *Biochem J* 2009 ; 418 : 29–37.

[84] Cieslak J.A. and Cullen J.J. Treatment of Pancreatic Cancer with Pharmacological Ascorbate. *Curr Pharm Biotechnol* 2015 ; 16 : 759–770.

[85] Farge T., Saland E., de Toni F., Aroua N., Hosseini M., Perry R, et al., Chemotherapy-resistant human acute myeloid leukemia cells are not enriched for leukemic stem cells but require oxidative metabolism. *Cancer Discov* 2017 ; 7 : 716–735.

[86] Holmstrom K.M. and Finkel T. Cellular mechanisms and physiological consequences of redox dependent signaling. *Nat Rev Mol Cell Biol* 2014 ; 15 : 411–421.

[87] Rani V., Deep G., Singh R.K., Palle K., Yadav U.C. Oxidative stress and metabolic disorders: pathogenesis and therapeutic strategies. *Life Sci* 2016 ; 148 : 183–193.

[88] Katz M., Amit I., and Yarden Y. Regulation of MAPKs by growth factors and receptor tyrosine kinases. *Biochim Biophys Acta* 2007 ; 1773 : 1161–1176.

[89] Carr A.C., Spencer E., Das A., Méier N., Lauren C., McPherson S., et al., Patients Undergoing Myeloablative Chemotherapy and Hematopoietic Stem Cell Transplantation Exhibit Depleted Vitamin C Status in Association with Febrile Neutropenia. *Nutrients* 2020 ; 12, 1879.

[90] Davies H.A.S, McLaren-Howard J., Gravett P., Finn M., Gueret-Wardle D. Lipoperoxides as an index of free radical activity in bone marrow transplant recipients. *Biol Trace Elem Res* 1995 ; 47 : 125–132.

[91] Nannya Y., Shinohara A., Ichikawa M., Kurokawa M. Serial Profile of Vitamins and Trace Elements during the Acute Phase of Allogeneic Stem Cell Transplantation. *Biol Blood Marrow Transplant* 2014 ; 20 : 430–434.

[92] Shenoy N., Bhagat T., Nieves E., Stenson M., Lawson J., Choudhary G.S., et al., Upregulation of TET activity with ascorbic acid induces epigenetic modulation of lymphoma cells. *Blood Cancer J* 2017 ; 7, e587.

[93] Klimant E., Wright H., Rubin D., Seely D., Markman M. Intravenous vitamin C in the supportive care of cancer patients: A review and rational approach. *Curr Oncol* 2018 ; 25, 139.

[94] Mayland C.R., Bennett M.I., Allan K. Vitamin C deficiency in cancers patients. *Palliate Med* 2005 ; 19 : 17–20.

[95] Riordan H.D., Riordan N.H., Jackson J.A., Casciari J.J, Hunninghake R, González MJ, et al., Intravenous vitamin C as a chemotherapy agent : A report on clinical cases. *PR Health Sci J* 2004 ; 23 : 115–118.

[96] Foyer C.F., Noctor G. Ascorbate and glutathione: the heart of the redox hub. *Plant Physiol* 2011 ; 155 : 2–18.

[97] McEligot A.J., Yang S., Meyskens F.L. Redox regulation by intrinsic species and extrinsic nutrients in normal and cancer cells. *Annu Rev Nutr* 2005 ; 25 : 261-295.

[98] Ngo B., van Riper J.M., Cantley L.C., Yun J. Targeting cancer vulnerabilities with high-dose vitamin C. *Nat Rev Cancer* 2019 ; 19(5) : 271-278.

[99] Abou-Jawde R.M., Reed J., Kelly M., Walker E., Andresen S., Baz R., et al., Efficacy and Safety Results with the Combination Therapy of Arsenic Trioxide, Dexamethasone, and Ascorbic Acid in Multiple Myeloma Patients: A Phase 2 Trial. *Med Oncol* 2006 ; 23 : 263–272.

[100] Wu K.L., Beksac M., Van Droogenbroeck J., Amadori S., Zweegman S., Sonneveld P. Phase II multicenter study of arsenic trioxide, ascorbic acid and dexamethasone in patients with relapsed or refractory multiple myeloma. *Haematologica* 2006 ; 91 : 1722–1723.

[101] Berenson J.R., Matous J., Swift R.A., Mapes R., Morrison B., Yeh H.S. A Phase I/II Study of Arsenic Trioxide/Bortezomib/Ascorbic Acid Combination Therapy for the Treatment of Relapsed or Refractory Multiple Myeloma. Clin. *Cancer Res* 2007 ; 13 : 1762–1768.

[102] Polireddy K., Dong R., Reed G., Chen P., Williamson S., Pessetto Z., et al., High dose parenteral ascorbate inhibited pancreatic cancer growth and metastasis: mechanisms and a phase I/IIa study. *Sci Rep* 2017 ; 7 : 17188.

[103] Zasowska-Nowak A., Nowak P.J., Cialkowska-Rysz A. High-dose vitamin C in advanced-stage cancer patients. *Nutrients* 2021 ; 13(3) : 735.

Chapter 3

Materials and Methods

Lunawati L. Bennett*, PhD, PharmD

Union University, College of Pharmacy, Jackson, Tennessee, USA

Abstract

This chapter describes the standardized materials and experimental procedures used throughout the studies presented in this book to investigate the anticancer effects of vitamin C alone and in combination with selected antineoplastic agents. The protocols include cell culture conditions, cytotoxicity assays, apoptosis and oxidative stress analyses, mitochondrial membrane potential assessment, Western blot analysis, and statistical evaluation. By centralizing these methods, consistency and reproducibility across different cancer models are ensured. Chapter-specific variations are described in the respective experimental chapters. This methodological framework provides a reliable foundation for interpreting mechanistic and therapeutic findings presented throughout the book. Unless otherwise noted, the protocols described here were consistently followed in subsequent chapters. For chapter-specific details, such as the use of different cell lines or unique experimental modifications, readers are referred to the respective chapters.

Keywords: vitamin C, anticancer mechanisms, cell culture methods, apoptosis and oxidative stress, western blot analysis

Abbreviations

AIF	Apoptosis inducing factor;
APAF	Apoptotic peptidase activating factor;
ATCC	American Type Culture Collection;
Bax	Bcl2 Associated X-protein;
Bcl2	B cell lymphoma 2;
Cas	Caspase;
CDK7	Cyclin dependent kinase 7;
Cyt C	Cytochrome C;
DMSO	Dimethyl sulfoxide;
DPBS	Dulbecco's phosphate-buffered saline;

* Corresponding Author's Email: llbennett@uu.edu

EGFR	Epidermal growth factor receptor;
EMEM	Eagle's minimum essential medium;
EMT	epithelial mesenchymal transition;
ER+	Estrogen receptor-positive;
ERK 1/2	Extracellular signal-regulated kinase 1/2;
FBS	Fetal bovine serum;
HER2	Human epidermal growth factor receptor 2;
IAP	Inhibitor of apoptosis protein;
MAPKs	Mitogen-activated protein kinases;
MEKs	Mitogen-activated protein kinase kinases;
MDM2	Mouse double minute 2 homolog;
MnSOD	Manganese superoxide dismutase;
MOMP	Mitochondrial outer membrane permeabilization;
p85	Phosphatidylinositol-3-kinase;
PR+	Progesterone receptor-positive;
PTEN	Phosphatase and tensin homolog;
ROCK	Rho-associated kinase;
ROS	Reactive oxygen species;
SAPK/JNK	Stress-activated protein kinase/c-Jun N-terminal kinase;
Smac/DIABLO	Second mitochondria-derived activator of caspases; Direct IAP-Binding protein with Low pI
SRB	Sulforhodamine B;
TNBC	Triple Negative Breast Cancer;
VC	Vitamin C;
Wnt	Wingless/integrated.

Note: these are commonly used abbreviations found in the following chapters.

Chemicals

Vitamin C and Antineoplastic Agents

- L-ascorbic acid (vitamin C): Sigma-Aldrich (St. Louis, MO, USA).
- Antineoplastic etoposide, doxorubicin, sorafenib, temsirolimus, paclitaxel, and afatinib: LC Laboratories (Woburn, MA, USA).

Culture Media and Reagents

- Cell cultures, fetal bovine serum (FBS), antibiotic-antimycotic solutions, McCoy's 5A medium, Iscove's Modified Dulbecco's Medium: American Type Culture Collection (ATCC, Manassas, VA, USA)

- Eagle's Minimum Essential medium (EMEM), Dulbecco Minimum Essential media (DMEM), Roswell Park Memorial Institute (RPMI) 1640: Thermo Fisher Scientific (Waltham, MA, USA).
- Plastic ware for cell culture: Greiner Bio-One (Monroe, NC, USA) and Corning (Corning, NY, USA).

Fluorescent Staining Dyes

- Rhodamine 123 (mitochondrial membrane potential): Sigma (St. Louis, MO, USA)
- Hoechst 33342 (nuclear stain): Life Technologies (Carlsbad, CA, USA)
- H2DCFDA (ROS detection): Invitrogen (Eugene, OR, USA).

Fluorescence imaging was performed using the FLoid™ Cell Imaging Station (Life Technologies, Carlsbad, CA, USA).

Reagents

- Sulforhodamine B (SRB), RIPA buffer (50 mM Tris-HCl, pH 8.0, 1% NP-40, 0.5% sodium deoxycholate, 150 mM NaCl, and 0.1% sodium dodecyl sulphate, protease and phosphatase inhibitor cocktail, Bradford Reagent, trichloroacetic acid: Sigma (Saint Louis, MO, USA)
- Dimethyl sulfoxide (DMSO): Ameresco (Solon, OH, USA).

Western Blot Materials

- SDS-PAGE gels, Enhanced Chemiluminescence (ECL) detection kit, PVDF transfer membranes: Bio-Rad (Hercules, CA, USA)
- Primary antibodies: PDL-1, Casp-3, Cas-7, Casp-8, Casp-9, Cyclin D1, Cyclin B1, Cytochrome c, PTEN, p53, p21, p38, Akt, CDK2, AIF-1, Apaf, mTOR, Smac/DIABLO, MnSOD, Vimentin, SAPK/JNK: Cell Signalling Technology (Beverley, MA, USA).
- Primary antibodies: β-actin, Bax, Bcl2, CDK7, EGFR, MEK-1, -2, -3 and -4: Santa Cruz Biotechnology, Inc (Santa Cruz, CA, USA)
- Dry milk: Santa Cruz (Santa Cruz, CA, USA)
- Secondary HRP-conjugated antibodies: Cell Signalling Technology (Beverley, MA, USA).

Procedure

Cell Culture and Treatment Conditions

Various human cancer cell lines and non-cancerous control cell lines were cultured in appropriate media supplemented with FBS and antibiotics, as recommended for each line per ATCC guidelines.

For each experiment, cells were plated at optimal seeding density to ensure logarithmic growth during treatment. Four treatment groups were applied consistently across all models:

1. Control (untreated cells),
2. Vitamin C (VC) at low to moderate millimolar concentration ranges,
3. Antineoplastic drug at sub-cytotoxic or minimally cytostatic dose, and
4. VC + drug combination administered simultaneously.

This standardized grouping allowed direct comparison of VC alone, drug alone, and synergistic or antagonistic effects in the combination.

Image Presentation and Contrast Standardization

Fluorescence and microscopy images were processed to optimize visibility for both digital and grayscale print formats. Depending on signal strength and background distribution, images were displayed either as **white-on-black** or **black-on-white** to best represent nuclear morphology, reactive oxygen species (ROS) signal intensity, and mitochondrial structural patterns.

All images within each experiment and within each cell line were processed using the **same contrast and inversion settings**, ensuring fair visual comparison among control, VC, drug, and combination groups. No selective enhancement, pixel removal, or artificial signal amplification was performed. Adjustments were limited to global brightness, contrast, and inversion when required for visual clarity.

Cytotoxicity Assay

Cells were seeded in 96-well flat-bottomed microplates at a volume of 100 μL per well, with a density of 1 × 10^5 cells/mL and allowed to adhere overnight in growth medium. The following day, the medium was replaced with fresh growth medium.

Cells were then treated with varying concentrations of VC, antineoplastic agents, or their combination, and incubated for 24 h at 37°C in a humidified atmosphere of 5% CO_2. The combination of VC and antineoplastics that produced a synergistic decrease in cell viability was selected for subsequent experiments.

The assay was performed according to the method described by Vichai and Kirtikara [1]. Briefly, cells were fixed with trichloroacetic acid (TCA) to a final concentration of 10% and incubated at 4°C for 1 h or longer. The plates were then gently washed with tap water and air-dried before staining with 50 μL of SRB solution (0.057% in 1% acetic acid). After 30 min, the plates were washed three times with 1% acetic acid to remove excess stain and dried for 30 min. Finally, 150 μL of TRIS buffer (10 mM, pH 10.5) was added, and the plates were placed on a shaker to dissolve the bound dye. Absorbance was measured at 590 nm using a spectrophotometer (Molecular Devices, CA, USA).

Morphology Analysis

To identify morphological changes, cells were observed at 0 h and 24 h under an inverted microscope (Motic AE31, Hong Kong). Cells were incubated in 12-well plates at a density of 1 × 10^5 cells/mL under standard culture conditions (37°C, 5% CO_2). The morphology of control and treated cells was examined and photographed at 40× magnification.

Wound-Healing (Migration) Assay

To assess cellular migration, cells were seeded in 12-well plates with a density of 1 × 10^5 cells/mL under standard culture conditions (37°C, 5% CO_2). After 24 h when cells reach 50-60% confluence, a single scratch was generated using a sterile pipette tip (100 μl) and cells were treated with VC, antineoplastics, or their combination. Images of the scratched were photographed (40X) under inverted microscope (Motic AE 31, Hong Kong) and the width of the scratch was measured by Image J software (NIH, USA).

Apoptosis Analysis

To identify the morphological changes of the nuclear chromatin inducing apoptosis of cells, Hoechst 33342 staining assay using fluorescent probe was performed as previously described [2]. Briefly, cells were seeded in 24-well plates with a density of 1 × 10^5 cells/mL under standard culture conditions (37°C, 5% CO_2) prior to treatment with VC, antineoplastics, or the combination for 24 h. The cells were then stained with Hoechst 33342 Cell Stain according to the manufacturer's protocol.

Intracellular ROS Analysis

To compare intracellular ROS generation of cells, H2DCF-DA staining assay using fluorescent probe was performed as previously described [2]. Briefly, cells were seeded in 24-well plates with a density of 1 × 10^5 cells/mL under standard culture conditions (37°C, 5% CO_2) prior to treatment with VC, antineoplastics, or the combination for 24 h. The cells were then stained with H2DCF-DA according to the manufacturer's protocol.

Mitochondrial Membrane Potential (Ψ_m) Analysis

To compare the mitochondrial membrane potential of cells, Rhodamine123 assay using fluorescent probe was performed as previously described [2]. Briefly, cells were seeded in 24-well plates with a density of 1 × 10^5 cells/mL under standard culture conditions (37°C, 5% CO_2) prior to treatment with VC, antineoplastics, or the combination for 24 h. The cells were then stained with Rhodamine 123 according to the manufacturer's protocol.

Western Blot Analysis

The Western blot technique was employed to assess the expressions of apoptotic signaling proteins and proteins associated with tumorigenesis, following the procedures outlined in previous studies [2]. Cells were treated with VC, antineoplastics, or their combination for 24 h. The proteins were extracted in RIPA buffer with protease and phosphate inhibitors and centrifuged at 12,000 rpm for 25 min at 4 °C. The protein concentrations were determined using the Bradford Protein Assay Reagent. Equivalent amounts of protein from each sample were loaded onto 10% polyacrylamide gels and separated by electrophoresis using PowerPac200 electrophoresis system (Bio-Rad).

The proteins were then transferred to PVDF membranes (Immuno-Blot PVDF, Bio-Rad). Blotting was performed using Trans Blot Turbo (Bio-Rad) for 30 min. The membranes were then blocked for 2 h at room temperature in 5% non-fat dry milk dissolved in Tris-buffered saline containing 0.1% Tween-20 (TBST). The milk was discharged following incubation of the membranes with different primary antibodies of interest diluted with 5% non-fat dry milk in TBST where the membranes were rocked on a multi shaker overnight at 4° C. The following day, the membranes were probed with horseradish peroxidase-conjugated anti-mouse IgG or anti-rabbit IgG antibody for 2 h in room temperature. The protein band was developed by ECL Western Blotting reagents (Bio Rad) and the pictures were taken using Bio-Rad ChemiDoc XRS+ (Bio-Rad). The band intensity was measured by Image J software (NIH, USA).

Statistical Analysis

All data are expressed as the mean ± SD of three independent experiments. Differences between individual and combination treatment groups were analyzed using one-way

ANOVA followed by Newman–Keuls post hoc test. Statistical significance was defined as $^{**}p < 0.01$, and $^{***}p < 0.001$.

Experimental Scope Statement

Certain assays, such as Western blot analyses or oxidative stress measurements, were performed selectively across models depending on preliminary findings and experimental feasibility. The presented results reflect representative and reproducible data that best illustrate the biological effects investigated.

References

[1] Vichai V., Kirtikara K. Sulforhodamine B colorimetric assay for cytotoxicity screening. *Nature Protocols* 2006 ; 1: 1112-1116.

[2] Bennett L.L., Mondal A. Curcumin and Afatinib synergistically inhibit growth of human osteosarcoma cells by inhibition of matrix metallo proteinases, mitogen activated kinases 1-4, and reactive oxygen species. *J of Pharm Drug Develop.* 2021 ; 3 : 1.

Chapter 4

High-Dose Vitamin C Does Not Induce Toxicity in Non-Cancerous Cells

Lunawati L. Bennett*, PhD, PharmD
Union University, College of Pharmacy, Jackson, Tennessee, USA

Abstract

High-dose vitamin C, also known as pharmacological concentration of vitamin C has been extensively investigated for its pro-oxidant cytotoxicity in malignant cells; however, its impact on normal cells is less well characterized. This chapter examines the cellular response of non-cancerous models, specifically human embryonic kidney epithelial cells (HEK 293) and normal lung fibroblasts (CCL 205), following exposure to pharmacological concentrations of vitamin C.
The results demonstrate that unlike cancerous cells which exhibit elevated susceptibility due to altered redox homeostasis, non-cancerous cells-maintained viability and did not display significant cytotoxic responses. These findings suggest that non-malignant cells possess more efficient antioxidant defense mechanisms, such as glutathione buffering and catalase activity, that mitigate the pro-oxidant effects of high-dose vitamin C. The absence of measurable cytotoxicity in HEK 293 and CCL 205 cells highlights the selectivity index of vitamin C and supports its therapeutic potential as an adjunctive anticancer strategy with a favorable safety margin for non-cancerous tissues.

Keywords: HEK 293, vitamin C, lung fibroblast, normal cells, redox

Abbreviations

VC	Vitamin C;
ROS	reactive oxygen species;
H_2O_2	hydrogen peroxide;
HEK	Human embryonic kidney;
H_2DCFDA	2,7-dichlorodihydrofluorescein diacetate;
MDR	multi drug resistance;
mTOR	mammalian target of rapamycin;
PD-L1	programmed death ligand;
MnSOD	Manganese Superoxide Dismutase;

* Corresponding Author's Email: llbennett@uu.edu

Smac/DIABLO	Second Mitochondria-derived Activator of Caspase Direct Inhibitor of Apoptosis-binding protein with Low pI;
p85	Phosphatidylinositol-3-kinase;
Bax	Bcl2 Associated X-protein;
Bcl2	B cell lymphoma 2.

Introduction

Vitamin C (VC) is a vital water-soluble micronutrient renowned for its antioxidant capacity, contribution to collagen biosynthesis, immune support, and maintenance of overall cellular health. Beyond these classical roles, recent research has highlighted its therapeutic potential in oncology, particularly when administered at pharmacological concentrations [1]. Unlike its normal dietary function as an antioxidant, high-dose VC exhibits pro-oxidant activity, generating reactive oxygen species (ROS) such as hydrogen peroxide (H_2O_2) in extracellular fluid. This pro-oxidant property has been shown to selectively induce cytotoxicity in cancer cells while sparing non-cancerous cells, offering a unique advantage over many conventional chemotherapeutics, which often damage both malignant and healthy tissues [2-4].

The selectivity of high-dose VC is rooted in intrinsic differences between normal and cancerous cells. Cancer cells typically display increased levels of labile iron and compromised antioxidant defenses, including reduced activity of catalase and glutathione peroxidase. These vulnerabilities render malignant cells highly susceptible to oxidative damage induced by ROS. In contrast, normal cells possess more robust detoxification systems, allowing them to neutralize ROS efficiently and maintain cellular integrity [4-6].

Another key mechanism involves the differential uptake of vitamin C. Certain cancer cells, especially those with KRAS or BRAF mutations, overexpress the glucose transporter GLUT1, which facilitates the transport of dehydroascorbic acid (DHA), the oxidized form of VC. Once inside the cell, DHA is converted back to ascorbate, consuming intracellular reducing equivalents such as glutathione (GSH) and NADPH. This leads to oxidative stress, inhibition of glycolysis through GAPDH inactivation, and subsequent energy depletion, culminating in selective cancer cell death [7].

High-dose VC has also been observed to enhance the efficacy of established chemotherapeutic agents, including sorafenib, paclitaxel, afatinib, doxorubicin, etoposide, and bortezomib, through synergistic induction of oxidative stress and mitochondrial dysfunction. Importantly, this synergy does not increase toxicity to normal cells, underscoring the potential for safer combination therapies [8-9].

The selective cytotoxicity of high-dose VC has far-reaching implications in cancer therapy. It offers a potential approach to reduce chemotherapy-associated toxicity, to improve patient outcomes, and to expand the repertoire of treatments available for resistant or aggressive cancers. Moreover, understanding the mechanisms by which normal cells resist high-dose VC-induced oxidative stress may reveal broader insights into cellular redox homeostasis and metabolism. Ongoing studies are exploring not only its role in combination therapy but also potential effects on epigenetic regulation, immune modulation, and tumor microenvironment remodeling, expanding the scope of VC as a multifunctional therapeutic agent [10].

To further examine the safety profile of high-dose VC and its cellular effects on non-cancerous cells, experiments were conducted using HEK 293 human embryonic kidney cells and CCL 205 fibroblasts cell lines as the models for the study under controlled culture conditions. Experimental methods were performed as described in Chapter 3 (Materials and Methods). Specific details unique to this study are described below.

Cell Cultures

Human embryonic kidney (HEK 293, ATCC CRL-1573) was isolated from kidney of an aborted embryo in the early 1970s by researcher Alex van der Eb, and were later immortalized by Frank Graham by transforming them with human adenovirus type 5 (Ad5) DNA, allowing for their continuous growth in culture. CCL 205 (ATCC CCD 18Lu) is fibroblast cells isolated in 1979 from the lung of a Black, two-and-a-half-month-old, female patient. They are cultured in Eagle's Minimum Essential Medium (EMEM) supplemented with 10% fetal bovine serum (FBS), 1% streptomycin/penicillin. The cells were cultured in T75 dishes and maintained in an incubator at 37°C in a 5% CO_2 humidified environment.

Results

Cell Viability

An increase in cell viability was observed in rat spleen cells treated with 2.5 mM and 8 mM VC, indicating that VC did not cause cell death in normal cells such as spleen.

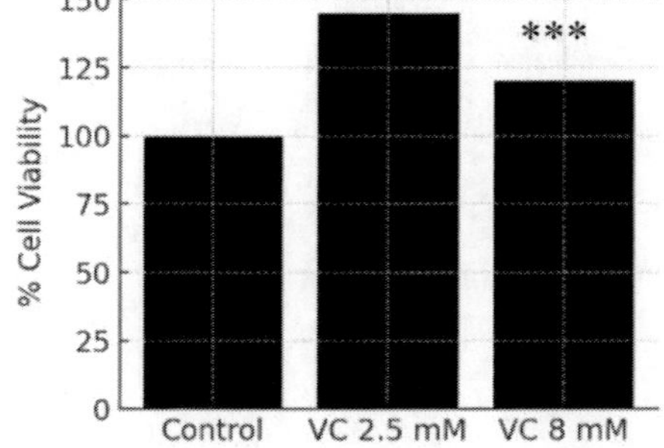

Figure 1. Rat spleen showed a high % cell viability compared to control showing non-cytotoxic effect of VC on normal cells. Statistical significance was determined using the post hoc Newman-Keuls test ***p < 0.01 compared to control.

Changes in Cell Morphology

Non-cancerous HEK 293 kidney cells exhibited increased growth when treated with 5 mM or 15 mM VC, as compared to the control, indicating that VC did not induce cell death in non-cancerous cells (see Fig.2).

Wound-Healing

Non-cancerous HEK 293 kidney cells treated with 5 mM or 15 mM VC for 24 h showed no significant changes in cell growth compared to the control, indicating that VC is non-cytotoxic to normal cells (see Fig.3).

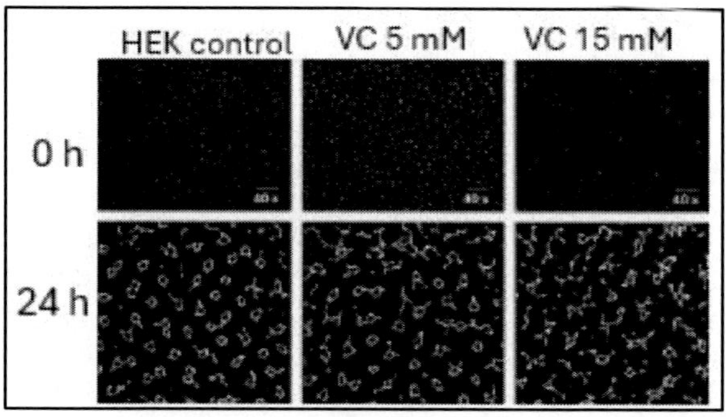

Figure 2. Inverted microscopic images VC at 5 mM and 15 mM showed promotion of cell growth in HEK-293 kidney cells. The scale bar represents 40X.

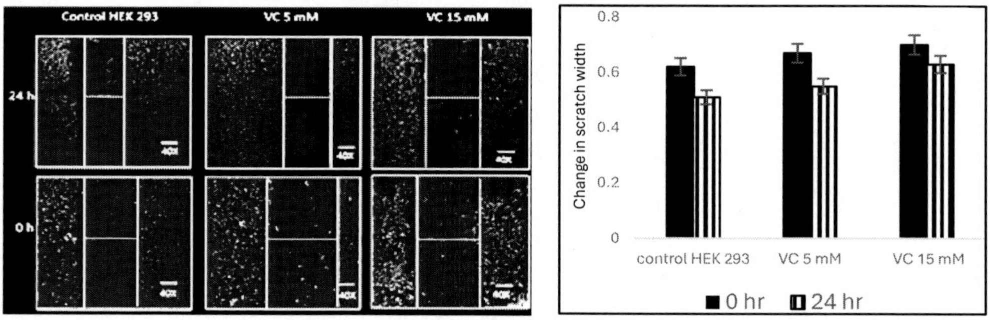

(a) (b)

Figure 3. (a). VC at 5 mM and 15 mM enhanced cell growth in non-cancerous HEK 293 kidney cells, as evidenced by a decreased scratch width with the corresponding histograms (b). Data are expressed as the mean ± SD (n = 3).

Induction of Apoptosis

Hoechst 33342 staining was used to evaluate intracellular ROS-induced nuclear damage in HEK 293 and CCL 205 cells following treatment with increasing concentrations of VC. Fluorescence microscopy showed uniformly stained, intact nuclei in control and VC-treated groups, with no evidence of nuclear condensation or fragmentation. The overall fluorescence intensity remained comparable across VC concentrations ranging from 5 mM to 15 mM, indicating the absence of oxidative stress–related chromatin alterations. These findings further confirm that high-dose VC does not exert cytotoxic or pro-oxidative effects on non-cancerous cells, supporting its safety profile in normal cellular systems.

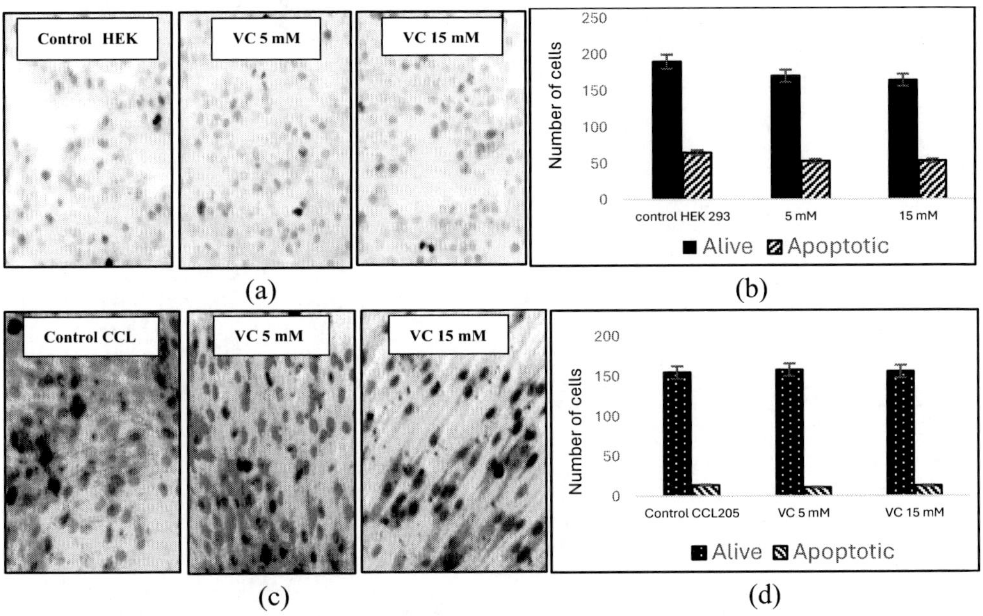

Figure 4. VC treatment at 5 mM and 15 mM in non-cancerous HEK 293 kidney cells or CCL 205 lung cells did not significantly affect ratio of apoptotic and alive cells as illustrated in histogram. VC didn't show cytotoxic effect on normal cells. The scale bar represents 100 μm.

Intracellular ROS Generation

The generation of intracellular ROS was assessed in HEK 293 and CCL 205 cells using H_2DCFDA staining. Fluorescence microscopy revealed no significant changes in fluorescence intensity with increasing VC concentrations between 5 mM and 15 mM. These findings suggest that VC does not induce oxidative stress in non-cancerous cells within this concentration range, supporting its relative safety and redox stability under physiological conditions (see Fig.5).

Mitochondrial Membrane Potential (Ψ_m)

Depletion of mitochondrial membrane potential is a hallmark of mitochondrial dysfunction and often signals cell stress or initiation of cell death pathways. Treatments of HEK 293 or CCL205 with high dose VC showed similar fluorescence intensity like control cells, indicating healthy mitochondria (see Fig. 6).

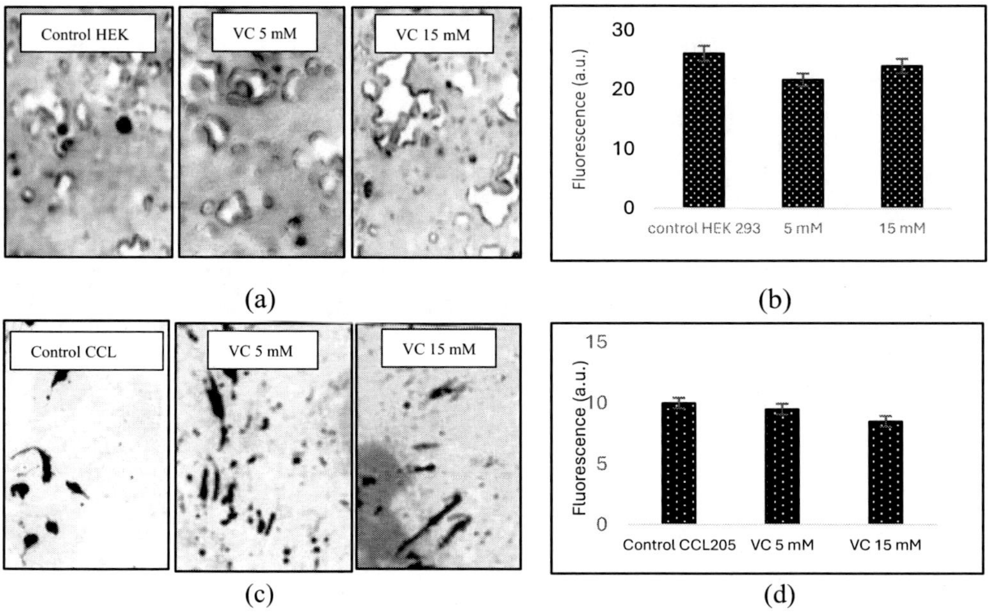

Figure 5. (a, c). Results of intracellular ROS generation assessed with H2DCF staining in HEK 293 and CCL 205 with a scale bar indicating 100 μm. (b, d) Presents a histogram illustrating the band intensity corresponding to treatments.

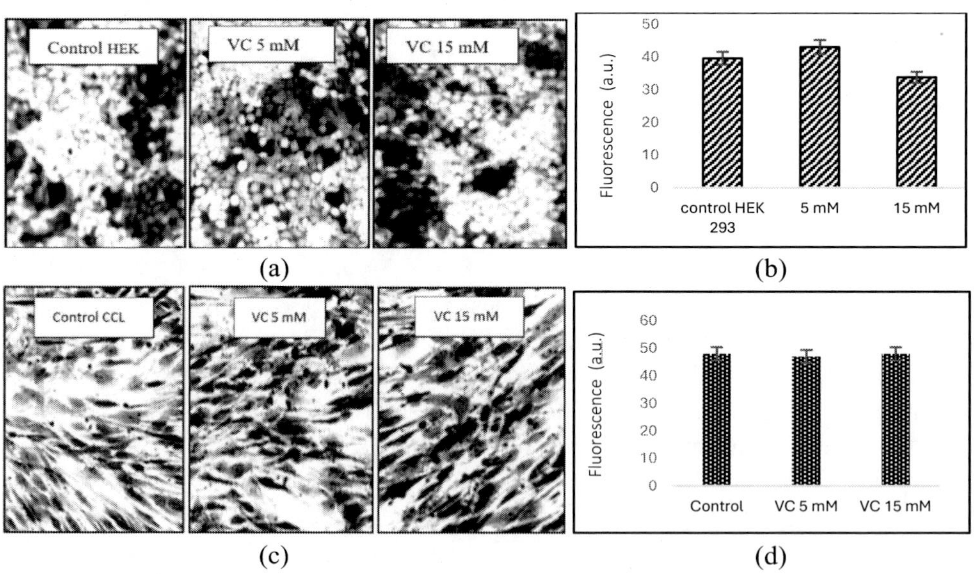

Figure 6. (a, c).VC treatment at 5 mM and 15 mM in non-cancerous HEK 293 and CCL 205 cells showed no significant change in membrane potential, showing VC has no effect on non-cancerous cells. The scale bar represents 100 μm. (b, d) Presents a histogram illustrating the band intensity corresponding to the treatments.

Induction of Cell Death

The viability of cells treated with VC was assessed using the nuclear-ID red/green staining method. Live cells were stained green, as the dye penetrated the cytoplasm of intact cell membrane, while dying or dead cells, with compromised membranes, were stained red. Cells that displayed a red or orange color when the red and green dye images were merged indicating dead cells while light green indicates alive cells. The green fluorescence in both HEK 293 and CCL 205 cells was predominant, signifying high cell viability in both control and VC-treated groups.

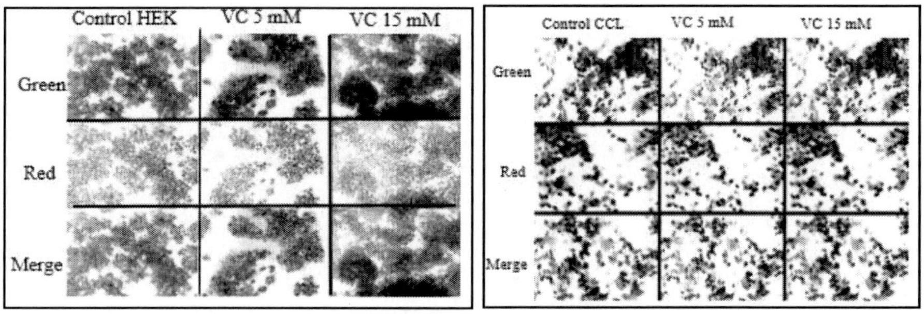

Figure 7. (a) (b). Showed HEK 293 and CCL 205 control versus treated cells with 5 mM or 15 mM VC displayed a similar proportion of live and dead cells, indicating that VC had no significant cytotoxic effect on these non-cancerous cell lines.

Modulation of p21, p53, PTEN, and MDM2

The impact of VC on the expression of key regulatory proteins, including p21, p53, PTEN, and MDM2, was assessed in HEK 293 and CCL 205. There was a significant increase in the expression levels of p21 and PTEN, indicating a positive regulatory effect on cell cycle control and tumor suppression. Conversely, the expression of MDM2 decreased, suggesting a potential inhibitory effect of VC on the MDM2 pathway.

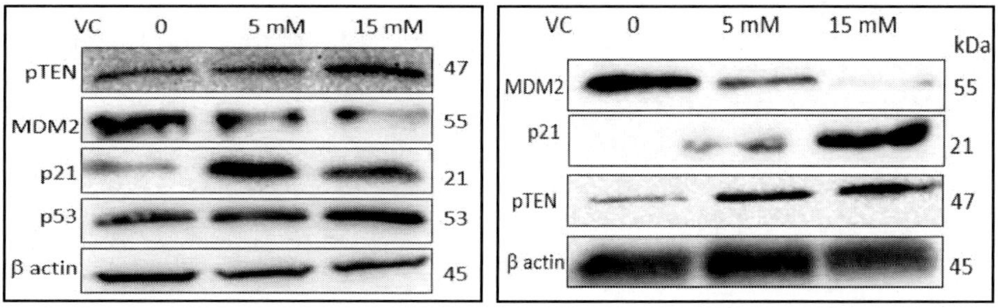

Figure 8. (a) Depicts the impact of VC on HEK 293 while (b) on CCL 205. Increase in p21, PTEN, and decrease in MDM2 expressions indicated a positive effect of VC on cell cycle control and tumor suppression proteins in both cell lines.

Modulation of MnSOD and Smac/DIABLO

The impact of VC on the expression of MnSOD and Smac/DIABLO showed a slight increase in Smac/DIABLO expression in HEK 293while significant increase in CCL 205. Increase in manganese superoxide dismutase MnSOD expressions, a key mitochondrial antioxidant enzyme, consistent with enhanced redox buffering capacity of VC. Increased expression of Smac/DIABLO, a mitochondrial protein that promotes apoptotic signaling by antagonizing inhibitor of apoptosis proteins (IAPs), shows positive effects of VC on non-cancerous cells.

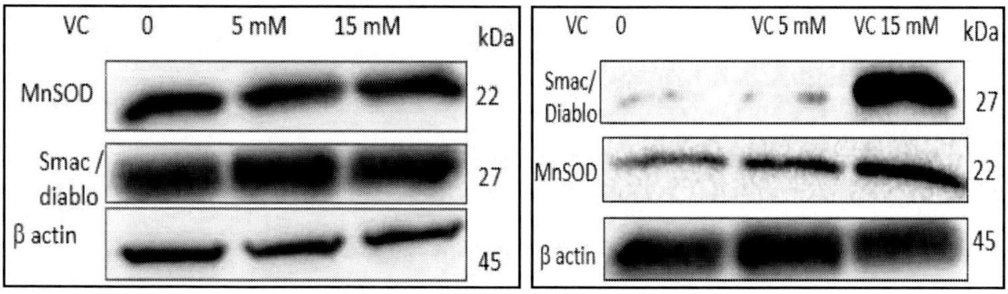

(a) (b)

Figure 9. Western blot analysis data showing the modulation of MnSOD and Smac/DIABLO in HEK 293 (a) and in CCL 205 cells (b).

Modulation of MDR-ABC, mTOR and PD-L1

The impact of VC on multi-drug resistance (MDR), mammalian target of rapamycin (mTOR) and programmed death-ligand (PD-L1) revealed that VC exposure caused decreased their protein expressions in HEK293 and CCL-205 cells, suggesting potential regulatory effects on growth, immune checkpoint, and drug transport mechanisms in non-cancerous cells.

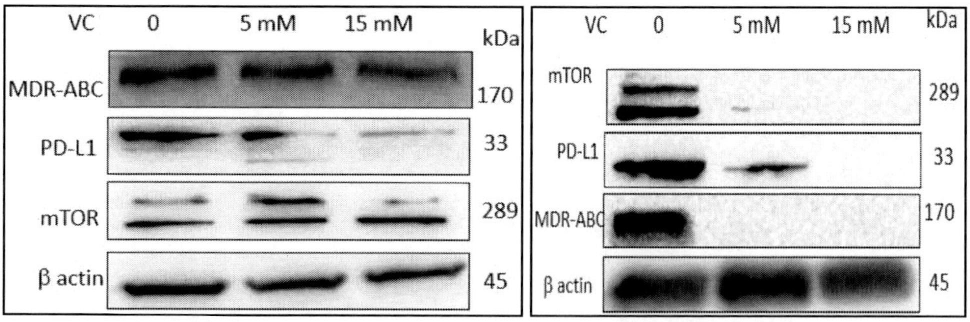

(a) (b)

Figure 10. Western blot analysis of HEK 293 (a) and CCL 205 (b) cells treated with VC. Treatment with VC at 5 mM or 15 mM resulted in decreased expression of mTOR, PD-L1, and MDR-ABC compared to control, indicating a favorable modulatory effect of VC on cellular signaling and drug-resistance–related proteins in non-cancerous cells.

Discussion

The present study was designed to evaluate the effects of PVC on non-cancerous cells to provide a baseline safety profile for comparison with malignant cell lines treated with VC and anticancer agents. Two different non-malignant human cell models were investigated: embryonic kidney (HEK293) and lung fibroblast (CCL205) cells. Across both models, VC at concentrations of 5 mM and 15 mM did not cause measurable cytotoxicity when compared to untreated controls. Normal cells generally maintain higher catalase activity and more efficient antioxidant systems, enabling them to detoxify extracellular hydrogen peroxide generated by high VC concentrations (5-6). This contrasts sharply with many cancer cells, which are often characterized by low catalase activity, dysregulated iron metabolism, and increased basal oxidative stress, rendering them selectively vulnerable to VC-induced oxidative damage.

Functional assays provided consistent evidence of cell preservation. Live/dead viability analysis showed no significant changes, indicating that membrane integrity and cell survival were maintained under VC treatment. Assessment of mitochondrial membrane potential using rhodamine and intracellular ROS with H2DCF revealed no major differences relative to control cells, suggesting that VC did not compromise mitochondrial function or induce oxidative stress in these normal cell types. Nuclear morphology assessed with Hoechst staining likewise showed no evidence of apoptosis or chromatin condensation. Together, these functional endpoints strongly indicate that non-cancerous HEK293 and CCL205 cells tolerate high-dose VC without undergoing cell death.

Pharmacologic concentration of VC can act as a pro-oxidant in tumor tissue while sparing normal cells. Preclinical and clinical investigations have demonstrated that high-dose intravenous VC can potentiate chemotherapy or radiotherapy without additional toxicity to healthy tissues [10]. The findings in HEK293 and CCL205 cells further reinforce this selectivity, showing that even at concentrations up to 15 mM, non-cancerous cells remain viable and metabolically stable.

Although overall cell viability was unaffected, western blot analysis revealed reproducible shifts in several signaling pathways, pointing toward adaptive or regulatory responses rather than cytotoxic injury. One notable change was the upregulation of MnSOD, a key mitochondrial antioxidant enzyme, consistent with enhanced redox buffering capacity. The increase in MnSOD aligns with the well-described role of VC as both an antioxidant and a redox modulator in normal tissues. This suggests that high-dose VC may strengthen, rather than overwhelm, antioxidant defenses in non-malignant cells.

Increased expression of Smac/DIABLO, a mitochondrial protein that promotes apoptotic signaling by antagonizing inhibitor of apoptosis proteins (IAPs), shows positive effects of VC. However, since no evidence of caspase activation or functional apoptosis was detected, Smac/DIABLO induction may reflect mitochondrial engagement in signaling without progression to cell death. Instead, it could represent a preparatory or stress-adaptive response that contributes to cellular homeostasis under high-dose VC conditions.

At the level of cell-cycle and growth regulation, both HEK293 and CCL205 displayed reductions in MDM2, along with modest increases in p21 and PTEN expression. These changes are consistent with stabilization of p53 activity, promotion of cell-cycle restraint, and reinforcement of tumor suppressive signaling. Such effects may be considered beneficial, as they are associated with enhanced genomic stability and protection against uncontrolled proliferation. In line with this, both cell types exhibited decreased expression of mTOR, a central regulator of cell growth and metabolism. Downregulation of mTOR in normal cells has been linked to metabolic moderation and increased stress resistance, suggesting that VC promotes a protective, energy-conserving state [11].

Interestingly, VC treatment was also associated with decreased expression of PD-L1 and MDR-ABC in both cell lines. These molecules are typically involved in immune evasion and drug efflux in cancer cells. While the biological relevance in non-malignant cells is less clear, their downregulation suggests that VC may modulate pathways associated with immune signaling and cellular defense, potentially reinforcing the selectivity of pharmacologic VC against malignant cells.

Taken together, the absence of cytotoxicity across multiple functional assays combined with these molecular adjustments suggests that pharmacologic VC does not damage non-cancerous cells but instead induces subtle adaptive responses [12]. These responses include enhanced antioxidant defenses, suppression of oncogenic and proliferative signaling, and reinforcement of tumor suppressive pathways. Importantly, the effects were consistent in two distinct non-malignant human cell models, strengthening the conclusion that high-dose VC is well tolerated in normal cellular contexts.

These findings are in line with earlier studies demonstrating that normal cells are resistant to the cytotoxic effects of pharmacologic VC, in contrast to cancer cells, which often undergo oxidative stress and apoptosis when exposed to similar concentrations. The results reinforce this model by showing that non-cancerous HEK293 and CCL205 cells remain viable and functionally intact even at 15 mM VC.

Conclusion

Pharmacologic VC appears safe in non-malignant cell models, producing no evidence of cytotoxicity while promoting molecular changes consistent with enhanced stress resistance and suppression of pro-growth signaling. These data provide a critical foundation for interpreting the effects of VC in cancer cell lines, where similar doses often induce apoptosis or synergize with chemotherapeutic agents. By demonstrating the lack of harm in normal cells, this study supports the therapeutic potential of high-dose VC as a selective anticancer strategy with minimal risk to healthy tissues.

Key Findings

High-dose VC (5–15 mM) did not induce cell death, oxidative stress, or mitochondrial dysfunction in non-cancerous HEK293 and CCL205 cells. Both cell types exhibited increased antioxidant defenses, particularly through MnSOD upregulation, and activated stress-adaptive signaling without triggering apoptosis. In parallel, VC treatment reduced the expression of MDM2, mTOR, PD-L1, and MDR-ABC transporters while modestly increasing tumor suppressors such as p21 and PTEN, suggesting reinforcement of protective regulatory mechanisms. Pharmacologic VC selectively spares normal cells while exerting cytotoxic or synergistic effects in cancer cells, underscoring their potential as a safe and effective adjunct in anticancer therapy.

Acknowledgments

The author thanks Union University for the source, support of research funding and colleagues and editing tools for assistance in improving the clarity of the manuscript. The author also thanks Dr. William Thierfelder for providing spleen rat.

References

[1] Betok K., Brozek-Pluska B. Vitamin C-protective role in oxidative stress conditions induced in human normal colon cells by label-free Raman spectroscopy and imaging. *Int J Mol Sci* 2021 ; 28 (13) : 6828.

[2] Karmierczak-Batanska J., Boguszewska K., Adamus-Grabicka A., Karwowski B.T. Two faces of vitamin C-antioxidant and pro-oxidative agent. *Nutrients* 2020, 12 (5) : 1501.

[3] Gregotek A., Skrzydlewska E. Ascorbic acid as antioxidant. *Vitam Horm* 2023 ; 121 : 247-270.

[4] Mehdi Z., Patronek M.S., Mapuskar K.A., Kalen A.L., Cullen J.J., Spitz D.R., et al., Utilization of pharmacological ascorbate to enhance hydrogen peroxide-mediated radiosensitivity in cancer therapy. *Int J Mol Sci* 2021 ; 22 (19), 10880.

[5] Chen Q., Espey M.G., Sun A.Y., Pooput C., Kirk K.L., Khosh D.B., et al., Pharmacological doses of ascorbate act as a prooxidant and decrease growth of aggressive tumor xerographs in mice. *PNAS* 2008 ; 32 :11105–11109.

[6] Yun Y., Mullarky E., Lu C., Bosch K.N., Kavalier A., Roper J., et al., Vitamin C selectively kills KRAS and BRAF mutant colorectal cancer cells by targeting GAPDH. *Science* 2015 ; 350 : 1391-1396.

[7] Hornung T.C., Biegalski H.K. Glut-1 explains the evolutionary advantage of the loss of endogenous vitamin C-synthesis: the electron transfer hypothesis. *Evol Med Public Health* 2019 ; 1 : 221-231.

[8] Hasan Khudhair D., Alokuraishy H.M., El-Kadem A.H., Negma W.A., Saber S., Cavalu S., et al., Combination of vitamin C and curcumin safeguards against methotrexate induced acute liver injury in mice by synergistic antioxidant effects. *Front Med (Lausanne)* 2022; 14:866343.

[9] Magri A., Garmano G., Lorenzato A., Lamba S., Monteno M., Arena S., et al., High-dose vitamin C enhances cancer immunotherapy. *Sci Trans Med* 2020 ; 12(532) : eaay8707.

[10] Huang W.Z., Liu T.M., Liu S.T., Chen S.Y., Huang S.M., Chen G.S. Oxidative status determines the cytotoxicity of ascorbic acid in human oral normal and cancer cells. *Int J Mol Sci* 2023 ; 24(5) : 4851.

[11] Saxton R.A., Sabatini D.M. mTOR signaling in growth, metabolism, and disease. *Cell* 2017; 18: 960-976. [12] Strand R., Orlicky D.J., Chen Y. Gene-dose effect of the glutathione biosynthesis gene on ascorbate deficiency in mice. *BBRC* 2025, 20 : 766 :151900.

Chapter 5

Combined Sorafenib and Vitamin C Triggers Mitochondria-Mediated Apoptosis and Suppresses Hepatocellular Carcinoma Cell Proliferation

Lunawati L. Bennett*, **PhD, PharmD**
Union University, College of Pharmacy, Jackson, Tennessee, USA

Abstract

Hepatocellular carcinoma, the most prevalent form of liver cancer, exhibits high levels of both inter- and intra-tumor heterogeneity, with significant genetic variations among patients. These factors affect the efficacy of the FDA-approved drug Sorafenib, leading to modest clinical benefits, severe side effects, and frequent development of drug resistance.

The goal of this study was to identify if vitamin C alone or in combination with a low dose of sorafenib is more effective in treating hepatocellular carcinoma, using HepG2 cells as the liver cancer model. Based on the results from the SRB assay, Rhodamine 123, Hoechst 33342, and Western blot assay, the addition of vitamin C to sorafenib inhibits the growth of cancerous cells by suppressing BCl-2, p38, SAPK/JNK, cyclin D1, cyclin B1, CDK2, CDK7, and MEK1-4. The combination also increases caspases -3, -7, -8, -9 and tumor suppressor proteins p21, p27, and PTEN. Collectively, these findings demonstrate that vitamin C enhances the anticancer efficacy of sorafenib by promoting mitochondrial-mediated apoptosis and disrupting key survival and cell-cycle regulatory pathways.

Keywords: liver cancer, caspases, vitamin C, sorafenib, HCC, tumor suppressor genes

Abbreviations

SF	sorafenib;
TKI	tyrosine kinase inhibitor;
PTEN	phosphatase and tensin homolog;
MAPK	mitogen activated protein kinase;
SAPK/JNK	stress-activated protein kinase/c-JUN N-terminal kinase;
HEPG2	hepatoblastoma;

* Corresponding Author's Email: llbennett@uu.edu

MEK	mitogen-activated protein kinase kinase;
Cas	caspase;
Bax	Bcl2 Associated X-protein;
Bcl2	B cell lymphoma 2;
Cas	Caspase;
CDK7	Cyclin dependent kinase 7;
Cyt C	Cytochrome C.

Introduction

Hepatocellular carcinoma (HCC) presents a significant global health challenge, ranking it as the seventh most common cancer and the second leading cause of cancer-related deaths [1-2].

Projections indicate a potential increase of over 55% in new cases and deaths from liver cancer by 2040, positioning it among the top three causes of cancer-related death in 46 countries [3]. The complexity of HCC treatment is further compounded by its diverse genetic variations among patients [3-4].

Sorafenib (SF), an oral multiple tyrosine kinase inhibitor (TKI), was FDA-approved in 2007 as the first-line standard therapy for HCC. SF targets angiogenesis, cell proliferation, and cell differentiation by inhibiting the RAF/MEK/ERK pathway and receptor tyrosine kinases [5]. Despite its role as a standard therapy, SF's clinical benefits are modest, and its use is limited by severe side effects and the frequent development of drug resistance [6-8].

Pharmacological ascorbate, achieved through high-dose intravenous vitamin C (VC) to attain plasma levels of ≥ 20 mM, has recently emerged as a potential non-toxic adjuvant to standard care radio-chemotherapy-based cancer therapies across various disease sites [9-10]. The proposed anti-cancer mechanism of pharmacological ascorbate involves redox-active metal-mediated or auto-oxidation of ascorbate, resulting in the formation of O_2 and H_2O_2 [11-13].

This study was designed to evaluate the chemo-enhancing potential of VC in combination with low-dose SF for treating HCC, using HepG2 cells as a model. This marks a novel discovery in the field.

To evaluate the cytotoxic potential of high-dose VC, various antineoplastic agents, including paclitaxel, doxorubicin, etoposide, temsirolimus, bortezomib, afatinib, and sorafenib - were tested on human hepatocellular cancer using the model HepG2 cell line. For combination studies, the lowest concentrations of each antineoplastic and high-dose VC that yielded a synergistic reduction in cell viability were selected. General experimental procedures followed the protocols outlined in Chapter 3 (Materials and Methods), while methodological details specific to this study are described below.

Cell Culture

The hepatocellular cell (HepG2, ATCC HB-8065) and cultured in EMEM media supplemented with 10% FBS and 1% streptomycin/penicillin. The cells were cultured in (T75) dish and maintained in incubator at 37 °C in 5% CO_2 humidified environment. HepG2, exhibits epithelial-like hepatocellular carcinoma from a 15-year-old white male youth with liver cancer, was used as model for liver cancer in the experiments.

Results

Cell Viability and Selection of Doses

VC treatment alone reduced HepG2 cell viability in a dose-dependent manner, while SF alone produced a pronounced cytotoxic effect, with ~50% reduction at mid-range concentrations. The combination of VC and SF produced a synergistic decrease in cell viability, and these conditions were selected for subsequent experiments.

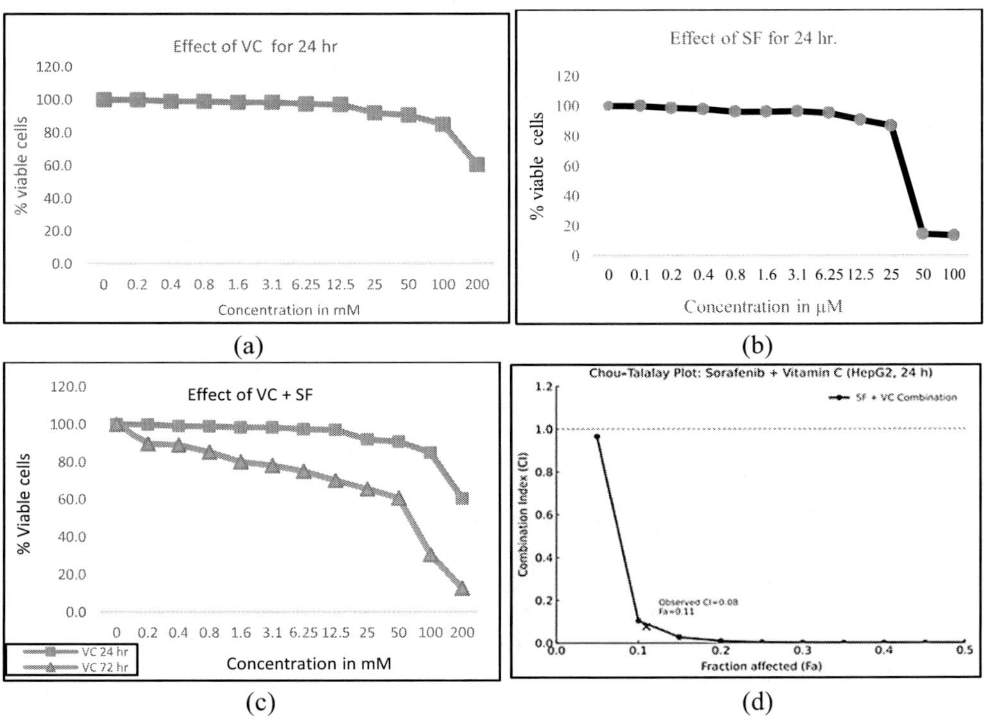

Figure 1. SRB assay results for HepG2 cells treated for 24 and 72 h with (a) VC (0–50 mM), showing decreased viability at concentration between 2.5 to 5 mM; (b) SF (0–100 μM), with ~50% reduction in viability between 25- 50 μM; and (c) combination treatment of 5 mM VC with 3 μM SF, demonstrating synergistic cytotoxicity. Data are expressed as mean ± SD (n = 3). (d)Chou–Talalay plot showing the combination index (CI) of SF and VC after 24 h. Values < 1 indicate synergism. At Fa = 0.11, the CI = 0.08, demonstrating strong synergy between VC and SF.

Changes in Cell Morphology

The morphological changes in HepG2 cells after 24 h treatment were observed with VC, SF, or their combination. Control cells exhibited healthy morphology with increased cell numbers and adherence to the culture dish. In contrast, cells treated with VC or SF alone showed reduced cell viability and altered morphology. The combination treatment with VC and SF resulted in further cell death, as indicated by the presence of floating cells on the culture dish.

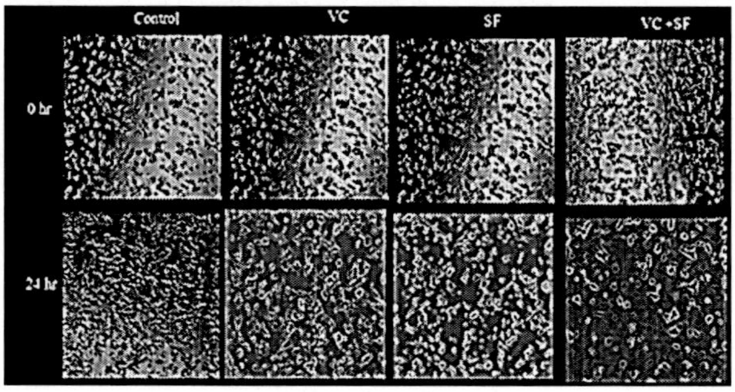

Figure 2. Results from inverted microscopic images of HepG2 cells (40x) after 24 h treatment with VC, SF, or their combination. Cells treated with VC or SF alone exhibited some morphological changes. Data are expressed as mean ± SD (n = 3).

Wound-Healing

After 24 h of treatment, the combination of VC and SF markedly reduced HepG2 cell migration, as evidenced by a wider wound gap compared to individual treatments or control. In contrast, control cells showed progressive re-closure, consistent with invasive potential. Quantitative analysis confirmed significantly reduced migration in the combination group relative to all other treatments.

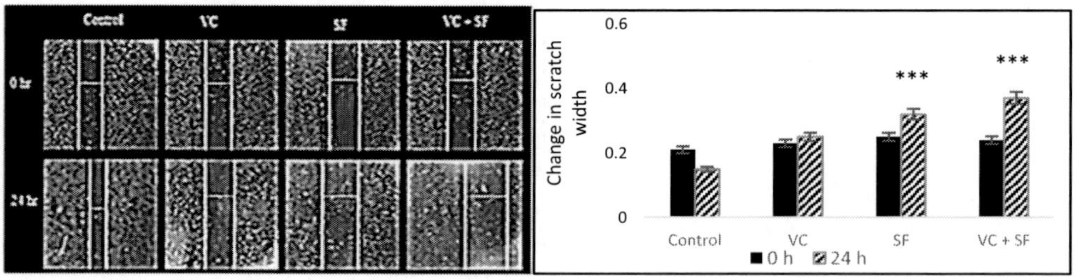

(a) (b)

Figure 3. Wound healing assay of HepG2 cells. (a) Representative images at 0 and 24 h for control, VC, SF, and combination treatments. (b) Histogram comparing wound width across treatment groups after 24 h. Data are expressed as mean ± SD (n = 3); significant differences are indicated by $^{**}p < 0.01$ and $^{***}p < 0.001$ (post hoc Newman–Keuls test).

Induction of Apoptosis

Hoechst 33342 staining revealed that apoptosis was most pronounced in HepG2 cells treated with the combination of VC and SF. Control cells maintained normal nuclear morphology with low fluorescence intensity, while apoptotic cells showed condensed and fragmented bright blue nuclei. Quantitative analysis confirmed a significantly lower percentage of viable cells in the VC-treated group compared to SF or combination treatments.

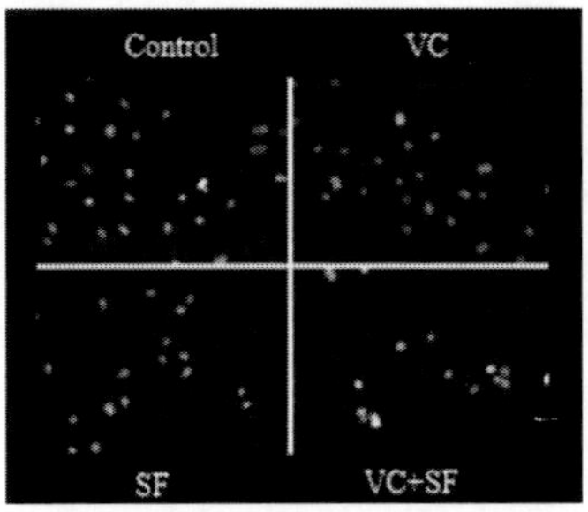

(a)

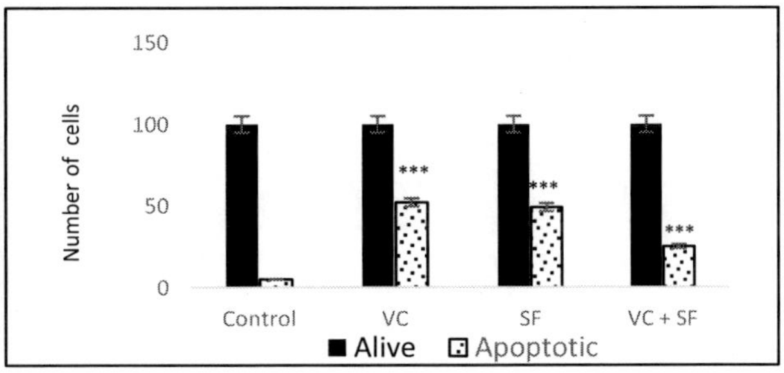

(b)

Figure 4. Apoptosis analysis in HepG2 cells after 24 h. of treatment. (a) Representative fluorescence microscopy images of control, VC, SF, and combination groups stained with Hoechst 33342. Apoptotic cells are characterized by condensed, brightly stained nuclei. Scale bar = 100 µm. (b) Histogram shows the percentage of apoptotic versus viable cells across treatment groups. Data are presented as mean ± SD (n = 3); ***$p < 0.001$ vs control (post hoc Newman–Keuls test).

Intracellular ROS Generation

ROS analysis demonstrated that all treatments induced a marked increase in intracellular ROS generation compared to control cells. This was evident from enhanced fluorescence intensity in VC, SF, and combination-treated groups, indicating elevated oxidative stress in HepG2 cells (see Fig.5).

Mitochondrial Membrane Potential (Ψ_m)

Assessment of mitochondrial membrane potential using Rhodamine 123 revealed a marked loss of fluorescence intensity in VC, SF, and combination-treated HepG2 cells compared to controls, consistent with mitochondrial depolarization and treatment-induced cell death. The results suggest that treatment disrupts mitochondrial $\Delta\Psi m$, impairing mitochondrial function and triggering downstream apoptotic/necrotic pathways (see Fig.6).

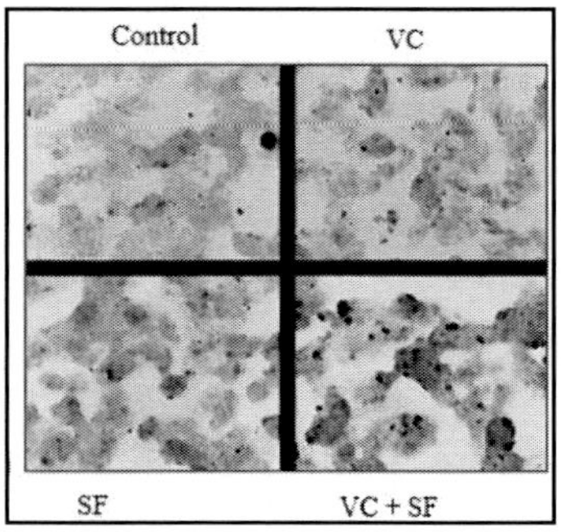

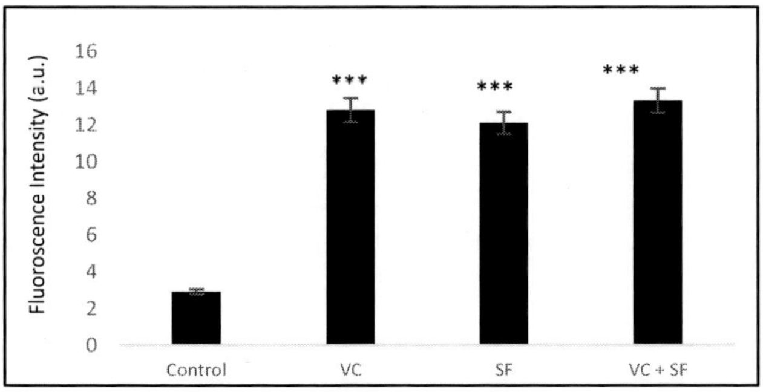

(a) (b)

Figure 5. Intracellular ROS generation in HepG2 cells after 24 h. of treatment.
(a) Representative fluorescence microscopy images following H2DCFDA staining. Increased fluorescence intensity corresponds to higher ROS levels. Scale bar = 100 μm. (b) Histogram of fluorescence intensity comparing control, VC, SF, and combination treatments. Data are expressed as mean ± SD (n = 3); ***p < 0.001 vs control (post hoc Newman–Keuls test).

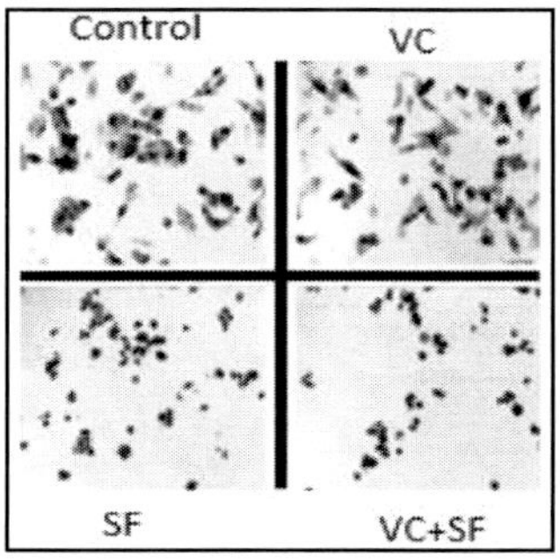

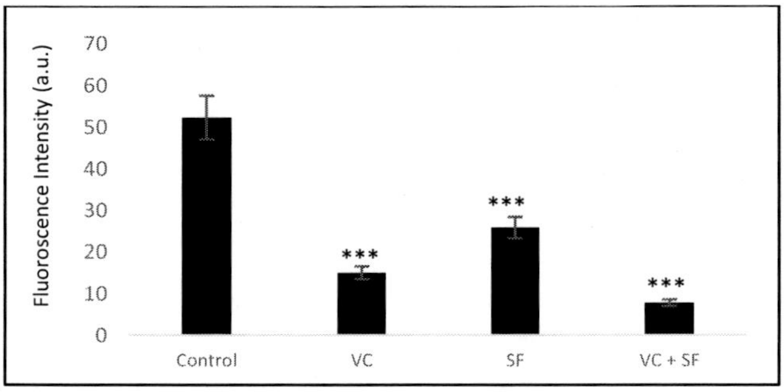

(a) (b)

Figure 6. Mitochondrial membrane potential in HepG2 cells after 24 h. of treatment.
(a) Representative fluorescence microscopy images stained with Rhodamine 123, showing reduced fluorescence intensity in VC, SF, and combination groups relative to control. Scale bar = 100 μm. (b) Histogram of fluorescence intensity quantifying mitochondrial depolarization across groups. Data are expressed as mean ± SD (n = 3); ***p < 0.001 vs control (post hoc Newman–Keuls test).

Modulation of Bax, Bcl2, Cytochrome C, and AIF

ROS generation was associated with modulation of mitochondrial apoptosis regulators. Combination treatment with VC and SF increased Bax expression and decreased BCl2 favoring a pro-apoptotic shift. In parallel, cytochrome c release was enhanced across treatments, consistent with mitochondrial membrane depolarization as well as AIF levels were increased compared to control.

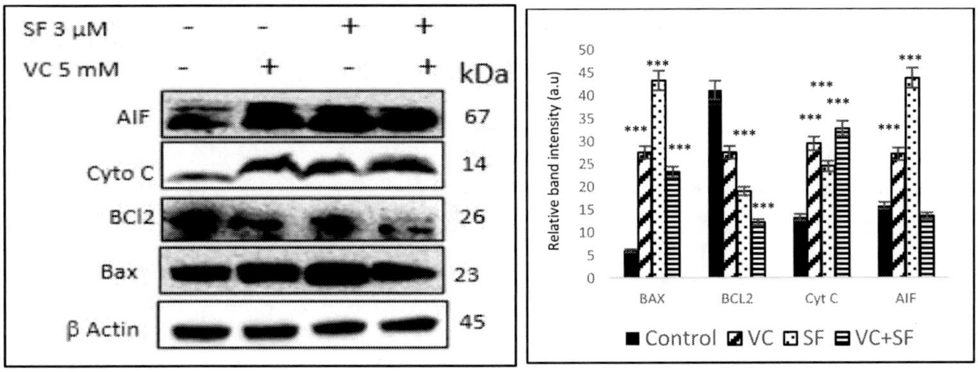

(a) (b)

Figure 7. Western blot analysis of apoptosis-related proteins in HepG2 cells after 24 h. of treatment. (a) Representative blots showing expression of Bax, Bcl-2, AIF, and cytochrome c in control, VC, SF, and combination groups. (b) Band intensity histogram quantifying protein expression relative to control. Data are presented as mean ± SD (n = 3); ***p < 0.001 vs control (post hoc Newman–Keuls test).

Modulation of Mitochondrial Signaling Proteins

Mitochondrial apoptosis, which involves activation of caspases in response to membrane depolarization, was evident following treatment with SF, VC, or their combination. Marked increases in caspase-9, -7, -3, -8, and Apaf-1 compared with the control indicate activation of both intrinsic and extrinsic apoptotic cascades. The combined SF and VC treatment produced the most pronounced response, demonstrating a synergistic induction of mitochondrial apoptosis.

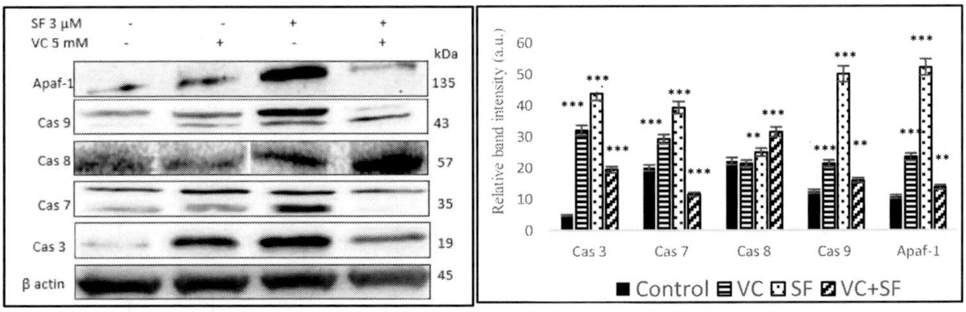

(a) (b)

Figure 8. Western blot analysis of mitochondrial apoptosis-related proteins in HepG2 cells after 24 h. of treatment. (a) Representative blots showing expression of caspases-3, -7, -8, and -9 in control, VC, SF, and combination groups. (b) Histogram of band intensity relative to control. Data are presented as mean ± SD (n = 3); **p< 0.01, ***p < 0.001 (post hoc Newman–Keuls test).

Modulation of MEK Kinase Pathway

To investigate the potential mechanism by which VC, SF, or their combination modulates aberrant cell signaling of mitogen-activated protein kinases (MAPKs), Western blot analysis was performed to assess the active and phosphorylated forms of mitogen-activated protein kinase kinase (MEK). Significant decreases in the expressions of MEK-1, MEK-2, MEK-3, and MEK-4 were observed with the combination of VC and SF.

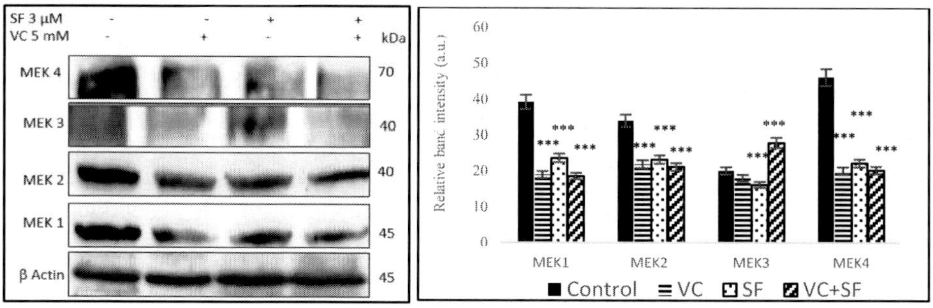

Figure 9. Western blot analysis of MEK isoforms in HepG2 cells after 24 h of treatment. (a) Representative blots showing MEK-1, -2, -3, and -4 expression in control, VC, SF, and combination groups. (b) Histogram of band intensity relative to control. Data are presented as mean ± SD; ***p < 0.001 vs control (post hoc Newman–Keuls test).

Modulation of Cell Cycle Regulatory Proteins

Inhibition of cell cycle progression is an important strategy in the management of HCC. Treatment with VC, SF, or their combination resulted in decreased expression of key cell cycle regulatory proteins, including cyclins (D1, E, and B1) and CDKs (2 and 7). These reductions suggest disruption of G1/S and G2/M checkpoints, with the combination treatment showing the greatest suppressive effect on HCC cell proliferation.

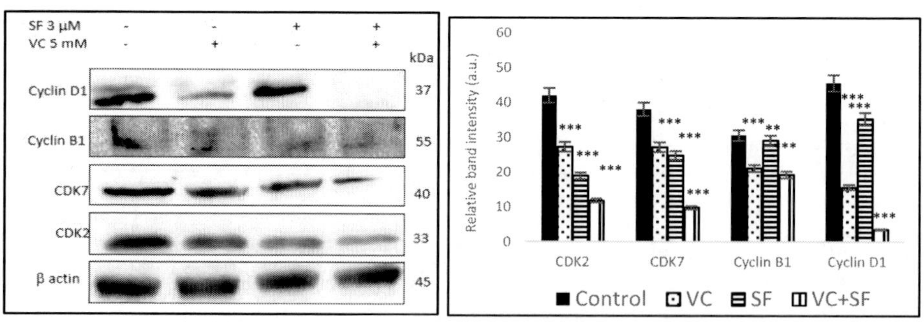

Figure 10. Western blot analysis of cell cycle regulatory proteins in HepG2 cells after 24 h of treatment. (a) Representative blots showing CDK2, CDK7, Cyclin D1, and Cyclin B1 expression in control, VC, SF, and combination groups. (b) Histogram of band intensity normalized to β-actin. Data are presented as mean ± SD (n = 3); significant differences are indicated as ***p < 0.001 (post hoc Newman–Keuls test).

Modulation of p21, p27, PTEN, and MDM2

The impact of VC, SF, and their combination on the expression of key regulatory proteins, including p21, p27, PTEN, and MDM2, was assessed. Treatment with VC, SF, or their combination resulted in notable modulation of these proteins. Specifically, there was a significant increase in the expression levels of p21, p27, and PTEN, indicating a positive regulatory effect on cell cycle control and tumor suppression. In contrast, the expression of MDM2 decreased, suggesting a potential inhibitory effect on the MDM2 pathway.

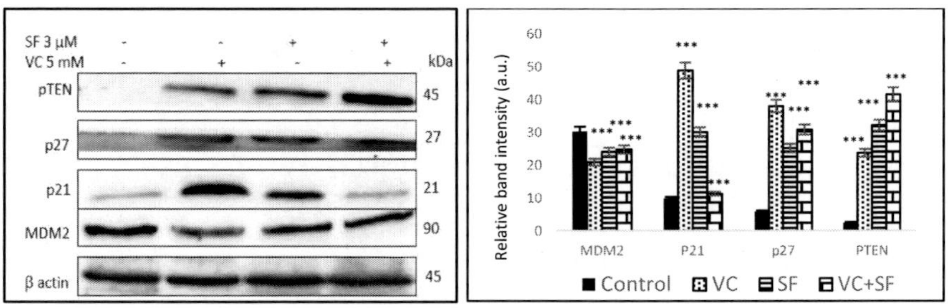

(a) (b)

Figure 11. Effect of VC, SF, and their combination on cell cycle regulatory proteins in HepG2 cells. (a) Representative Western blots showing the expression of p21, p27, PTEN, and MDM2 following treatment with VC, SF, or their combination. (b) Densitometric analysis demonstrates upregulation of p21, p27, and PTEN, alongside a decrease in MDM2 expression, normalized to β-actin. Data are expressed as mean ± SD (n = 3). Significant differences are indicated as $^{**}p < 0.01$, $^{***}p < 0.001$, post hoc Newman–Keuls test.

Modulation of Akt/p85/mTOR

The effect of VC, SF, and their combination on Akt, mTOR, and p85 proteins were assessed. Decreased Akt, p85, and mTOR expression were observed in VC or combination treatment, while increase in p85 or Akt expression was noted in SF only treatment. The Akt and p85 pathways are interconnected, and alterations in one component can influence the other through feedback mechanisms. Histogram represents the changes in protein expressions.

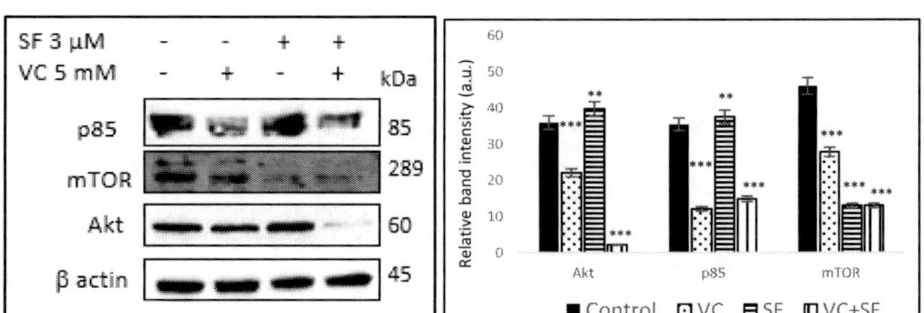

(a) (b)

Figure 12. Effect of VC, SF, and their combination on Akt, p85, mTOR in HepG2 cells. (a) Representative Western blots showing the expression of these proteins following treatment with VC, SF, or their combination. (b) Densitometric analysis demonstrates upregulation of Akt/p85/mTOR expression, normalized to β-actin. Data are expressed as mean ± SD (n = 3). Significant differences are indicated as $^{**}p < 0.01$, $^{***}p < 0.001$, post hoc Newman–Keuls test.

Modulation of SAPK/JNK and p38

The impact of VC, SF, and their combined treatment on SAPK/JNK and p38 proteins was evaluated. The combination of VC and SF resulted in a marked decrease in both p38 and SAPK/JNK protein expressions, whereas individual treatments with either VC or SF caused a moderate increase in these stress-activated kinases. This differential regulation suggests that the combination treatment effectively suppresses stress-induced signaling pathways, potentially contributing to enhanced apoptotic sensitivity in HepG2 cells.

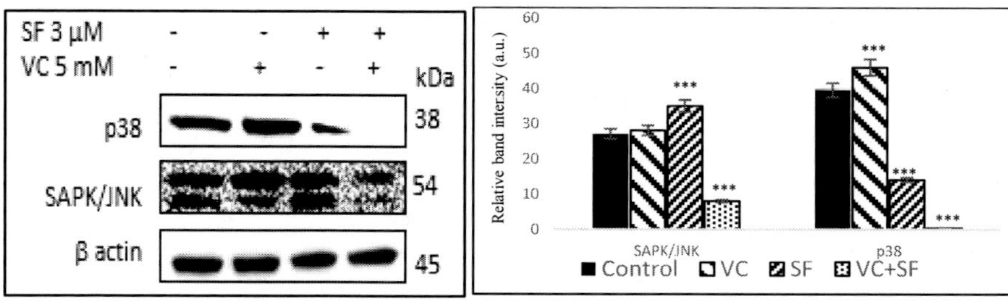

(a) (b)

Figure 13. Effect of VC, SF, and their combination on SAPK/JNK and p38 in HepG2 cells. (a) Representative Western blot analysis data showing the modulation of these proteins compared to control. (b) Densitometric histogram comparing relative protein levels normalized to β-actin. Data are expressed as mean ± SD ($n = 3$). Significant differences are indicated as $^{**}p < 0.01$, $^{***}p < 0.001$, post hoc Newman–Keuls test.

Modulation of ERK 1/2 and EGFR

The impact of VC, SF, and their combined treatment on ERK1/2 and EGFR proteins was assessed. Treatment with VC, SF, or their combination led to increased expression of both ERK1/2 and EGFR proteins, with the combination showing the most pronounced effect. The accompanying histogram clearly illustrates these expression patterns, indicating that activation of the ERK–EGFR axis may contribute to the cellular response observed in HepG2 cells.

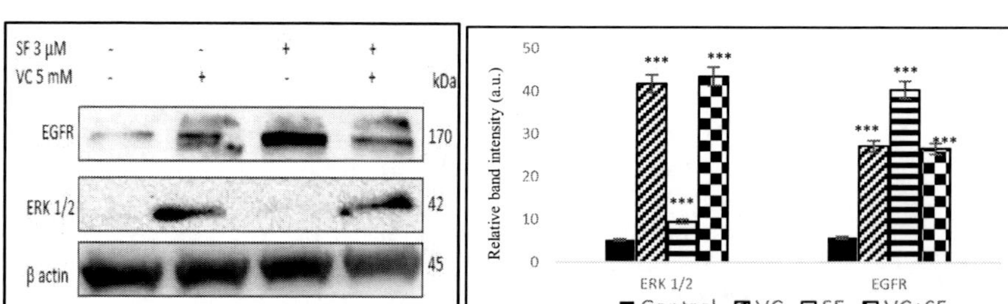

(a) (b)

Figure 14. Effect of VC, SF, and their combination on ERK1/2 and EGFR in HepG2 cells. (a) Representative Western blot analysis data showing the modulation of these proteins compared to control. (b) Densitometric histogram comparing relative protein levels normalized to β-actin. Data are expressed as mean ± SD ($n = 3$). Significant differences are indicated as $^{**}p < 0.01$, $^{***}p < 0.001$, post hoc Newman–Keuls test.

Modulation of Wnt, β-catenin, and ROCK

The impact of VC, SF, and their combined treatment on Wnt, β-catenin, and Rho-associated protein kinase (ROCK) proteins was assessed. A decrease in Wnt and β-catenin expression was observed across all treatments, while an increase in ROCK expression was noted with VC or SF alone. In contrast, the combined treatment of VC and SF resulted in a simultaneous decrease in ROCK, Wnt, and β-catenin levels, indicating enhanced suppression of the Wnt/β-catenin signaling pathway. These findings suggest that the combination treatment may inhibit cell migration and epithelial–mesenchymal transition (EMT), contributing to reduced metastatic potential in HepG2 cells.

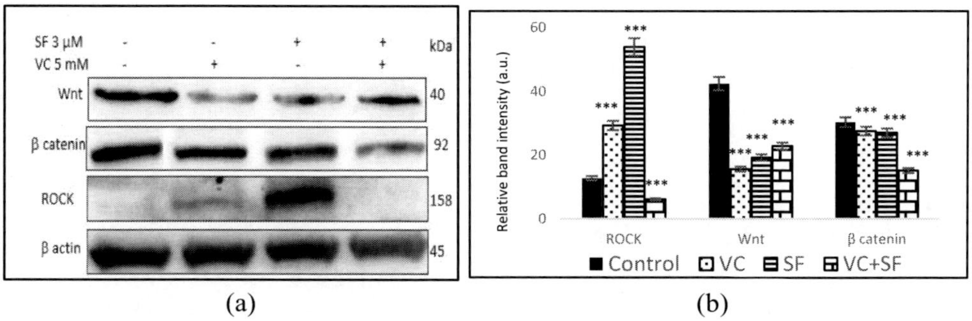

Figure 15. Western blot analysis data showing the modulation of ROCK, Wnt, and β-catenin expression after treatment of HepG2 cells with VC, SF, or their combination.
(a) Representative Western blot analysis data showing the modulation of these proteins compared to control. (b) Densitometric histogram comparing relative protein levels normalized to β-actin. Data are expressed as mean ± SD (n = 3). Significant differences are indicated as $^{**}p < 0.01$, $^{***}p < 0.001$, post hoc Newman–Keuls test.

Modulation of MnSOD, Smac/Diablo, and E-Cadherin

The impact of VC, SF, and their combined treatment on MnSOD, Smac/Diablo, and E-cadherin proteins was assessed. All three proteins showed increased expression following treatment with VC, SF, or their combination, with the greatest elevation observed in the combined group. Upregulation of MnSOD indicates enhanced oxidative stress response, while increased Smac/Diablo and E-cadherin levels suggest activation of pro-apoptotic signaling and restoration of epithelial characteristics, collectively supporting the cytoprotective and anti-metastatic effects of the treatment.

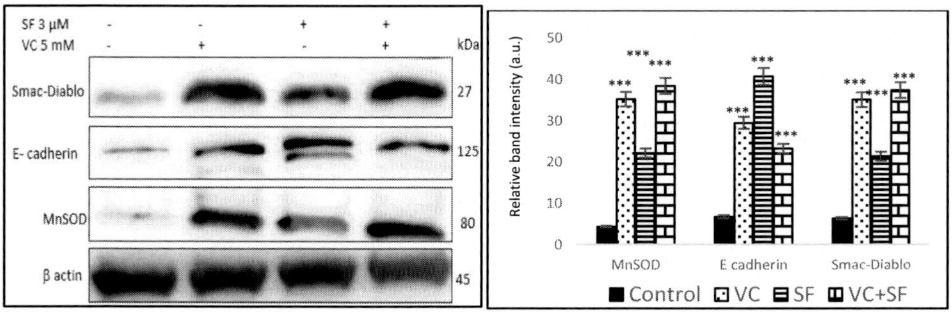

(a) (b)

Figure 16. Western blot analysis of MnSOD, E-cadherin, vimentin, and Smac/DIABLO expression in HepG2 cells following treatment with VC, SF, or their combination. (a) Representative blots showing differential modulation of apoptotic and EMT-related proteins. (b) Densitometric histogram comparing relative protein levels normalized to β-actin. Data are expressed as mean ± SD (n = 3). Statistical significance was determined using the Newman–Keuls post hoc test (**p < 0.001).

Discussion

As illustration in Figure 17, the mechanism involves in the interplay between SF, VC, and their combination in HepG2 hepatocellular carcinoma cells are complex including oxidative stress, mitochondrial dysfunction, stress compensatory feedback, and apoptosis. Across all treatments, significant induction of intrinsic apoptosis, suppression of cell cycle progression, inhibition of pro-survival signaling pathways, and modulation of oxidative stress–related proteins were observed.

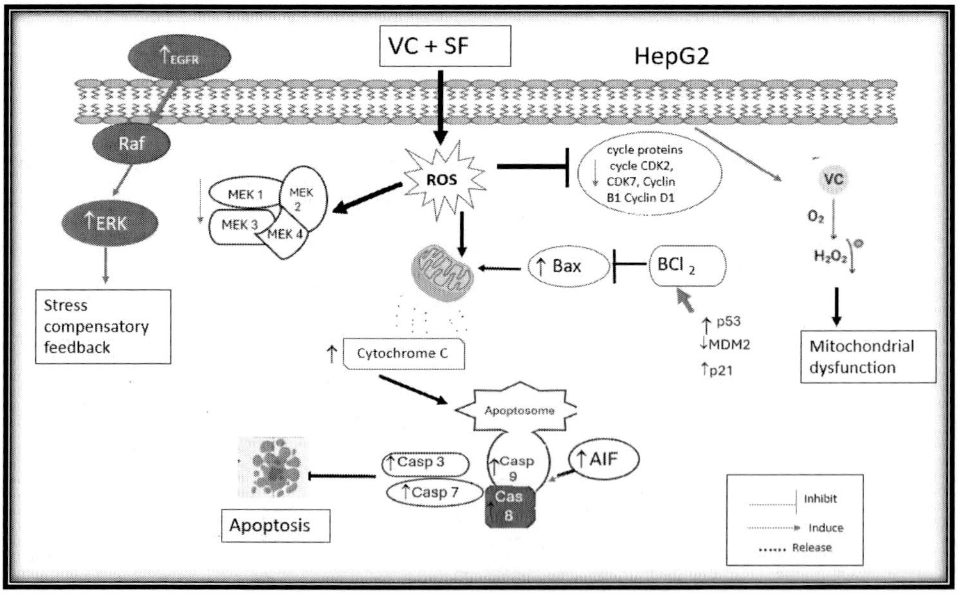

Figure 17. Proposed Mechanistic Model of VC and SF Interaction in Liver cancer.

All treatments significantly increased pro-apoptotic markers (Bax, cytochrome C, AIF) while decreasing anti-apoptotic Bcl-2, indicating potent activation of the intrinsic (mitochondrial) apoptotic cascade. This is consistent with prior reports in HepG2 and other HCC lines where SF triggered Bax/BAK activation and mitochondrial cytochrome C release, leading to caspase-3 activation and PARP cleavage [14]. Similarly, pharmacological doses of VC generate ROS, causing mitochondrial stress and apoptosis, often working synergistically with SF [15].

Caspase profiling revealed consistent increases in initiator cas-8 and -9 and executioner cas-3 across treatments. The exception was cas-7, which decreased in the combination group - suggesting a complex interplay where casp-3 may compensate or casp-7 is degraded via feedback mechanisms. Study showed SF was known to induce cas-3 strongly, while cas-8 activation remains variable [16].

This study demonstrated a consistent downregulation of cyclins D1 and B1, as well as cyclin-dependent kinases CDK2 and CDK7, across all treatment groups. These molecular changes are indicative of cell cycle arrest at both the G1/S and G2/M checkpoints, key regulatory transitions that control cell proliferation [17]. The observed reduction in cyclin D1 aligns with previous findings on SF, which is well-documented to exert antiproliferative effects in hepatocellular carcinoma (HCC) cells primarily through the suppression of cyclin D1 expression [14, 17]. This suppression contributes to a blockade at the G1/S transition, preventing the initiation of DNA replication and cell cycle progression.

While the direct influence of VC on cyclins and CDKs is less extensively characterized in current literature, there is emerging evidence suggesting that its antiproliferative effects may occur through alternative, indirect mechanisms. VC is known to elevate intracellular oxidative stress in cancer cells, particularly by disrupting redox homeostasis, which can lead to DNA damage and activation of cell cycle checkpoints [18]. In addition, VC has been reported to inhibit the mTOR signaling pathway, a critical regulator of cell growth and protein synthesis. mTOR inhibition can result in reduced expression of cyclins and CDKs, thereby contributing to cell cycle disruption [18] Although the mechanistic pathways differ between SF and VC, they appear to converge on key regulatory modes of the cell cycle, ultimately impairing HCC cell proliferation.

The observed upregulation of CDK inhibitors p21and p27 in this study, in conjunction with increased expression of the tumor suppressor PTEN and a concomitant reduction in MDM2 levels, strongly suggests the induction of sustained cell cycle arrest. This molecular profile also implies a potential enhancement of p53-mediated apoptotic signaling. Both p21 and p27 are key regulators of cell cycle progression, functioning primarily to inhibit CDK activity, thereby halting the transition from G1 to S phase [19]. Their induction is frequently associated with cellular responses to stress and DNA damage, often mediated through p53-dependent transcriptional activation [20].

Sorafenib, a multi kinase inhibitor used in this study, has been previously reported to promote the expression of both p21 and p27 [21]. This contributes to its antiproliferative effects by reinforcing the cell's natural checkpoints and preventing uncontrolled progression through the cell cycle. Additionally, the observed downregulation of MDM2 - an E3 ubiquitin ligase that negatively regulates p53 by targeting it for degradation - may further stabilize and activate p53 [22]. This stabilization amplifies the transcription of downstream targets involved in cell cycle inhibition and apoptosis, enhancing the therapeutic impact of treatment.

Although there are fewer direct studies specifically detailing VC effect on MDM2 expression, VC is known to modulate several upstream signaling pathways that converge on cell survival and growth. Notably, VC has been shown to upregulate PTEN, a lipid phosphatase that antagonizes PI3K activity and thereby downregulates the AKT/mTOR signaling cascade [23]. Through PTEN induction and mTOR inhibition, VC may synergize with SF in suppressing the PI3K/AKT/mTOR pathway, a central axis frequently dysregulated in cancer that supports proliferation and survival. This combinatorial targeting may not only enhance cytostatic effects but could also be prime tumor cells for apoptotic elimination by tipping the balance in favor of p53 activity [24].

Differential modulation of the MAPK signaling cascade was observed in this study. Specifically, a decrease in MEK1 through MEK4 levels was noted, except for MEK3, which exhibited a marked increase in the combo of SF and VC. This suggests a selective regulation within the MAPK family, with MEK3 potentially playing a unique compensatory or context-specific role, possibly tied to p38 activation pathways under stress conditions. The heterogeneous modulation of MEK isoforms highlights the complexity of MAPK signaling dynamics in response to multi-agent therapies [25].

Interestingly, both EGFR and ERK levels were paradoxically elevated despite upstream inhibition, particularly in the combination treatment. This is likely indicative of compensatory proliferative signaling - a well-documented feedback mechanism in which blockade of upstream nodes such as RAF or MEK prompts cells to activate alternative proliferative routes to maintain survival [26]. Such rebound effects underscore the inherent adaptability of cancer signaling networks, where therapeutic targeting of one axis (e.g., RAF-MEK) may inadvertently relieve negative feedback loops, leading to hyperactivation of others (e.g., ERK or EGFR). This phenomenon supports the need for combinatorial strategies that simultaneously address multiple signaling arms [21, 27].

Consistent reductions in Akt and mTOR were observed across treatment conditions, aligning with VC's established ability to suppress both mTORC1 and mTORC2 complexes. This suppression is thought to occur through ROS-mediated degradation of Rictor, a defining component of mTORC2, thereby disrupting AKT phosphorylation and downstream survival signaling [15]. These effects are particularly significant given the central role of the PI3K/AKT/MTOR axis in regulating cell growth, metabolism, and resistance to apoptosis.

Notably, in the SF-only treatment group, levels of p85 - the regulatory subunit of PI3K - increased, which may reflect an adaptive upregulation aimed at restoring PI3K activity due to mTOR inhibition. In contrast, p85 levels declined in both the VC-only and combination treatments, suggesting that VC exerts a more robust suppressive effect on the PI3K pathway, possibly through combined oxidative stress and PTEN activation. This reinforces the concept that VC enhances pathway inhibition when used with SF, potentially reducing the opportunity for escape signaling in HCC. Moreover, stress-associated kinases p38 MAPK and SAPK/JNK were downregulated under all treatment conditions. Given their dual roles in both apoptosis and cell survival, this downregulation may signify an attenuation of stress-induced pro-survival responses [28]. In cancers that rely on these pathways for adaptation to therapeutic pressure or oxidative stress, their suppression could contribute to sensitization to apoptosis and reduced tumor viability.

The consistent downregulation of Wnt signaling components, including β-catenin, across all treatment groups signifies effective suppression of a critical oncogenic pathway frequently implicated in HCC progression. The Wnt/β-catenin pathway plays a central role in regulating cell proliferation, differentiation, and survival, and its aberrant activation is associated with tumorigenesis, metastasis, and therapy resistance. Thus, its inhibition by SF and VC, individually and in combination, underscores a favorable therapeutic effect targeting one of the core proliferative axes in HCC [29-30].

Interestingly, the expression of showed divergent regulation depending on treatment modality. ROCK levels were elevated in response to single-agent treatments with either SF or VC, suggesting a potential stress or compensatory response aimed at maintaining cytoskeletal dynamics and cell contractility. ROCK is a known downstream effector of Rho GTPases and plays a key role in actin cytoskeleton organization, cell motility, and epithelial-mesenchymal transition (EMT) processes intimately linked to cancer cell invasion and metastasis [31]. However, in the combination treatment group, ROCK expression was notably decreased. This differential pattern hints at a synergistic interference with cytoskeletal regulation when SF and VC are administered together. The reduction in ROCK under the combinatorial regimen may reflect a more profound disruption of cell motility machinery, potentially leading to diminished migratory and invasive capabilities of HCC cells. This is particularly relevant given the role of ROCK in facilitating tumor cell contractility, invasion through extracellular matrices, and metastatic dissemination. By concurrently targeting multiple signaling and structural components, the combined treatment may offer a dual benefit: suppressing both proliferative and invasive phenotypes.

All treatments led to increased expression of manganese superoxide dismutase (MnSOD), second mitochondria-derived activator of caspases/direct IAP binding protein with low pI (Smac/DIABLO), and E-cadherin. The upregulation of MnSOD suggests a heightened mitochondrial antioxidant defense in response to elevated ROS, indicating activation of a ROS-mediated stress pathway. MnSOD plays a crucial role in mitigating oxidative damage by converting superoxide radicals into hydrogen peroxide, which can then be further detoxified by catalase or glutathione peroxidase [32]. Simultaneously, the elevation of Smac/DIABLO implies mitochondrial outer membrane permeabilization (MOMP) and release of pro-apoptotic factors. Smac/DIABLO neutralizes inhibitors of apoptosis proteins (IAPs) thereby facilitating caspase activation and apoptotic progression [33]. This aligns with a pro-death signaling cascade typically observed in response to mitochondrial dysfunction or genotoxic stress. Furthermore, increased expression of E-cadherin, a hallmark epithelial marker, may signify a reversal of the epithelial-to-mesenchymal transition (EMT) [34]. This reversal, sometimes referred to as mesenchymal-to-epithelial transition (MET), is associated with the suppression of cellular motility and invasiveness, thereby reducing the metastatic potential of cancer cells [35-36]. Restoration of E-cadherin-mediated cell-cell adhesion could indicate a re-establishment of epithelial phenotype and tumor suppressive characteristics [37]. The combination of SF and VC suggest that the treatments not only induce mitochondrial-mediated apoptosis but may also attenuate metastatic progression by reinforcing epithelial traits in the current study.

Vitamin C enhances SF cytotoxicity by generating H_2O_2 and perturbing mitochondrial calcium buffering capacity, potentiating mitochondrial-mediated apoptosis [11]. SF itself inhibits mitochondrial respiration and promotes ROS accumulation. Together, SF and VC robustly drive down cell survival pathways (PI3K/AKT/mTOR, Wnt) and cycle regulators (cyclins/CDKs/MDM2), while activating multiple apoptosis axes. The selective increase in MEK3 and EGFR/ERK in the combo suggests survival feedback - indicative of potential drug resistance mechanisms that could be therapeutically targeted.

Conclusion

This study suggests that VC potentiates the anti-cancer activity of SF in HepG2 cells by augmenting apoptosis, inhibiting proliferation, disrupting oncogenic signaling, and inducing oxidative and mitochondrial stress. These mechanistic insights support the therapeutic potential of combining VC with kinase inhibitors like SF and warrant further in vivo validation and clinical investigation.

Key Findings

VC, SF, and their combination exert strong anti-tumor effects in HepG2 by inducing intrinsic apoptosis, cell cycle arrest, and suppression of key oncogenic pathways. Treatments increased pro-apoptotic markers (Bax, cytochrome C, AIF) and caspases while reducing Bcl-2 and cyclins/CDKs, indicating mitochondrial-mediated apoptosis and blockade of cell cycle progression. Upregulation of p21, p27, and PTEN with MDM2 downregulation reinforced p53-dependent inhibition of proliferation. Combined treatment further suppressed PI3K/AKT/mTOR and Wnt/β-catenin signaling, decreased ROCK expression, and elevated MnSOD, Smac/DIABLO, and E-cadherin, reflecting enhanced oxidative stress, caspase activation, and reduced invasiveness. Overall, VC potentiated SF cytotoxicity through synergistic oxidative and mitochondrial stress, leading to amplified apoptosis and growth inhibition in HCC cells.

Acknowledgments

The author thanks Union University for the source and support of research funding as well as colleagues and editing tools for assistance with improving the clarity of the manuscript.

References

[1] Choi S., Kim B.K., Yon D.K., Lee S.W., Chang H.H., Park S., et al., Global burden of primary liver cancer and its association with underlying etiologies, sociodemographic status, and sex differences from 1990-2019: A DALY-based analysis of the Global Burden of Disease 2019 study. *Clin Mol Hepatology* 2023; 29 :433-452.

[2] Bray F., Ferlay J., Soerjomataram I., Siegel R.L., Torre L.A., Jemal A. Global cancer statistic 2018: GLOBOCAN estimates of incidence and mortality worldwide for 36 cancers in 185 countries. *CA Cancer J Clin* 2020 ; 70 :313.

[3] Rumgay H., Arnold M., Ferlay J., Vignat J., McGlynn K.A., Soerjomataram I. Global burden of primary liver cancer in 2020 and predictions to 2040. *J Hepatol* 2022 ; 77 : 1598-1606.

[4] Jiang S.H., Dong F.Y., Yang J.Y., Liu D.J., Wang J.H. Increased serotonin signaling contributes to the Warburg effect in pancreatic tumor cells under metabolic stress and promotes growth of pancreatic tumors in mice. *Gastroenterology* 2017 ; 153 : 277-291.

[5] Abdelgalil A.A., Alkahtani H.M., Al-Jenoobi F.I. Sorafenib. *Profile Drug Subst Excip Relat Methodol* 2019 ; 44 : 239–266.

[6] Zhang X., Zhu X.J., Zhong Z., Du J.C., Cui X.L., Hu Y.H, et al., Small molecule-induced differentiation as a potential therapy for liver cancer. *Adv Sci* 2022 ; 9 : 2103619.

[7] Mousa A.B. Sorafenib in the treatment of advanced hepatocellular carcinoma. *Saudi J Gastroenterol* 2008 ; 14 : 40-42.

[8] Zhu Y.J., Zheng B., Wang H.Y., Chen L. New knowledge of the mechanisms of sorafenib resistance in liver cancer. *Acta Pharmacol Sin* 2017 ; 38 : 614–622.

[9] Schoenfeld J.D., Sibenaller Z.A., Wagner B.A., Spitz D.R., Allen B.G. Redox active metals and H2O2 mediate the increased efficacy of pharmacological ascorbate in combination with gemcitabine or radiation in pre-clinical sarcoma models. *Redox Biology* 2018 ; 14 : 417-422.

[10] Du J, Martin SM, Levine BA, Wang S, Knudsen CM, Cullen JJ. Mechanism of ascorbate-induced cytotoxicity in pancreatic cancer. J Am. Assoc. Cancer Res. 2010 ; 16 :509-520.

[11] Chen Q., Espey M.G., Krishna M.C., Mitchell J.B., Corpe C.P., Buettner G.R., et al., Pharmacological ascorbic acid concentrations selectively kill cancer cells: action as a pro-drug to deliver hydrogen peroxide to tissues. *PNAS* 2005 ; 102 : 13604-13609.

[12] Chen Q., Espey M.G., Sun A.Y., Lee J.H., Buettner G.R., Levine M. Ascorbate in pharmacologic concentration selectively generate ascorbate radical and hydrogen peroxide in extracellular fluid *in vivo*. *PNAS* 2007 ; 104 : 8749-8754.

[13] Olney K.E., Du J., Van Erve T.J., Witmer J.R., Wagner B.A., Buettner G.R., et al., Inhibitors of hydroperoxide metabolism enhance ascorbate-induce cytotoxicity. *Free Radic Res* 2013 ; 47 :154-163.

[14] Fernando J., Sancho P., Lledo J., Caja L., Fausto N., Fabregat I. Sorafenib sensitizes hepatocellular carcinoma cells to physiological apoptotic stimuli. *J cell Physio* 2012 ; 227 (4): 1319-1325.

[15] Du J., Cullen J.J., Buettner G.R. Synergistic effects of ascorbate and sorafenib in hepatocellular carcinoma: New insights into ascorbate cytotoxicity. *Free Radic Biol Med* 2016; 95:44–65.

[16] Rodríguez-Hernández M.A., González R., de la Rosa A.J., Gallego P., Ordóñez R., Navarro-Villarán E., et al., Molecular characterization of autophagic and apoptotic signaling induced by sorafenib in liver cancer cells. *J Cellular Physiol* 2018 ; 234 : 692-708

[17] Hu W., Yuan Q., Liu X.H., Zhu H.C., Lv S.Q., Wang X.H. Cyclophilin D-mediated apoptosis attributes to sorafenib-induced cytotoxicity in clear cell-renal carcinoma. *Eur J Pharmacol* 2015 ; 749 : 142-150.

[18] Szarka A., Kapuy O., Lorinz T., Banhegyi G. Vitamin C and cell death. *Antioxidants and Redox Signaling* 2021 ;34 : 11.

[19] Qin S., Wang G., Chen L., Geng H., Zheng Y., Xia C., et al., Pharmacological vitamin C inhibits mTOR signaling and tumor growth by degrading Rictor and inducing HMOX1 expression. *PLOS Genetics* 2023 ; e1010629.

[20] Wei J., Meng F., Qu K., Wang Z., Zhang L. Sorafenib inhibits proliferation and invasion of human hepatocellular carcinoma cells via up-regulation of p53 and suppression of FoxM1. *Acta Pharmacologica Sinica* 2015; 36: 241-251.

[21] Rouleau L., Antony A.N., Bisetto S., Newberg A., Doria C., Levine M., et al., Synergic effects of ascorbate and sorafenib in hepatocellular carcinoma: New insights into ascorbate toxicity. *Free Radic Biol Med* 2016 ; 95 : 308-322.

[22] Tang W., Chen Z., Zhang W., Zhang B., Wu F., Wang Q., et al., The mechanism of sorafenib resistance in hepatocellular carcinoma theoretical basis and therapeutic aspects. *Sig Transduct Target Ther* 2020 ; 87 : 5.

[23] Wang K., Qiu X., Zhang Z., Xu H., Su R., Gao F., et al., ATRA sensitized the response of hepatocellular carcinoma in sorafenib by downregulation of p21-activated kinase-1. *Cell Commun Signal* 2023 ; 21 : 193.

[24] Shen X., Wang J., Kong W., John C., Deng B., Zhang H., et al., High-dose ascorbate exhibits anti-proliferative and anti-invasive effects dependent on PTEN/Akt/mTOR pathway in endometrial cancer *in vitro* and *in vivo*. *Int J Biol Sci* 2025 ; 21 (4) : 1545 – 1565.

[25] Kim J., Lee S.D., Jin D.H., Jung S.I., Han Y., Yang Y., et al., Enhanced antitumor activity of vitamin C via p53 in cancer cells. *Free Rad Biol Med* 2012 ; 53 : 1607-1615.

[26] Hou W., Xia H., Zhou S., Xu H., Gong Q., Nie Y., et al., The MEK inhibitors enhance the efficacy of sorafenib against hepatocellular carcinoma cells through reducing p-ERK rebound. *Trans Cancer Res* 2019 ; 8(4) : 1224-1232.

[27] Ezzoukhry Z., Louandre C., Trecherel E., Godin C., Dupont S., Barbare J.C., et al., EGFR activation is a potential determinant of primary resistance of hepatocellular carcinoma cells to sorafenib. *Int J Cancer* 2012 ; 131 : 2961-2969.

[28] Wang X., Qian S., Wang S., Jia S., Zheng N., Yao Q., et al., Combination of vitamin C and lenvatinib potentiates antitumor effects in hepatocellular carcinoma cells in *vitro*. *Peer J* 2023 ; 11 : e14610.

[29] Vilchez V., Turcios L., Marti F., Gedaly R. Targeting Wnt/β-catenin pathways in hepatocellular carcinoma treatment. *World J Gastroenterol* 2016 ; 22 : 823-832.

[30] Khalaf A.M., Fuentes D., Morshid A.I., Burke M.R., Kaseb A.O., Hassan M. Role of Wnt/β-catenin signaling in hepatocellular carcinoma pathogenesis, and clinical significance. *J Hepatocellular Carcinoma* 2018 ; 5 : 61-73.

[31] Vennin C., Rath N., Pajic M., Olson M.F., Timpson P. Targeting ROCK activity to disrupt and prime pancreatic cancer for chemotherapy. *Small GTPases* 2020 ; 11(1): 45-52.

[32] Ozden O., Park S.H., Kim H.S., Jiang H., Coleman M.C., Spitz D.R., et al., Acetylation of MnSOD directs enzymatic activity responding to cellular nutrient status or oxidative stress. *Aging (Albany NY)* 2011 ; 3(2): 102-107.

[33] Paul A., Krelin Y., Arif T., Jeger R., Shoshan-Barmatz V. A new role for the mitochondrial pro-apoptotic protein SMAC/DIABLO in phospholipid synthesis associated with tumorigenesis. *Mol Ther* 2018 ; 26 (3) : 680-694.

[34] Holley A.K., Bhakthavatsala V., Velez-Roman J.M., St. Clair D.K. Manganese superoxide dismutase: guardian of the powerhouse. *Int J Mol Sci* 2011 ; 12(10) : 7114-7162.

[35] Grujic J., Allen A.R. MnSOD mimetics in therapy: exploring their role in combating oxidative stress-related diseases. *Antioxidants* 2024 ; 13 (12), 1444.

[36] Bansal M.P. Cancer metastasis, ROS/redox signaling, and PCD resistance/redox metabolism. In *Redox Regulation and Therapeutic Approaches in Cancer*. Springer, Singapore. 2023 ; 173-206.

[37] Rubtsova S.N., Zhitnyak I.Y., Gloushankova N.A. Dual role of E-cadherin in cancer cells. *Tissue Barriers* 2022 ; 10 : e2005420.

Chapter 6

How Vitamin C Enhances Paclitaxel Induced Toxicity in Malignant Pleural Mesothelioma Cells via Oxidative Stress, Mitochondrial Dysfunction, and Multi-Pathway Modulation

Lunawati L. Bennett*, **PhD, PharmD**
Union University, College of Pharmacy, Jackson, Tennessee, USA

Abstract

Malignant pleural mesothelioma is an aggressive cancer caused by asbestos exposure. This carcinogen is still present in industrial buildings and housing in various regions, including developing countries. Without treatment, mesothelioma has a median survival time of 12 months, with most patients succumb to death within 24 months.
This study aims to identify effective treatment options for MPM by using the lowest effective concentrations of anticancer agents to kill cancer cells and to determine whether vitamin C can enhance the efficacy of these agents for synergistic treatment of this cancer. Based on results from SRB assays, Rhodamine 123, Hoechst 33342 staining, and Western blot analysis, treatment of MSTO-211H a lung model for mesothelioma cells with paclitaxel at 1 μM and vitamin C at 3 mM effectively kills mesothelioma cells. The observed accumulation of reactive oxygen species following treatment led to increased expression of p21, p53, and caspases-3, -7, and -9, accompanied by a marked downregulation of MEK-1, -2, -3, and -4. This coordinated shift reflects enhanced activation of mitochondrial-dependent apoptosis and suppression of pro-survival signaling pathways. Together, these findings suggest that the addition of vitamin C may potentiate therapeutic response and improve treatment management of malignant pleural mesothelioma.

Keywords: lung cancer, malignant pleural mesothelioma, caspases, paclitaxel, vitamin C

---

* Corresponding Author's Email: llbennett@uu.edu

Abbreviations

MPM	Malignant pleural mesothelioma;
MSTO	Misato mitochondrial distribution and morphology regulator;
PX	Paclitaxel;
MDM2	Murine Double Minute 2;
ERK	extracellular signal-regulated kinase;
EGFR	epidermal growth factor receptor;
AIF	apoptosis inducing factor.

Introduction

Malignant pleural mesothelioma (MPM) is a rare and aggressive cancer originating in the pleural cavity, impacting the outer lining of the lungs [1-2]. Both genders are equally susceptible to MPM when exposed to asbestos. Approximately 80% of male workers are affected due to occupational or environmental asbestos exposure [3-5]. Asbestos, a group of fibrous minerals used in over 3,000 products for commercial buildings over the centuries, contains carcinogenic fibers that can cause cancer [2]. Although asbestos use is currently banned in Western countries, MPM incidence is still expected to rise in countries where asbestos use has not been banned or where it is still prevalent, such as in rural areas or industrialized countries undergoing building renovations with asbestos [5-6]. Environmental exposure remains widespread due to natural deposits disturbed by human activities, and many homes are located near asbestos deposits, such as underground rocks [4]. A significant milestone was achieved on March 19, 2024, when the United States Environmental Protection Agency (EPA) issued a landmark ruling to ban chrysotile asbestos, the only form of asbestos used in the U.S. [7].

Mesothelioma has a poor prognosis, with a median survival of 6 to 18 months and a 5-year survival rate of less than 5% [4]. Due to the disease's latency of 20 to 60 years post-asbestos exposure, patients with MPM are often diagnosed at an advanced stage [4, 8-10]. The poor prognosis of MPM is partly due to the lack of reliable screening tools, specific biomarkers, and effective systemic therapies [8-10].

Current standard care for MPM includes surgery with the intent to cure if diagnosed at an early stage or palliative care using a combination of chemotherapy agents such as platinum-based drugs (carboplatin or cisplatin) and anti-folates (pemetrexed) [11]. There is no clear evidence supporting the use of neo-adjuvant or adjuvant chemotherapy, or the use of second or third-line agents to treat MPM; thus, any new treatment options are highly valuable for this aggressive and lethal cancer [10-13].

Paclitaxel (PX), a compound isolated from *Taxus brevifolia*, is an anticancer drug that promotes tubulin polymerization and stabilizes microtubules, preventing their depolymerization, which leads to mitotic arrest and cell death [14-16]. This taxane has been approved by the Food and Drug Administration (FDA) for the treatment of ovarian, breast, and lung cancers [16].

Pharmacological dose of vitamin C (VC) has recently emerged as potential non-toxic adjuvants to standard radio-chemotherapy-based cancer therapies [17-18]. To achieve pharmacological doses, intravenous VC should be administered to attain plasma levels of $\geq$ 20 mM. The proposed anti-cancer mechanism of pharmacological VC involves redox-active metal-mediated or auto-oxidation of ascorbate, resulting in the formation of O_2 and H_2O_2 [19-21].

This study aims to evaluate the chemo-enhancing potential of VC in combination with low-dose PX for treating human MPM, using MSTO cells as a model. The findings of this study reveal that VC synergistically works with PX inhibiting cell cycle regulatory proteins marking a novel discovery in the field.

To evaluate the cytotoxic potential of high-dose VC, various antineoplastic agents - including paclitaxel, doxorubicin, etoposide, temsirolimus, bortezomib, afatinib, and sorafenib - were tested on human MPM using the model MSTO cell line. For combination studies, the lowest concentrations of each antineoplastic and high-dose VC that yielded a synergistic reduction in cell viability were selected. General experimental procedures followed the protocols outlined in Chapter 3 (Materials and Methods), while methodological details specific to this study are described below.

Cell Culture

The mesothelioma lung cancer cell line MSTO-211H (ATCC CRL-2081) was cultured in RPMI-1640 medium supplemented with 10% FBS and 1% penicillin-streptomycin. Cells were maintained in T75 flasks at 37°C in a humidified atmosphere containing 5% CO_2. MSTO-211H, which exhibits fibroblast-like morphology, was originally derived in 1985 from the lung of a 62-year-old Caucasian male with biphasic mesothelioma.

Results

Cell Viability and Selection of Doses

VC treatment alone reduced MSTO cell viability in a dose-dependent manner, while PX alone produced a pronounced cytotoxic effect, with ~50% reduction at mid-range concentrations. The combination treatment of 3 mM VC and 1 μM PX produced a synergistic decrease in cell viability, and these conditions were selected for subsequent experiments.

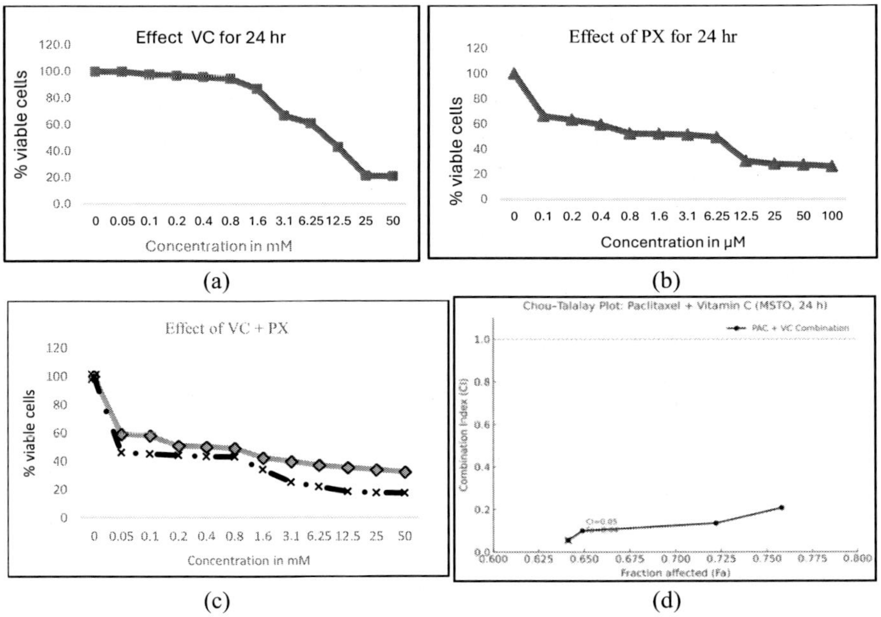

Figure 1. SRB assay results for MSTO cells treated for 24 h with (a) VC (0–50 mM), showing decreased viability at higher concentrations than 3 mM; (b) PX (0–100 μM), with ~50% reduction in viability between 0.8 and 1.6 μM; and (c) combination treatment of 3 mM VC with 1 μM PX, demonstrating synergistic cytotoxicity at 24 hr. and 48 hr. (d) Fraction affected (Fa) values between 0.64–0.76 correspond to combination indices (CI) between 0.05 and 0.21, confirming a strong synergistic interaction. The combination enhances cytotoxic efficacy at substantially lower concentrations than either agent alone, suggesting translational potential for VC to sensitize mesothelioma cells to PX. Data are expressed as mean ± SD (n = 3).

Changes in Cells Morphology

The morphological changes in MSTO cells after 24 h treatment were observed with VC, PX, or their combination. Control cells exhibited healthy morphology with increased cell numbers and adherence to the culture dish. In contrast, cells treated with VC or PX alone showed reduced cell viability and altered morphology. The combination treatment with VC and PX resulted in further cell death, as indicated by the presence of floating cells on the culture dish.

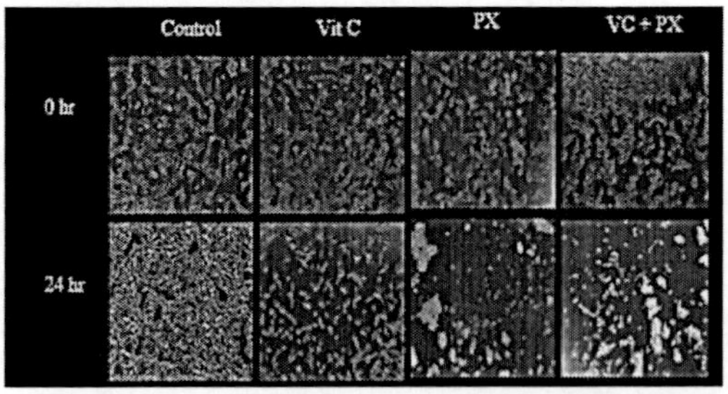

Figure 2. Results from inverted microscopic images of MSTO cells (40x) after 24 h of treatment with VC, PX, or their combination. In the combination treatment, most cells became detached from the dish, with only a few remaining attached. Data are expressed as mean ± SD (n = 3).

Wound-Healing

After 24 h of treatment, the combination of VC and PX markedly reduced MSTO cell migration, as evidenced by a wider wound gap compared to individual treatments or control. In contrast, control cells showed progressive re-closure, consistent with invasive potential. Quantitative analysis confirmed significantly reduced migration in the combination group relative to all other treatments.

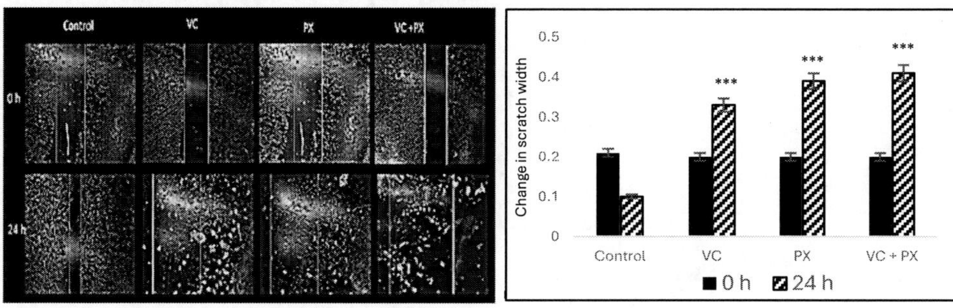

(a) (b)

Figure 3. Wound healing assay of MSTO cells. (a) Representative images at 0 and 24 h for control, VC, PX, and combination treatments. (b) Histogram comparing wound width across treatment groups after 24 h. Data are expressed as mean ± SD (n = 3); significant differences are indicated by ***$p < 0.001$ (post hoc Newman–Keuls test).

Induction of Apoptosis

Hoechst 33342 staining revealed that apoptosis was most pronounced in MSTO cells treated with VC alone, whereas PX or the combination induced relatively fewer apoptotic events. Control cells maintained normal nuclear morphology with low fluorescence intensity, while apoptotic cells showed condensed and fragmented bright blue nuclei. Quantitative analysis confirmed a significantly higher percentage of viable cells in the VC-treated group compared to PX or combination treatments.

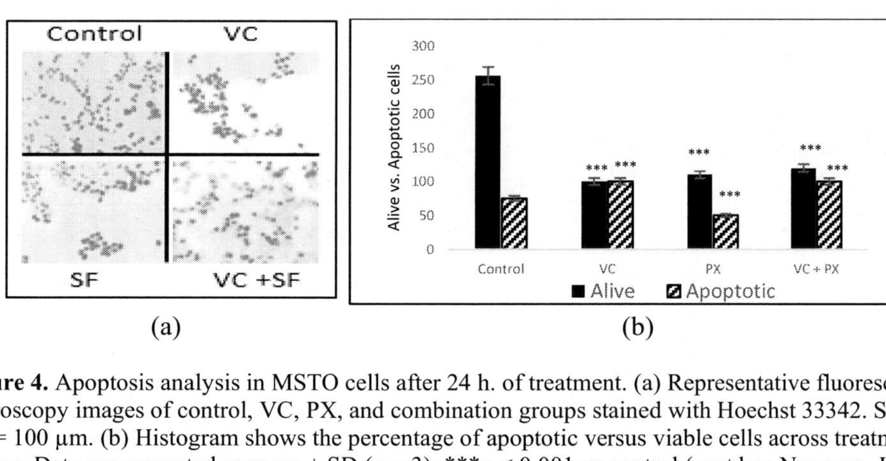

(a) (b)

Figure 4. Apoptosis analysis in MSTO cells after 24 h. of treatment. (a) Representative fluorescence microscopy images of control, VC, PX, and combination groups stained with Hoechst 33342. Scale bar = 100 μm. (b) Histogram shows the percentage of apoptotic versus viable cells across treatment groups. Data are presented as mean ± SD (n = 3); ***$p < 0.001$ vs control (post hoc Newman–Keuls test).

Intracellular ROS Generation

ROS analysis demonstrated that all treatments induced a marked increase in intracellular ROS generation using H2DCFDA staining, compared to control cells. This was evident from the enhanced fluorescence intensity observed in VC-, PX-, and combination-treated groups, indicating elevated oxidative stress levels. The combination treatment produced the brightest fluorescence, reflecting the highest ROS accumulation and suggesting a synergistic enhancement of oxidative damage in MSTO cells.

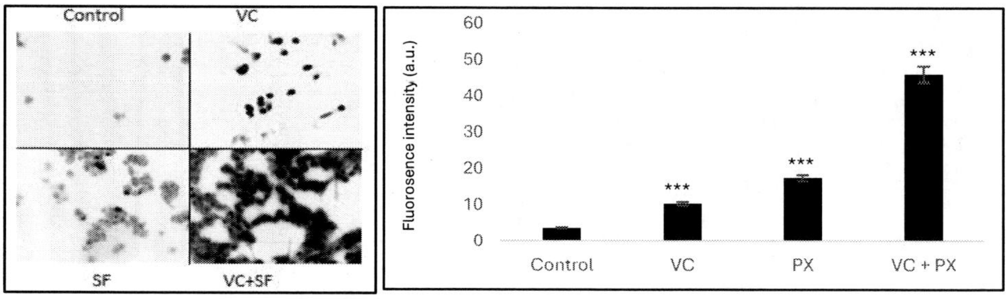

(a) (b)

Figure 5. Intracellular ROS generation in MSTO cells after 24 h. of treatment. (a) Representative fluorescence microscopy images following H2DCFDA staining. Scale bar = 100 μm. (b) Histogram of fluorescence intensity comparing control, VC, PX, and combination treatments. Data are expressed as mean ± SD (n = 3); ***p < 0.001 vs control (post hoc Newman–Keuls test).

Mitochondrial Membrane Potential (Ψ_m)

Assessment of mitochondrial membrane potential using Rhodamine 123 revealed a marked loss of fluorescence intensity in VC, PX, and combination-treated MSTO cells compared to controls, consistent with mitochondrial depolarization and treatment-induced cell death showing as darker color.

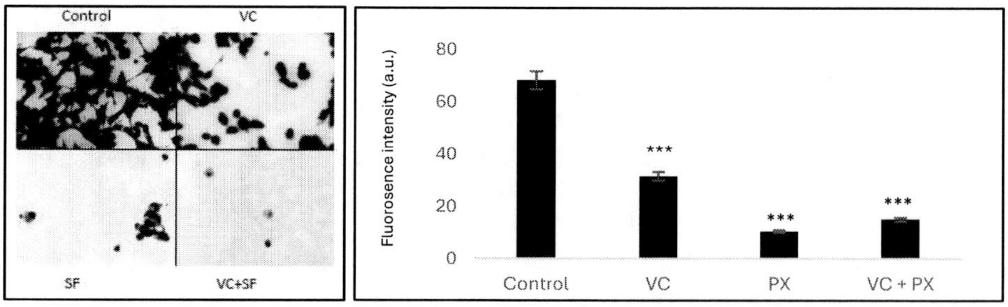

(a) (b)

Figure 6. Mitochondrial membrane potential in MSTO cells after 24 h. of treatment. (a) Representative fluorescence microscopy images. Scale bar = 100 μm. (b) Histogram of fluorescence intensity quantifying mitochondrial depolarization across groups. Data are expressed as mean ± SD (n = 3); ***p < 0.001 vs control (post hoc Newman–Keuls test).

Modulation Bax, Bcl2, AIF, and Cytochrome C

ROS generation was associated with modulation of mitochondrial apoptosis regulators. Combination treatment with VC and PX increased Bax expression and decreased BCl2 favoring a pro-apoptotic shift. In parallel, cytochrome c release was enhanced across treatments, consistent with mitochondrial membrane depolarization as well as AIF levels were increased compared to control.

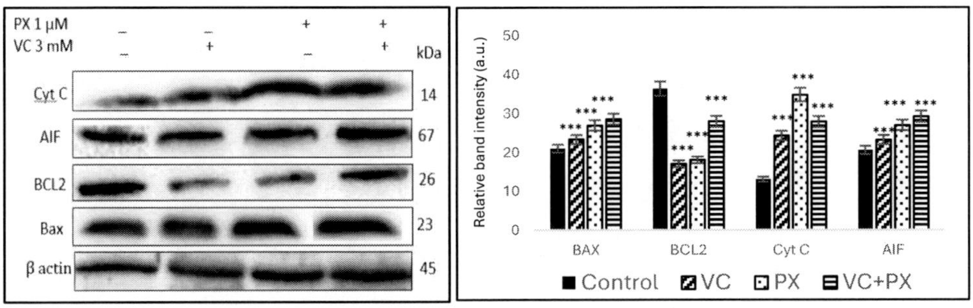

(a) (b)

Figure 7. Western blot analysis of apoptosis-related proteins in MSTO cells after 24 h. of treatment. (a) Representative blots showing expression of Bax, Bcl-2, AIF, and cytochrome c in different groups. (b) Densitometric histogram compares relative protein levels normalized to β-actin. Data are presented as mean ± SD (n = 3); ***p < 0.001 vs control (post hoc Newman–Keuls test).

Modulation of Mitochondrial Signaling Proteins

Mitochondrial apoptosis involves activation of caspases in response to membrane depolarization showed treatment with PX or VC alone led to a reduction in cas-9, cas-7, and cas-3 compared with the control. Combined PX and VC treatment markedly enhanced the activation of cas -3, -7, and -9, indicating a synergistic induction of mitochondrial apoptosis.

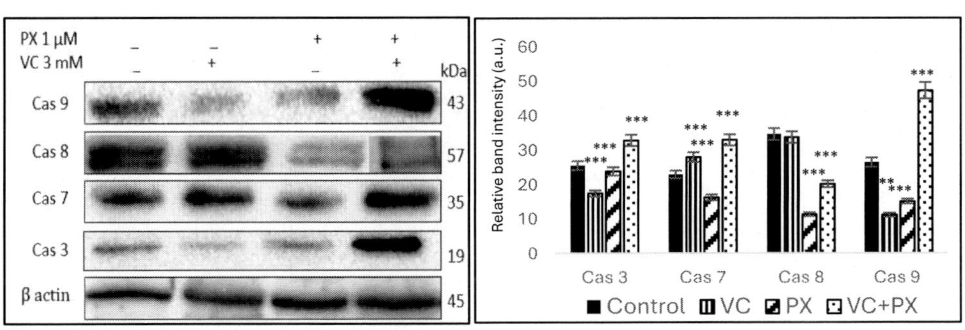

(a) (b)

Figure 8. Western blot analysis of mitochondrial apoptosis-related proteins in MSTO cells after 24 h. of treatment. (a) Representative blots showing expression of cas-3, -7, -8, and -9 in control, VC, PX, and combination groups. (b) Densitometric histogram compares relative protein levels normalized to β-actin. Data are presented as mean ± SD (n = 3); ***p < 0.001 (post hoc Newman–Keuls test).

Modulation of MEK Kinase Pathway

To explore the effect of VC, PX, and their combination on MAPK signaling, the expression of MEK isoforms was assessed. Most treatments resulted in downregulation of MEK-1, -2, -3, and -4, suggesting deactivation of pro-survival signaling pathways. However, VC treatment alone caused an increase in MEK-1 and -3 expression, indicating a partial activation of the MAPK cascade and an unfavorable response compared with the pronounced inhibitory effect observed under combination treatment.

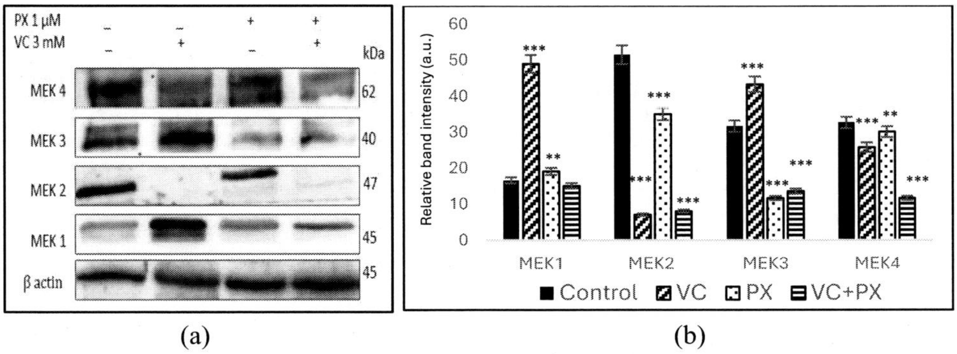

Figure 9. Western blot analysis of MEK isoforms in MSTO cells after 24 h of treatment. (a) Representative blots showing MEK-1, -2, -3, and -4 expression in control, VC, PX, and combination groups. (b) Densitometric histogram compares relative protein levels normalized to β-actin. Data are presented as mean ± SD (n = 3). ** $p < 0.01$, ***$p < 0.001$ vs control (post hoc Newman–Keuls test).

Modulation of Cell Cycle Regulatory Proteins

Treatment with VC, PX, or their combination disrupted the expression of key cell cycle regulatory proteins, with decreased levels of CDK2, CDK7, cyclin B1, and cyclin D1 observed across all treatment groups. These proteins play critical roles in driving cell cycle progression through the G1/S and G2/M transitions; thus, their downregulation indicates inhibition of cell proliferation and induction of cell cycle arrest. The observed reductions reflect a favorable effect of VC or PX alone, further enhanced by their combination, suggesting cooperative suppression of cell cycle advancement in MSTO cells.

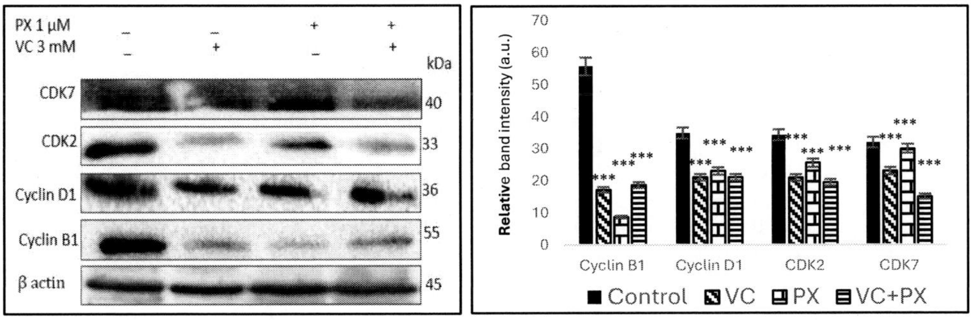

(a) (b)

Figure 10. Western blot analysis of cell cycle regulatory proteins in MSTO cells after 24 h of treatment. (a) Representative blots showing CDK2, CDK7, Cyclin D1, and Cyclin B1 expression in treatment group. (b) Densitometric histogram compares relative protein levels normalized to β-actin. Data are presented as mean ± SD (n = 3); with significant differences indicated as ***p < 0.001 (post hoc Newman–Keuls test).

Modulation of p21, p27, PTEN, MDM2 and p53

The effect of VC, PX, and their combination on the expression of critical cell cycle regulatory proteins was examined. Treatment with VC, PX, or their combination led to a pronounced upregulation of p21, p27, p53, and PTEN, supporting their role in promoting cell cycle arrest and tumor suppression. In contrast, MDM2 expression was significantly reduced across treatment groups, consistent with diminished negative regulation of p53. These findings suggest that VC and PX, either alone or in combination, enhance cell cycle checkpoint control and tumor suppressive genes signaling while attenuating oncogenic regulators.

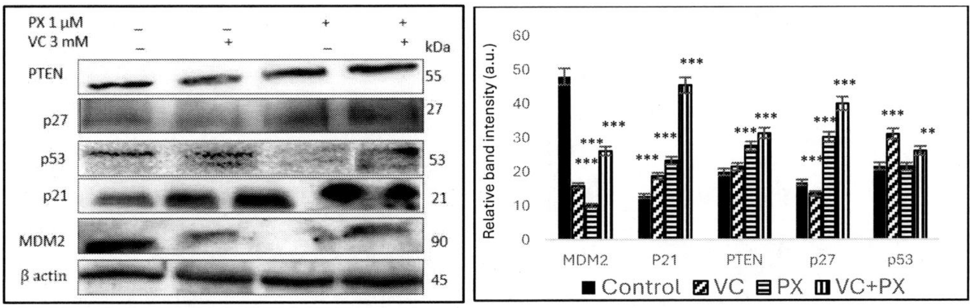

(a) (b)

Figure 11. Western blot analysis of MDM2, p21, p53, p27, PTEN expressions in MSTO cells following treatment with VC, PX, or their combination. (a) Representative blots showing the expression of these proteins. (b) Densitometric histogram compares relative protein levels normalized to β-actin. Data are expressed as ± SD (n = 3). Significant differences are indicated as **p < 0.01, ***p < 0.001, post hoc Newman–Keuls test.

Modulation of Akt/p85/mTOR

The effect of VC, PX, and their combination on the P85/Akt/mTOR signaling axis was assessed in MSTO cells. VC treatment led to a marked reduction in Akt expression, whereas PX or the combination caused a moderate increase compared to control. In contrast, p85, also known as p13k, expression was consistently elevated across all treatment groups, with the strongest induction observed in PX- and combination-treated cells. mTOR expression was also increased, most prominently in PX-treated cells. The increased expressions of these proteins indicated disadvantage of using VC in combination to PX in MSTO cells.

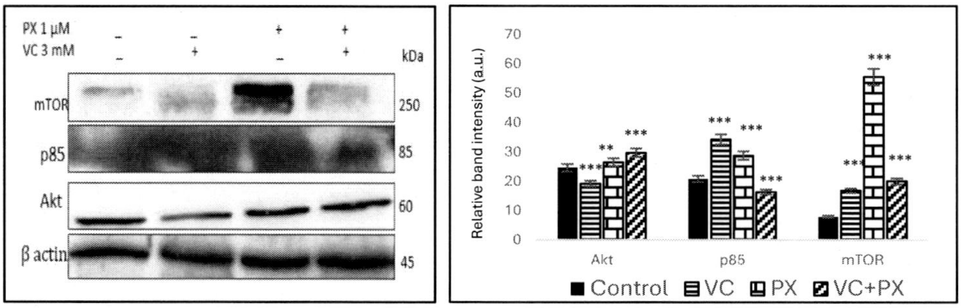

(a) (b)

Figure 12. Western analysis of pI3K/Akt/mTOR signaling proteins in MSTO cells. (a) Representative blots image showing different modulations of these proteins. (b) Densitometric histogram compares relative protein levels normalized to β-actin. Data represent mean ± SD of three independent experiments. Significant differences compared with the control are indicated as **$p < 0.01$, ***$p < 0.001$ determined by post hoc Newman–Keuls test.

Modulation of SAPK/JNK and p38

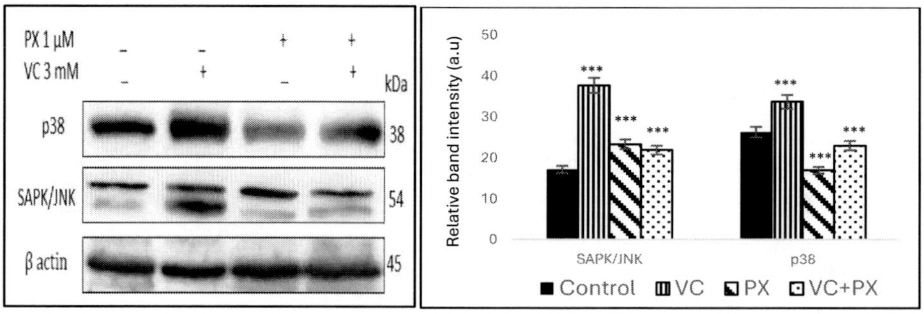

(a) (b)

Figure 13. Western blot analysis of SAPK/JNK and p38 protein expression in MSTO cells following treatment with VC, PX, and the combination. (a) Representative blot images of these proteins. (b) Densitometric histogram compares relative protein levels normalized to β-actin. Data is expressed as mean ± SD of three independent experiments. Significant differences compared with the control are indicated as **$p < 0.01$ and ***$p < 0.001$, determined by post hoc Newman–Keuls test.

The impact of VC, PX, and their combination on stress-activated protein kinases was examined by measuring SAPK/JNK and p38 expression. Treatment with VC, PX, or their combination resulted in an overall increase in SAPK/JNK expression compared to the control. VC only treatment caused increase expression of p38, while PX alone or in combination with VC reduced p38 levels.

Modulation of ERK 1/2 and EGFR

The effect of VC, PX, and their combination on ERK1/2 and EGFR expression was also evaluated. All treatments led to an increase in ERK1/2, and EGFR protein levels compared with the control, indicating consistent upregulation of this pathway by VC, PX, or their combination. Activation of the ERK1/2–EGFR signaling axis is commonly associated with enhanced cell survival and proliferation; however, the concurrent activation with elevated ROS and apoptotic markers suggests a compensatory stress response.

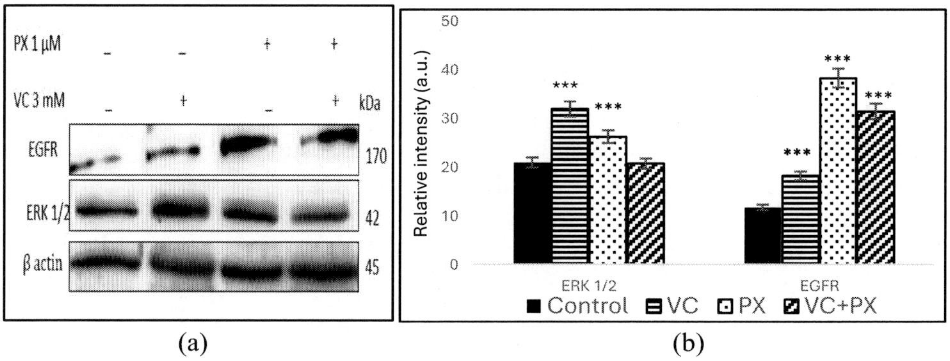

Figure 14. Western blot analysis of ERK1/2 and EGFR expressions after VC, PX, and their combination in MSTO cells. (a) Representative blot images of these proteins. (b) Densitometric histogram compares relative protein levels normalized to β-actin. Data is expressed as mean ± SD of three independent experiments. Significant increases are indicated as $^{**}p < 0.01$ and $^{***}p < 0.001$, determined by post hoc Newman–Keuls test.

Modulation of Wnt/β-catenin/ROCK

The effect of VC, PX, and their combination on Wnt, β-catenin, and ROCK expression were evaluated in MSTO cells. The proteins are key components of signaling systems that regulate cell polarity, cytoskeletal organization, and epithelial–mesenchymal transition (EMT). Wnt levels were increase following treatment with VC, PX or the combination. Notably, a slight reduction in β-catenin expression was observed with the combined treatment relative to single agent. In contrast, ROCK expression was decreased across all treatment groups, indicating consistent suppression of this protein by VC, PX, or their combination.

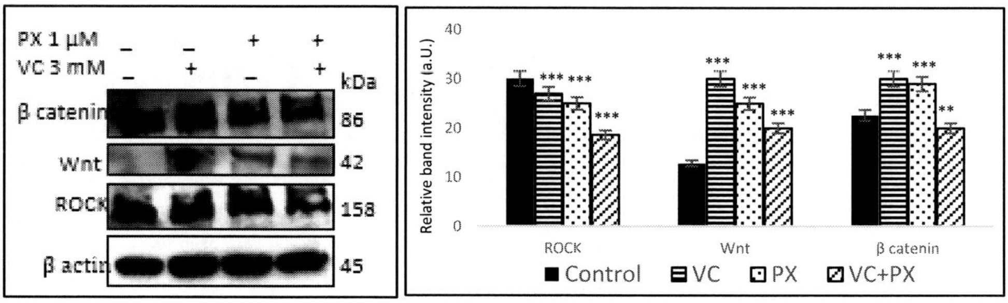

(a) (b)

Figure 15. Western blot analysis of Wnt/β-catenin/ROCK expressions after VC, PX and their combination in MSTO cells. (a) Representative blot images across all groups. (b) Densitometric histogram compares relative protein levels normalized to β-actin. Data is expressed as mean ± SD of three independent experiments. Significant changes are indicated as ** p< 0.01, ***p < 0.001 determined by post hoc Newman–Keuls test.

Modulation of MnSOD, Smac/Diablo, and Vimentin

The effect of VC, PX, and their combination on MnSOD, Smac-Diablo, and Vimentin expression were examined in MSTO cells. Treatment with VC, PX, or their combination resulted in increased expression of MnSOD and Smac-Diablo compared with the control. In contrast, Vimentin overexpression observed only in cells treated with PX, while VC or the combination had negligible effect on Vimentin levels.

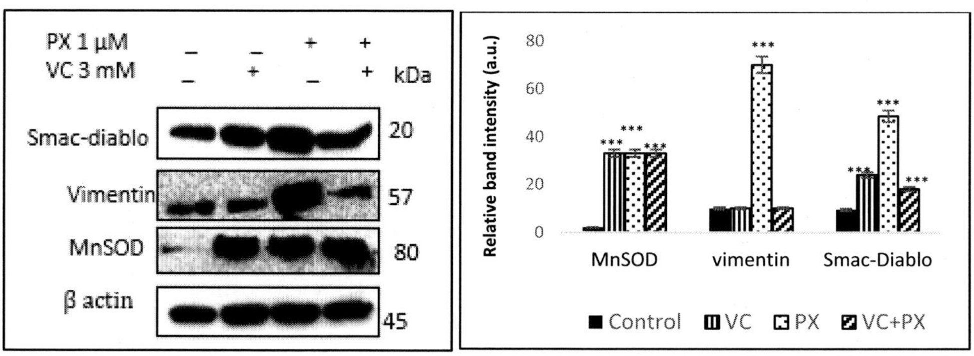

(a) (b)

Figure 16. Western blot analysis of MnSOD, Smac-Diablo, and Vimentin expressions after VC, PX and their combination in MSTO cells. (a) Representative blot images across all groups, (b) Densitometric histogram compares relative protein levels normalized to β-actin. Data is expressed as mean ± SD of three independent experiments. Significant increases are indicated as ***p < 0.001, determined by post hoc Newman–Keuls test.

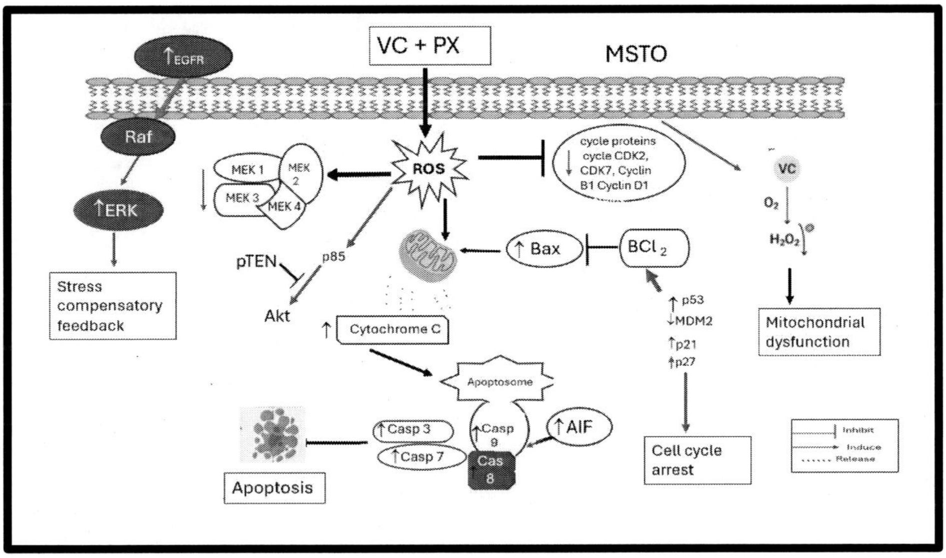

Figure 17. Proposed mechanistic model of VC and PX in MPM cells.

Discussion

As illustrated in Figure 17, the proposed mechanism involves in the interplay between VC and PX provides compelling evidence that when used in combination, they exert synergistic cytotoxic effects against MPM cells. Both agents individually reduced cell viability, yet the combination produced a more profound suppression, accompanied by extensive cell detachment and morphological features consistent with apoptosis. These findings support the concept of combinatorial regimens incorporating antioxidants or pro-oxidant agents with established chemotherapeutics to maximize cancer cell killing.

A key mechanistic insight from this study is the prominent role of oxidative stress. Both VC and PX independently elevated intracellular ROS levels, and their combination markedly intensified this effect, in line with previous reports that excessive ROS can overwhelm cellular antioxidant defenses and drive apoptosis [22-24]. The downstream consequences of ROS accumulation - loss of mitochondrial membrane potential and cytochrome c release - confirm that mitochondria act as a pivotal hub in mediating drug-induced death. The observed upregulation of Bax and downregulation of Bcl-2 further establish mitochondrial permeabilization as an initiating event, consistent with the intrinsic apoptotic pathway.

Activation of the caspase cascade reinforces this interpretation. The significant increases in caspases-3, -7, -8, and -9, alongside Smac/DIABLO upregulation, suggest that both intrinsic and extrinsic apoptotic networks remain functionally engaged [25-26]. Interestingly, MnSOD upregulation may reflect an adaptive cellular attempt to buffer against oxidative stress; however, the magnitude of ROS generation likely surpassed these protective responses, culminating in apoptosis.

The current findings also highlight complex crosstalk between stress and survival pathways. Upregulation of EGFR and ERK1/2, coupled with decreased MEK1-4, suggests a disrupted but still partially active ERK/EGFR axis. Such activation is frequently associated with compensatory survival signaling under chemotherapeutic stress. Similarly, the PI3K/Akt/mTOR pathway was activated which may represent another adaptive pro-survival response [27-28]. This paradox - where pro-apoptotic and pro-survival signaling are concurrently engaged - reflects the intricate balance that determines cell fate under drug exposure. Sustained oxidative stress and mitochondrial dysfunction may ultimately tip this balance toward apoptosis despite activation of pro-survival cascades.

Stress-activated protein kinases (SAPK/JNK and p38) were also induced, consistent with ROS-mediated signaling. While these kinases are classically linked to stress and apoptotic outcomes, they may transiently contribute to adaptive responses before prolonged activation enforces cell death.

Cell-cycle analysis further underscores the inhibitory potential of VC and PX. Upregulation of tumor suppressors (p21, p27, p53, and PTEN) and concurrent downregulation of cyclins (B1, D1) and CDK2 indicate robust checkpoint activation and suppression of proliferative drive. These changes suggest that the treatments not only induce apoptosis but also impair the proliferative capacity of surviving cells, thereby reducing the likelihood of cancer regrowth [29-30].

Pathways linked to metastasis and drug resistance were also modulated. The downregulation of ROCK implies compromised cytoskeletal organization and reduced migratory potential, which may translate into impaired invasive behavior. In contrast, Wnt and β-catenin signaling were largely upregulated, although combination treatment partially attenuated β-catenin expression. This nuanced modulation highlights a potential limitation: while ROS-driven apoptosis is pronounced, compensatory oncogenic pathways such as Wnt/β-catenin may remain active, representing a possible mechanism of residual resistance.

Future studies should aim to dissect these dualistic signaling outcomes more precisely, with particular focus on the interplay between pro-apoptotic mitochondrial damage and compensatory pro-survival pathways such as PI3K/Akt/mTOR and Wnt/β-catenin. In-depth time-course and dose-response analyses could clarify whether survival signaling represents a transient adaptation or a sustained mechanism of resistance. Additionally, evaluating combination strategies that pair VC and PX with inhibitors of EGFR, Akt/mTOR, or Wnt/β-catenin may help overcome residual resistance and further enhance therapeutic efficacy. Extending these findings into in vivo MPM models will be essential to validate translational potential, while investigating biomarkers of oxidative stress and mitochondrial dysfunction could identify patient subgroups most likely to benefit from such combinatorial regimens.

Conclusion

These findings reveal a dualistic cellular response: strong activation of apoptosis via mitochondrial and caspase-dependent pathways, counterbalanced by induction of survival and oncogenic signaling (EGFR/ERK, PI3K/Akt/mTOR, Wnt/β-catenin). The synergy observed between VC and PX likely reflects the ability of ROS and mitochondrial dysfunction to overwhelm compensatory pro-survival signaling, thereby committing cells to apoptosis

Key Findings

VC, PX, and their combination act synergistically in MSTO to induce strong cytotoxic effects through excessive ROS generation and mitochondrial dysfunction. This leads to cytochrome c release, Bax upregulation, Bcl-2 downregulation, and activation of caspases-3, -7, -8, and -9, with Smac/DIABLO reinforcing apoptotic signaling. In addition, cell-cycle arrest was observed through upregulation of p21, p27, p53, and PTEN alongside suppression of cyclins and CDK2, indicating reduced proliferative capacity. Notably, compensatory survival pathways (PI3K/Akt/mTOR, EGFR/ERK, Wnt/β-catenin) were also activated, reflecting a dual response; however, sustained oxidative stress and mitochondrial damage ultimately tipped the balance toward apoptosis.

Acknowledgments

The author thanks Union University for the source and support of research funding. The author thanks colleagues and editing tools for assistance with improving the clarity of the manuscript.

References

[1] Karunakaran K.B., Yanamala N., Boyce G., Ganapathiraju M.K. Malignant pleural mesothelioma interactions with 364 novel protein-protein interactions. *Cancer* 2021 ;13 : 1660.

[2] Mutti L., Peikert L., Robinson B.W.S., Carbone M., Thomas A., Hassan R. Scientific advances and new frontiers in mesothelioma therapeutics. *J Thorac Oncol* 2018 ; 13 : 1269-1283.

[3] Roe O.D., Stella G.M. Malignant pleural mesothelioma: history, controversy and future of a man-made epidemic. *Eur Respir Rev* 2015 ; 24, 115–131.

[4] Gray S.G. Emerging avenues in immunotherapy for the management of malignant pleural mesothelioma. *BMC Pulmonary Med* 2021 ; 21 : 148.

[5] Carbone M., Baris Y.I., Bertino P., Way S., Yang H., Miller A. Erionite exposure in North Dakota and Turkish villages with mesothelioma. *PNAS* 2011 ; 108 : 13618–13623.

[6] Baumann F., Buck B.J., Metcalf R.V., Merkler D.J., Carbone M. The presence of asbestos in the natural environment is likely related to mesothelioma in young individuals and women from Southern Nevada. *J Thorac Oncol* 2015 ; 10 : 731–737.

[7] Callis L. EPA makes 'historic' ruling to ban hazardous material: a symbol of how [the] law can and must be used. *http://www. msn.com*. Retrieved April 13, 2024.

[8] Fennell D.A., Gaudino G., O'Byrne K.J., van Meer Beeck J. Advances in the systemic therapy of malignant pleural mesothelioma. *Nat Clin Pract Oncol* 2008 ; 5: 136–147.

[9] Schrepel A., Astoul P., Baas P. Guidelines of the European Respiratory Society and the European Society of Thoracic Surgeons for the management of malignant pleural mesothelioma. *Eur Respir J* 2010 ; 35 : 479–495.

[10] Creaney J., Robinson B.W. Malignant mesothelioma biomarkers - from discovery to use in clinical practice for diagnosis, monitoring, screening and treatment. *Chest* 2017; 152: 143–149.

[11] Ceresoli G., Zucali P.A., Favaretto A.G., Morenghi E., Cavina R., Parra H.J., et al., Phase II study of pemetrexed plus carboplatin in malignant pleural mesothelioma. *J Clin Oncol* 2006 ; 24 : 1443–1448.

[12] Schulte J.J., Husain A.N. Update on the pathologic diagnosis of malignant mesothelioma. *Trans Lung Cancer Res* 2020 ; 9 : 917-923.

[13] Kindler H.L., Ismalia N., Armato III S.G., Jahan T., Jones C.M., Pass H., et al., R Treatment of malignant pleural mesothelioma: American Society of Clinical Oncology Clinical Practice Guideline. *J Clin Oncol* 2018 ; 36 : 1343-1373.

[14] Meng A., Ly Q., Lu J. Prodrug strategies for paclitaxel. *Int J Mol Sci* 17 2016 ; 5.

[15] De Furia M.D. Paclitaxel (Taxol): A new natural product with major anticancer activity. *Phytomedicine* 1997 ; 4 : 273–282.

[16] Weaver B.A. How Taxol/paclitaxel kills cancer cells. *Mol Biol Cell* 2014 ; 25 : 2677-2681.

[17] Schoenfeld J.D., Sibenaller Z.A., Wagner B.A., Spitz D.R., Allen B.G. Redox active metals and H2O2 mediate the increased efficacy of pharmacological ascorbate in combination with gemcitabine or radiation in pre-clinical sarcoma models. *Redox Biology* 2018 ; 14 : 417-422.

[18] Du J., Martin S.M., Levine B.A., Wang S., Knudsen C.M., Cullen J.J. Mechanism of ascorbate-induced cytotoxicity in pancreatic cancer. *J Am Assoc Cancer Res* 2010 ; 16 :509-520.

[19] Chen Q., Espey M.G., Krishna M.C., Mitchell J.B., Corpe C.P., Buettner G.R., et al., Pharmacological ascorbic acid concentrations selectively kill cancer cells: action as a pro-drug to deliver hydrogen peroxide to tissues. *PNAS* 205 ; 102 : 13604-13609.

[20] Chen Q., Espey M.G., Sun A.Y., Lee J.H., Buettner G.R., Levine M. Ascorbate in pharmacologic concentration selectively generate ascorbate radical and hydrogen peroxide in extracellular fluid *in vivo*. *PNAS* 2007 ; 104 : 8749-8754.

[21] Olney K.E., Du J., Van Erve T.J., Witmer J.R., Wagner B.A., Buettner G.R., et al., Inhibitors of hydroperoxide metabolism enhance ascorbate-induce cytotoxicity. *Free Radic Res* 2013 ; 47 :154-163.

[22] Shen X., Wang J., Kong W., Deng B., Chen S., Haag J.M., et al., High-dose ascorbate exhibits anti-proliferative and anti-invasive effects dependent on PTEN/AKT/mTOR pathway in endometrial cancer *in vitro* and *in vivo*. *Int J Biol Sci* 2025 ; 27 : 21 (4) : 1545-1565.

[23] Park J.H., Davis K.R., Lee G., Jung Y., Park J., Lee M.A., et al., Ascorbic acid alleviates toxicity of paclitaxel without interfering with its anticancer effect. *Nutrition Res* 2012 ; 32 : 873-883.

[24] Bennett L.L. Synergistic effect of resveratrol and paclitaxel in the treatment of malignant pleural mesothelioma. *OBM Genetics* 2024 ; 8(4) : 268.

[25] Böttger F., Valles-Marti A., Cahn L., Jimenez C.R. High-dose intravenous vitamin C, a promising multi-targeting agent in the treatment of cancer. *Frontiers in Pharmacology* 2021 ; 40 : 343.

[26] Fandy T.E., Shankar S., Srivastava R.K. Smac/DIABLO enhances the therapeutic potential of chemotherapeutic drugs and irradiation and sensitizes TRAIL-resistant breast cancer cells. *Mol Cancer* 2008 ; 30 :60.

[27] Dong C., Wu J., Nie J., Chen C. Activation of P13K/AKT/mTOR pathway causes drug resistance in breast cancer. *Front Pharmocol* 2021 ; 15 : 628690.

[28] Rong C., Muller M.F., Xiang F., Jensen A., Plinkert P.K., Hess J., et al., Adaptive ERK signaling activation in response to therapy and in silico prognostic evaluation of EGFR-MAPK in HNSCC. *British J of Cancer* 2020 ; 123: 288-297.

[29] Satheesh N.J., Samuel S.M., Busseelberg D. Combination therapy with vitamin C could eradicate cancer stem cells. *Frontiers in Pharmacology* 2020 ; 11 : 1–12.

[30] Wu F., Yang J., Wang Y., Zeng Q., Deng S, Zhou H. Signaling pathways in cancer-associated fibroblasts and their therapeutic implications. *Signal Transduct Targeted Ther* 2021 ; 6(1) : 1–20.

Chapter 7

How Vitamin C Enhances Afatinib Cytotoxicity in Osteosarcoma Cells by Modulating Apoptotic and Epithelial-Mesenchymal Transition Pathways

Lunawati L. Bennett*, **PhD, PharmD**
Union University, College of Pharmacy, Jackson, Tennessee, USA

Abstract

Osteosarcoma is the most common form of bone cancer affecting children and adolescents that can metastasize other parts of the body such as the lungs. The five-year survival rate is about 55-70%. This rate drops to just 20% if the cancer has metastasized. Chemotherapeutic drugs like doxorubicin and cisplatin have been used, but these drugs also cause high toxicity to normal cells. Therefore, alternative therapies are needed to treat this bone cancer.

This study specifically investigates whether vitamin C alone or in combination with a low dose of afatinib is more effective in treating osteosarcoma, using SaOS-2 as the model for bone cancer cells. Based on the results from SRB assays, Rhodamine 123, H2DCFDA, and Hoechst 33342 staining, and Western blot assays, the addition of vitamin C to afatinib inhibits the growth of cancerous cells by suppressing epidermal receptor kinase, epidermal growth factor receptor, p38, SAPK/JNK, Akt, and cell cycle proteins. In addition, suppression of mitogen activated protein kinases -1, -2, -3, and -4 and downregulation of matrix metalloproteinase -2, and -9 showed that vitamin C enhances afatinib's cytotoxic effect on osteosarcoma. Taken together, these findings indicate that vitamin C not only reinforces afatinib's inhibition of proliferative and invasive signaling pathways but also promotes mitochondrial-mediated apoptosis, supporting the therapeutic potential of combining vitamin C with afatinib in osteosarcoma treatment strategies.

Keywords: bone cancer, vitamin C, afatinib, osteosarcoma, childhood cancer

Abbreviations

AF	afatinib;
OS	Osteosarcoma;
Wnt-1	Wingless integration site -1;

* Corresponding Author's Email: llbennett@uu.edu

ROCK	rock associated coiled containing kinase;
Apaf	apoptotic protease activating factor;
SAPK/JNK	stress-activated protein kinase/c-Jun N-terminal kinase.

Introduction

Osteosarcoma (OS) is a primary malignant bone tumor derived from bone-forming mesenchymal cells to bone surface, joints, or any part within the bone. It can cause local invasion in 85% of OS patients with distant metastasis to the lungs in 74% of cases [1]. Children and adolescents are the most affected, with annual incidence of 0.2-3 cases per 100,000 and 0.8-11 cases per 100,000, respectively [2-4]. In the U.S., there are an estimated 3,600 new cases of OS each year, resulting in approximately 1,720 deaths [5]. Worldwide, the incidence of OS is about 3.4 per million people per year [6].

Treatment OS includes surgical amputation, radiation, and chemotherapy. Radiation treatment is controversial due to its questionable effectiveness and its causing increased risk of infection [7]. Surgery combined with chemotherapies using cisplatin, adriamycin, methotrexate, and cyclophosphamide has significantly improved overall survival and quality of life and is recognized as the standard treatment [7]. However, changes in genetic and epigenetic characteristics can cause drug resistance through increased drug metabolism, evasion of apoptosis, or reduced drug uptake [1].

Afatinib (AF) is a second-generation tyrosine kinase inhibitor (TKI) that inhibits the epidermal growth factor receptor (EGFR) and human epidermal growth factor receptor 2 (HER-2/neu) [8-10]. AF was approved by the Food and Drug Administration for the treatment of non-small cell lung cancer with mutated EGFR. This drug inhibits downstream oncogenic signaling pathways related to cancer proliferation, invasion, metastasis, and angiogenesis and binds to the Erb family, blocking signaling of EGFR family dimers [10-13].

High-dose intravenous vitamin C (VC) to attain plasma levels of $\geq$ 20 mM, has recently emerged as a potential non-toxic adjuvant to standard care radio-chemotherapy-based cancer therapies across various disease sites [14-15]. The proposed anti-cancer mechanism of pharmacological of VC involves redox-active metal-mediated or auto-oxidation of ascorbate, resulting in the formation of O_2 and H_2O_2 [16-18].

This study was designed to evaluate the chemo-enhancing potential of VC in combination with low-dose AF for treating OS, utilizing SaOS-2 cells as a model. The findings of this investigation reveal that the use of VC synergistically with Afatinib inhibits several signaling pathways in OS cells, marking a novel discovery in the field.

To evaluate the cytotoxic potential of high-dose VC, various antineoplastic agents - including paclitaxel, doxorubicin, etoposide, temsirolimus, bortezomib, afatinib, and sorafenib - were tested on human osteosarcoma using the model SaOS-2 cell line. For combination studies, the lowest concentrations of each antineoplastic and high-dose VC that yielded a synergistic reduction in cell viability were selected. General experimental procedures followed the protocols outlined in Chapter 3 (Materials and Methods), while methodological details specific to this study are described below.

Cell Culture

Osteosarcoma (SaOS-2, ATCC HTB-85) and cultured in McCoy's 5A media supplemented with 15% FBS and 1% streptomycin/penicillin. The cells were cultured in T75 and maintained in incubator at 37° C in 5% CO_2 humidified environment. Saos-2 cell exhibits epithelial morphology that was isolated from the bone of an 11-year-old white female patient, was used as the model for bone cancer in the experiments.

Results

Cell Viability and Selection of Doses

Cells treated with VC alone displayed no significant reduction in viability at concentrations below 2.5 mM. Similarly, AF treatment did not alter viability at concentrations below 3 μM. Based on these findings, 3 μM of AF was selected for combination studies with VC to assess potential synergistic effects. Co-treatment with VC and AF markedly decreased cell viability compared to either agent alone, indicating a synergistic cytotoxic interaction. Chou–Talalay analysis demonstrated that combined treatment of SaOS-2 cells with afatinib (AF) and vitamin C (VC) produced dose-dependent synergy. The combination achieved the strongest synergy (CI ≈ 0.55) at VC 5 mM + AF 3 μM, where cytotoxicity was maximized. This trend indicates that pharmacologic VC augments AF efficacy, consistent with oxidative stress-mediated sensitization and disruption of cell-survival signaling.

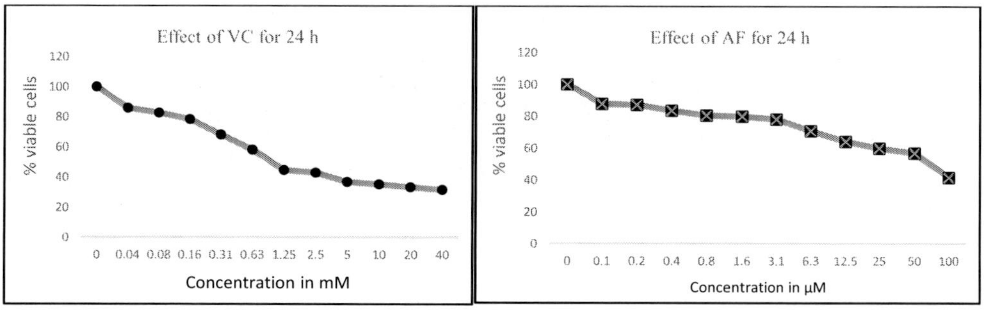

(a) (b)

Figure 1. (Continued).

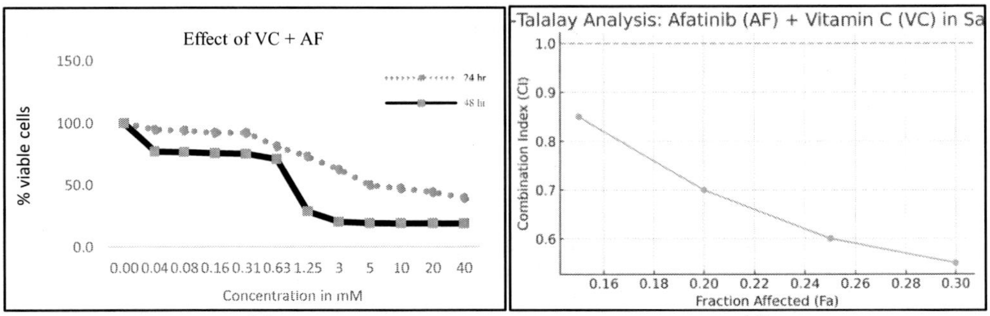

(c) (d)

Figure 1. SRB assay results for Saos-2 cells treated for 24 h with (a) VC (0–40 mM), showing decreased viability at higher concentrations than 3 mM; (b) AF (0–100 μM), with ~50% reduction in viability between 6 and 12.5 μM; and (c) combination treatment of 5 mM VC with 3 μM AF, demonstrating synergistic cytotoxicity at 24 hr. and 48 hr. (d) Dose-dependent synergistic profile, with the greatest synergy observed at VC 5 mM + AF 3 μM (CI ≈ 0.55, Fa = 0.3).

Changes in Cell Morphology

The morphology of SaOS-2 cells changed in all treatment groups compared to the control. It is evident that control cells remained healthy after 24 h, exhibiting increased cell numbers and adherence to the culture dish. However, cells treated with VC or AF alone showed a reduced number of viable cells with altered morphologies. Furthermore, the combination of VC and AF resulted in additional cell death, as evidenced by the presence of floating cells on the culture dish.

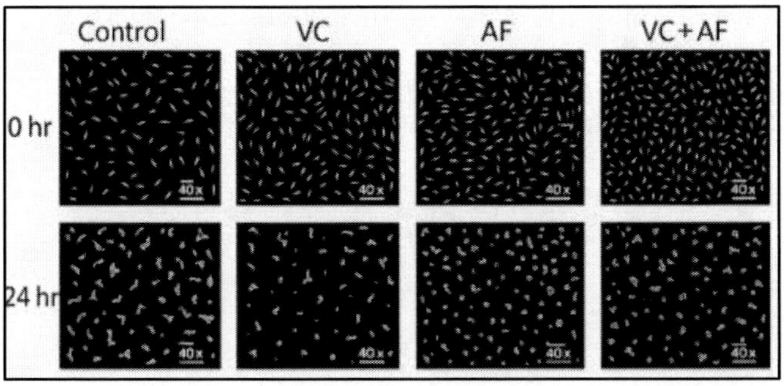

Figure 2. Inverted microscopic images of SaOS-2 cells (40X) after 24 h. treatment with VC, AF, or combination of VC and AF revealed alterations in cell morphology. Cells treated with VC or AF exhibited some changes in morphology, while in the combination treatment, most cells were detached from the dish, with only a few remaining attached.

Wound-Healing

After 24 h treatment, the combination of VC and AF resulted in less migration of SaOS-2 cells, leading to a wider gap in the wound compared to cells treated with VC or AF alone. In the control group, cells migrated closer after 24 h. The remigration in the control group suggests signs of invasion, marking an initial step in cancer metastasis. The histogram in compared the wound width among SaOS-2 cells in the control, VC or AF treatments individually, and the combination treatment.

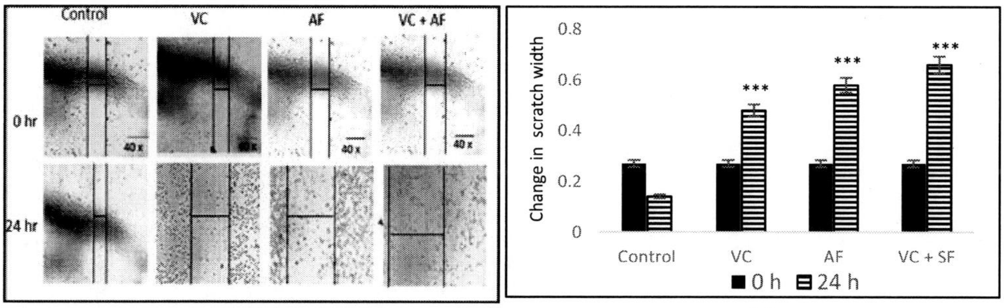

(a) (b)

Figure 3. Wound healing assay of SaOs-2 cells. (a) Representative images at 0 and 24 h for control, VC, AF, and combination treatments. (b) Histogram comparing wound width across treatment groups after 24 h. Data are expressed as mean ± SD (n = 3). Significant differences are indicated by ***p < 0.001 (post hoc Newman–Keuls test).

Induction of Apoptosis

The combination of VC and AF induced a lower rate of apoptosis in SaOS-2 cells compared to cells treated with VC or AF alone. This was confirmed through Hoechst 33342 staining, as observed in the fluorescence microscopic images depicted. The nuclei of control cells exhibited lower fluorescence intensity, indicating normal and healthy. In contrast, cells undergoing apoptosis displayed a bright blue color due to nuclear condensation and fragmentation, with histogram comparing normal and apoptotic cells.

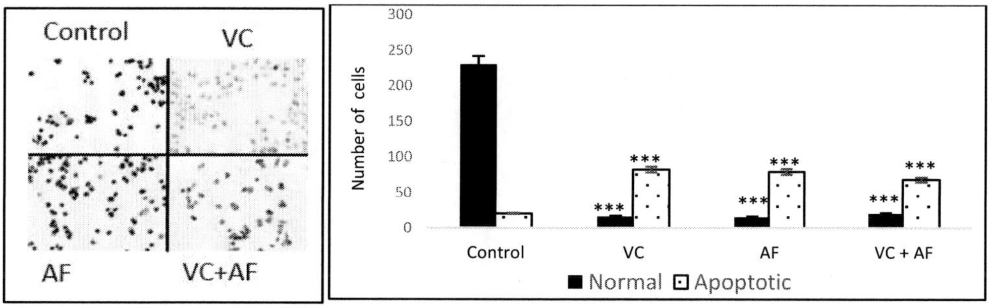

(a) (b)

Figure 4. Apoptosis analysis in SaOs-2 cells after 24 h. of treatment. (a) Representative fluorescence microscopy images of control, VC, AF, and combination groups stained with Hoechst 33342. Scale bar = 100 μm. (b) Histogram shows the percentage of apoptotic versus viable cells across treatment groups. Data are presented as mean ± SD (n = 3). Significant changes are indicated as *** p < 0.001, post hoc Newman-Keuls test.

Intracellular ROS Generation

ROS analysis demonstrated that all treatments induced a marked increase in intracellular ROS generation compared to control cells. This was evident from enhanced fluorescence intensity in VC, AF, and combination-treated groups, indicating elevated oxidative stress in SaOS-2 cells.

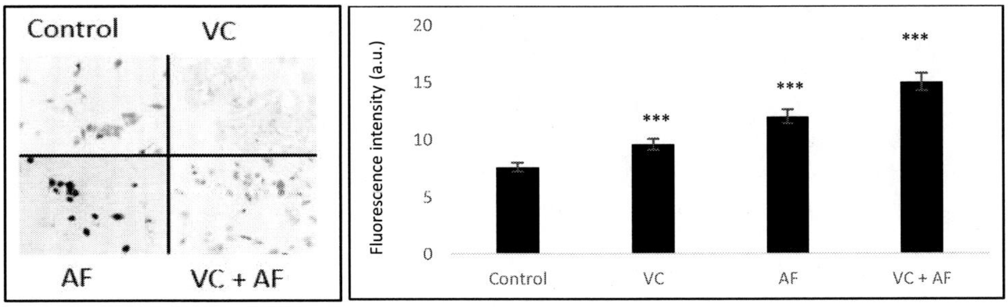

(a) (b)

Figure 5. Intracellular ROS generation in SaOS-2 cells after 24 h. of treatment. (a) Representative fluorescence microscopy images following H2DCFDA staining. Increased fluorescence intensity corresponds to higher ROS levels. Scale bar = 100 μm. (b) Histogram of fluorescence intensity comparing VC, AF, and combination to control. Data are expressed as mean ± SD (n = 3); significant ***p < 0.001 vs control (post hoc Newman–Keuls test).

Mitochondrial Membrane Potential (Ψ_m)

Assessment of mitochondrial membrane potential using Rhodamine 123 revealed a marked loss of fluorescence intensity in VC, AF, and combination-treated SaOS-2 cells compared to controls, consistent with mitochondrial depolarization and treatment-induced cell death. The results suggest that treatment disrupts mitochondrial ΔΨm, impairing mitochondrial function and triggering downstream apoptotic/necrotic pathways (see Fig. 6).

Modulation of Bax, Bcl2, Cytochrome C, and Apaf-1

ROS generation was associated with modulation of mitochondrial apoptosis regulators. Combination treatment with VC and AF increased Bax and Apaf-1 expressions and decreased BCl2 favoring a pro-apoptotic shift. In parallel, cytochrome c release was enhanced across treatments, consistent with mitochondrial membrane depolarization (see Fig.7).

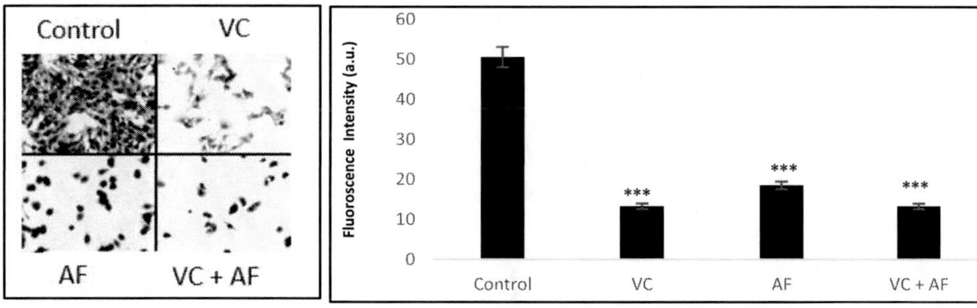

(a) (b)

Figure 6. Mitochondrial membrane potential in SaOS-2 cells after 24 h of treatment. (a) Representative fluorescence microscopy images stained with Rhodamine 123, showing reduced fluorescence intensity in VC, AF, and combination groups relative to control. Scale bar = 100 µm. (b) Histogram of fluorescence intensity quantifying mitochondrial depolarization across groups. Data are expressed as mean ± SD; ***p < 0.001 vs control (post hoc Newman–Keuls test).

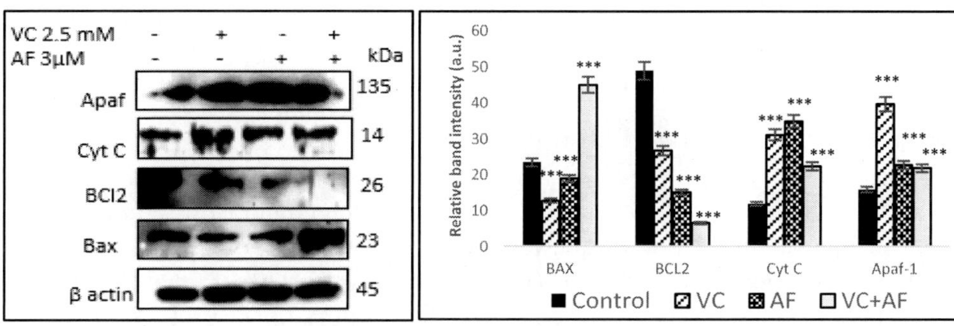

(a) (b)

Figure 7. Western blot analysis of Bax, Bcl2, Apaf, and cytochrome C expressions following treatment with VC, AF, or their combination. (a). Representative blots showing differential modulation of apoptotic and EMT-related proteins. (b) Densitometric histogram compares relative protein levels normalized to β-actin. Data are expressed as mean ± SD (n = 3). Statistical significance was indicated as *** p < 0.001, post hoc Newman-Keuls test.

Modulation Mitochondrial Signaling Proteins

Mitochondrial apoptosis, resulting from a decline in mitochondrial membrane potential ($\Delta\Psi$m), is a tightly regulated process that involves the sequential activation of initiator and effector caspases, including caspases-9, -3, -8, and -7. These enzymes serve as central executioners of the intrinsic and extrinsic apoptotic pathways, mediating the cleavage of vital cellular substrates and leading to controlled cell death. However, in the present study, the expressions of caspases -9, -3, -8, and -7 were lower in all treatment groups compared with the control, suggesting that VC, AF, or their combination did not induce apoptotic signaling through caspase activation. This observation indicates that the cytotoxic response elicited by these treatments may be mediated through non-apoptotic or alternative stress-related mechanisms, such as oxidative stress–driven growth inhibition or modulation of survival pathways, rather than classical caspase-dependent mitochondrial apoptosis.

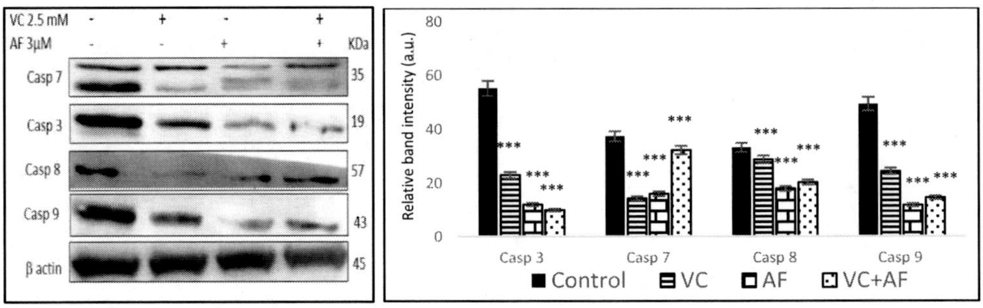

(a) (b)

Figure 8. Western blot analysis results from various mitochondrial signaling proteins in SaOS-2 cells. (a). Representative blots expression of these proteins. (b) Densitometric histogram compares relative protein levels normalized to β-actin. Data are expressed as mean ± SD (n = 3). Statistical significance was determined using the Newman–Keuls post hoc test (**p < 0.001).

Modulation of MEK Kinase Pathway

To investigate the potential mechanism of VC, AF, or their combination in modulating aberrant cell signaling of mitogen-activated protein kinases (MAPKs), Western blot analysis was conducted to assess the active and phosphorylated forms of mitogen-activated protein kinase (MEK). Decrease in the expressions of MEK- 1, -2, -3, and -4 was observed across all treatment indicating favorable effect of VC, AF, or their combination.

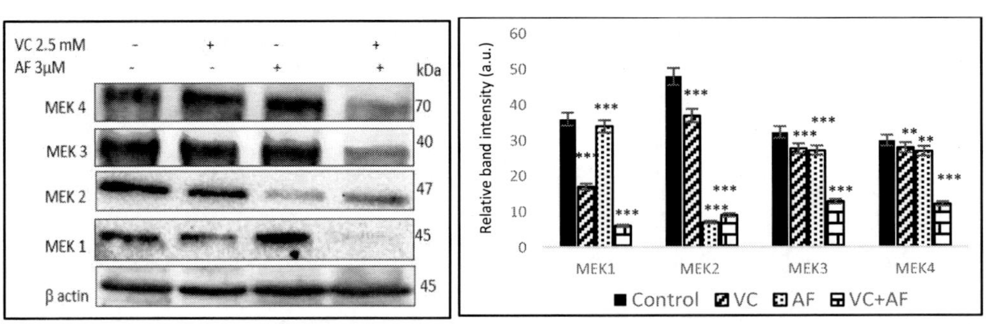

(a) (b)

Figure 9. Western blot analysis MEK-1, -2, -3, and -4 expressions in SaOS-2 after VC, AF, and their combination. (a) Representative blot analysis of these proteins. (b) Densitometric histogram compares relative protein levels normalized to β-actin. Data are expressed as mean ± SD (n = 3). Significant change indicated by ***p < 0.001, according to the post hoc Newman-Keuls test.

Modulation of Cell Cycle Regulatory Proteins

Inhibition of cell cycle progression is also an important strategy in the management of osteosarcoma. Decreases in proteins involved in cell cycle regulation CDK7, CDK2, cyclin B, and cyclin D1 were seen in SaOS-2 cells treated with VC, AF, or their combination. These proteins play critical roles in driving cell cycle progression through the G1/S and G2/M transitions; thus, their downregulation indicates inhibition of cell proliferation and induction of cell cycle arrest.

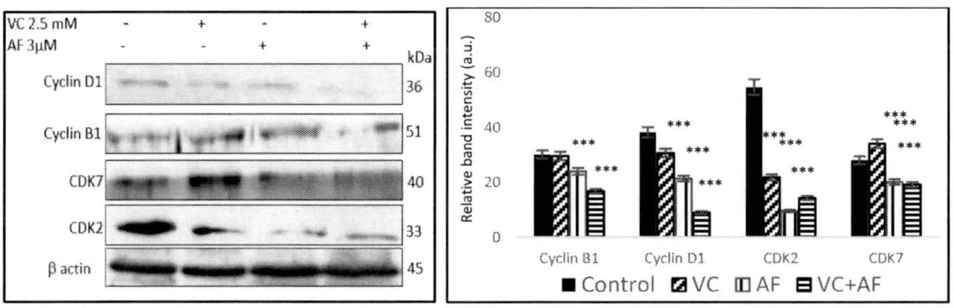

(a) (b)

Figure 10. Western blot analysis of cell cycle proteins in SaOS-2 cells after treatment with VC, AF, or their combination. (a) Representative blot analysis of all treatment groups. (b) Densitometric histogram compares relative protein levels normalized to β-actin. Data are expressed as mean ± SD (n = 3). Significant change indicated by ***$p < 0.001$, according to the post hoc Newman-Keuls test.

Modulation of p21, p53, PTEN, and MDM2

The impact of VC, AF, and their combination on the expression of key regulatory proteins, including p21, p53, PTEN, and MDM2, was assessed. A significant increase in the expression levels of p21, PTEN and p53 was observed in all treatment groups compared to the control. These tumor suppressor proteins showed favorable effect of VC, AF and their combination. In addition, decrease in MDM2 indicated favorable treatment outcome with VC and AF in SaOS-2 cells.

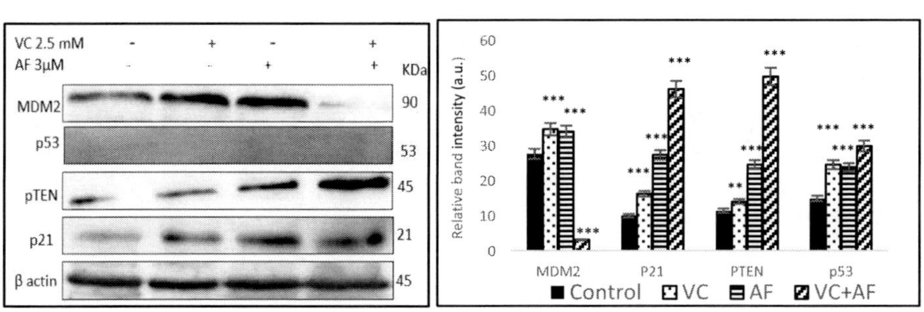

(a) (b)

Figure 11. Western blot analysis of p21, PTEN, p53, and MDM2 expression after VC, AF, and their combination treatment in SaOS-2 cells. (a) Representative blot analysis of these protein expressions. (b) Densitometric histogram compares relative protein levels normalized to β-actin. Data are expressed as mean ± SD (n = 3). Significant changes are marked as **$p < 0.01$ and ***$p < 0.001$, according to the post hoc Newman-Keuls test.

Modulation of Akt/p85

The effect of VC, AF, and their combination on Akt and p85 (also known as p13) proteins was assessed. Decreased levels of Akt were observed in all treatment groups, with a notable decrease in p85 in cells treated with the combination of VC and AF only. The decreased expressions of Akt and p85 suggest a favorable effect of the VC and AF combination on SaOS-2 cells.

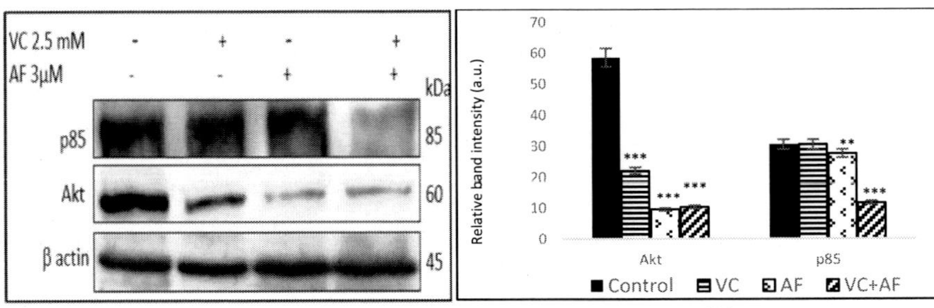

(a) (b)

Figure 12. Western blot analysis of PI3K and Akt in SaOS-2 cells after VC, AF, or their combination. (a) Representative blot analysis of these proteins expressions. (b) Densitometric histogram compares relative protein levels normalized to β-actin. Data are expressed as mean ± SD (n = 3). Significant changes are indicated as **p < 0.01 and ***p < 0.001, according to the post hoc Newman-Keuls test.

Modulation of SAPK/JNK and p38

The impact of VC, AF, and their combination on SAPK/JNK and p38 protein expression was evaluated in SaOS-2 cells. All treatment groups showed decreased levels of both p38 and SAPK/JNK proteins, with the most pronounced downregulation observed in cells treated with the combination of VC and AF. This reduction in stress-activated kinases suggests that VC, either alone or in combination with AF, effectively suppresses stress-induced signaling pathways, thereby attenuating cellular responses associated with oxidative or mitogenic stress.

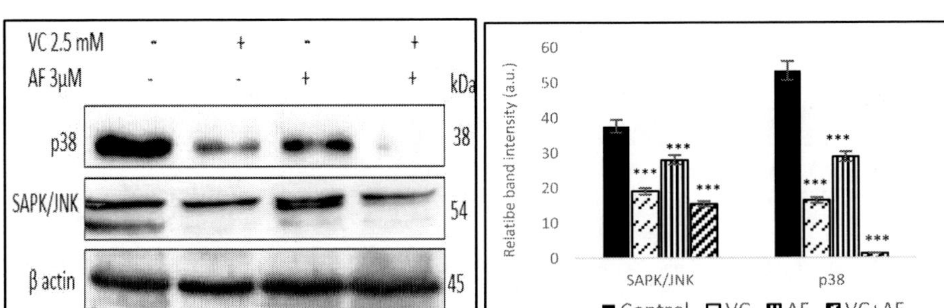

(a) (b)

Figure 13. (a) Western blot analysis of SAPK/JNK and p38 data after treating SaOS-2 cells with VC, AF, or their combination. (a) Representative blots of these proteins. (b) Densitometric histogram compares relative protein levels normalized to β-actin. Data are expressed as mean ± SD (n = 3). Significant decreases are indicated as *** p < 0.001, post hoc Newman-Keuls test.

Modulation of ERK 1/2, SRC, and EGFR

The impact of VC, AF, and their combination on ERK1/2, SRC, and EGFR proteins was assessed in SaOS-2 cells. These proteins are central components of the MAPK and tyrosine kinase signaling cascades that regulate cell proliferation, differentiation, and survival. Aberrant activation of these pathways has been strongly associated with tumor growth and therapeutic resistance in osteosarcoma and other cancers. Treatment of SaOS-2 cells with VC, AF, or their combination led to a marked decrease in ERK1/2 and EGFR expression, indicating a favorable inhibitory effect on proliferative signaling. Only slight changes in SRC expression were observed following VC, AF, or combination treatments, suggesting that the major modulatory effect of these agents was directed toward ERK1/2–EGFR–mediated pathways rather than SRC-dependent signaling.

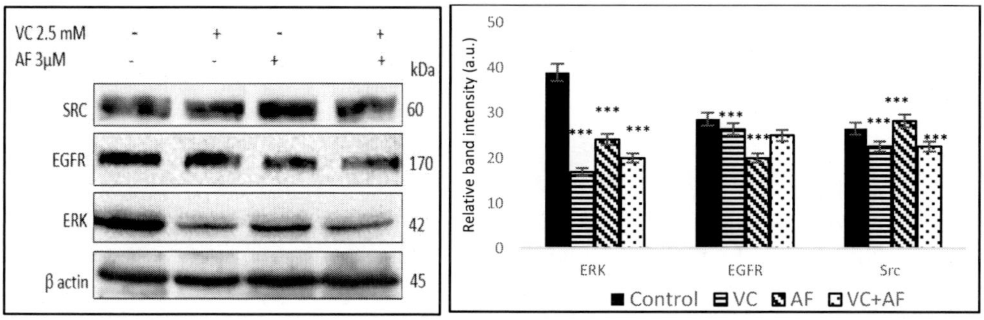

(a) (b)

Figure14. Western blot analysis of ERK, SRC, and EGFR expressions in SaOS-2 after cells after treatment with VC, AF, or their combination. (a) Representative blots showing expression of these proteins. (b) Densitometric histogram compares relative protein levels normalized to β-actin. Data are expressed as mean ± SD (n = 3). Significant changes are indicated as *** $p < 0.001$, post hoc Newman-Keuls test.

Modulation of Wnt/β-catenin/ROCK

The effects of VC, AF, and their combination on Wnt, ROCK, and β-catenin proteins were examined in SaOS-2 cells, showing their expressions were significantly increased across all treatment groups. This upregulation suggests that VC and AF may modulate cytoskeletal remodeling and cell adhesion through activation of the Wnt/β-catenin–ROCK axis, potentially reflecting compensatory or differentiation-related cellular responses.

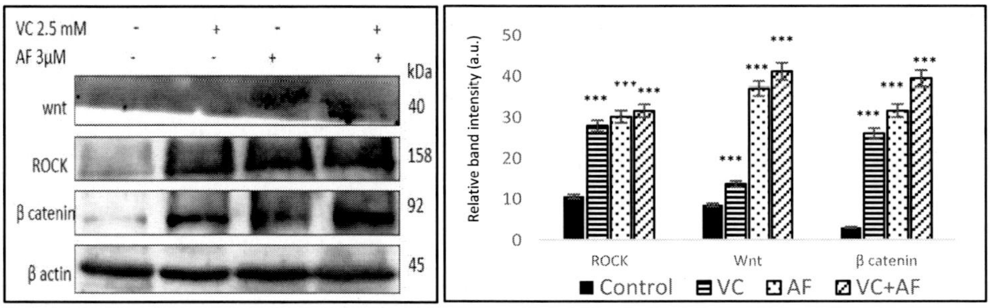

(a) (b)

Figure 15. Western blot analysis of ROCK, Wnt, and β-catenin expressions after treatment of SaOS-2 cells with VC, AF, or their combination. (b) Densitometric histogram compares relative protein levels normalized to β-actin. Data is expressed as mean + SD of three independent experiments significant changes are indicated as *** $p < 0.001$, post hoc Newman-Keuls test.

Modulation of MnSOD, Smac/Diablo, and Vimentin

The impact of VC, AF, and their combination on MnSOD, Smac/Diablo, and Vimentin proteins was assessed, showing an increase in MnSOD expression in SaOS-2 cells treated with the combination of VC and AF, while increased Smac/Diablo expression was noted only with VC treatment. Increased expression of Vimentin was observed in all treatment groups. These findings suggest that VC and AF may enhance oxidative stress defense (via MnSOD), promote pro-apoptotic signaling (via Smac/Diablo), and influence cytoskeletal dynamics or EMT processes (via Vimentin).

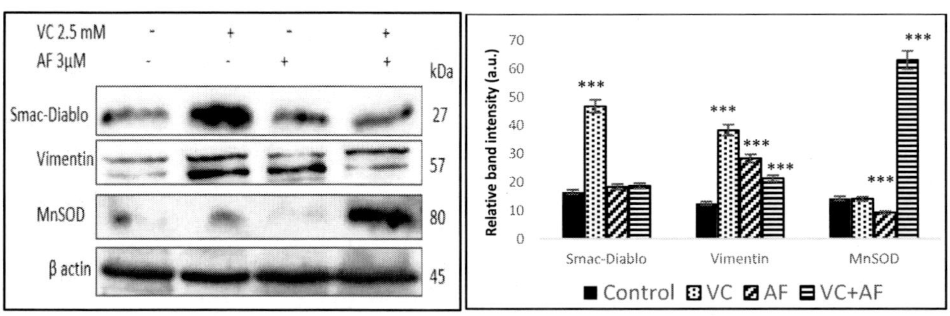

(a) (b)

Figure 16. Western blot analysis data of MnSOD, Smac/Diablo, and Vimentin after treatment with VC, AF, or their combination. (b) Densitometric histogram compares relative protein levels normalized to β-actin. Data are expressed as mean ± SD ($n = 3$). Significant changes are indicated as *** $p < 0.001$, post hoc Newman-Keuls test.

Modulation of MMP 2 and MMP 9

The impact of VC, AF, and their combination on MnSOD, Smac/Diablo, and Vimentin proteins was assessed, showing an increase in MnSOD expression in SaOS-2 cells treated with the combination of VC and AF, while increased Smac/Diablo expression was noted only with VC treatment. Increased expression of Vimentin was observed in all treatment groups. The effect of VC, AF, and their combination on the decreased expression of matrix metalloproteinases-2 and -9 further demonstrated the favorable impact of combining AF and VC in SaOS-2 cells. A slight increase in MMP-2 expression, accompanied by a decrease in MMP-9, was observed with AF alone, suggesting differential modulation of extracellular matrix remodeling enzymes. Collectively, these findings imply that VC and AF not only enhance oxidative and apoptotic regulatory mechanisms but may also suppress metastatic potential through inhibition of MMP activity.

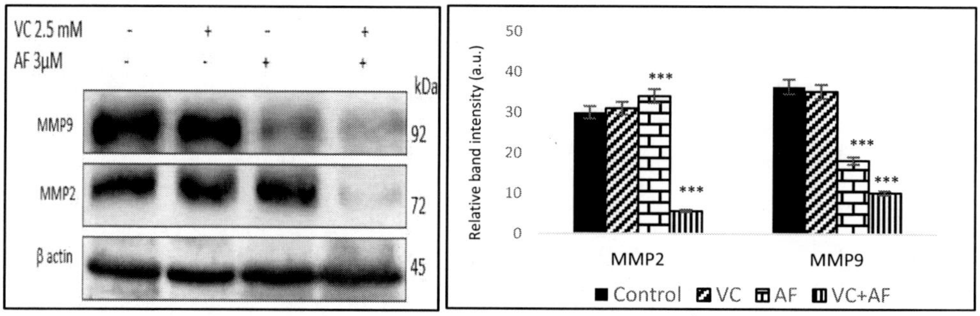

(a) (b)

Figure 17. Western blot analysis of MMP -2 and -9 after treatment of SaOS-2 with VC, AF, and their combination. (a) Representative blots showing expression of these proteins. (b) Densitometric histogram compares relative protein levels normalized to β-actin. Data are expressed as mean ± SD ($n = 3$). Significant changes are indicated as $^{**}p < 0.01$, $^{***}p < 0.001$, post hoc Newman-Keuls test.

Discussion

As illustrated in Figure 18, the proposed mechanism involves AF and VC effect on SaOS-2 osteosarcoma cells include apoptosis, oxidative stress, mitochondrial integrity, cell cycle regulation, and inhibition of angiogenesis. The rationale stemmed from the known inhibitory action of AF on the Erb family of tyrosine kinases and the pro-oxidant, apoptosis-inducing effects of high-dose VC in cancer cells [12, 16]. The hypothesize is by combining these agents, augmentation of apoptotic pathways and disruption of key oncogenic signaling cascades are more efficient than when either agent alone. The findings indicate that the combination treatment potentiates apoptosis and cell death compared to monotherapy, supporting the hypothesis of a synergistic interaction between AF and VC in osteosarcoma treatment.

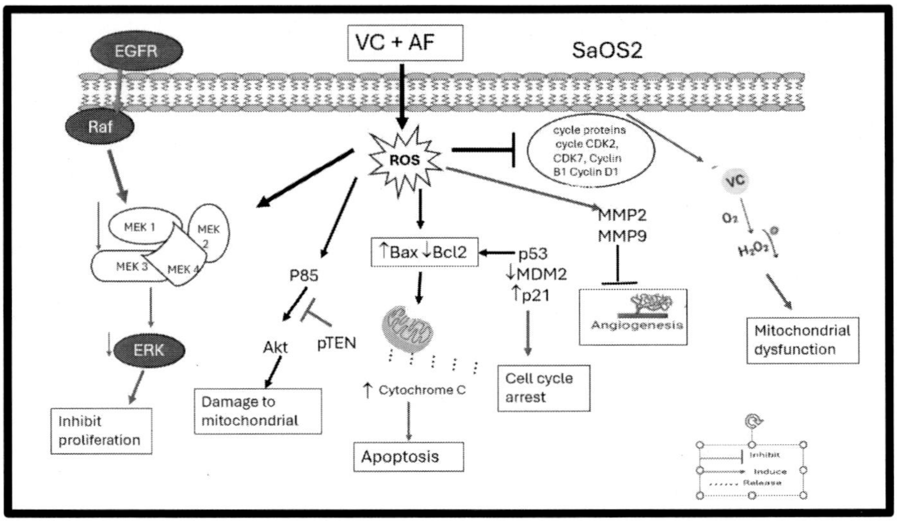

Figure 18. Proposed mechanistic model of VC and AF synergy in osteosarcoma.

The observed increase in apoptosis, as indicated by Hoechst 3342 staining, is corroborated by increased ROS generation (H2DCFDA assay) and disrupted mitochondrial membrane potential (Rhodamine 123). Notably, the combination of AF and VC caused a marked increase in pro-apoptotic Bax and a reduction in anti-apoptotic Bcl-2 levels, consistent with activation of the intrinsic apoptotic pathway. This aligns with previous findings reporting that AF induces mitochondrial-mediated apoptosis in lung cancer cells by modulating Bax/Bcl-2 ratios [19]. Interestingly, VC alone did not significantly elevate Bax, suggesting that the synergistic enhancement of mitochondrial apoptosis is specific to the combination. However, Bcl-2 decreased across all groups, indicating enhanced mitochondrial outer membrane permeabilization (MOMP) and promoting intrinsic apoptosis [20]. These findings align with prior studies that showed high-dose VC can sensitize cancer cells to apoptosis by altering Bcl-2 family protein balance [21].

Despite elevated cytochrome c and Apaf release, a paradoxical decrease in caspases -3, -7, -8, and -9 was observed across all treatments, including the combination. This may suggest a caspase-independent cell death mechanism, potentially mediated via Apaf-1 and Smac/Diablo, which was uniquely upregulated in VC-treated cells. These findings echo reports demonstrated Apaf-mediated, caspase-independent apoptosis in response to VC in neuroblastoma cells [22-23]. The increase in Apaf-1 despite decreased caspases further supports a deviation from classical caspase-dependent apoptosis, indicating a shift in apoptotic signaling pathways under oxidative stress conditions.

Consistent downregulation of CDK2, CDK7, Cyclin B1, and Cyclin D1 suggests robust inhibition of cell cycle progression, with the combination treatment exerting the strongest effect. The decline in cyclin D1, a hallmark of G1 phase transition, is noteworthy, as AF is known to induce G1 arrest in various cancers via EGFR blockade [24-25].

Moreover, p21 upregulation across all treatments, including a moderate increase in p53, supports a tumor suppressive response, likely mediated by oxidative stress and EGFR inhibition [26]. Although p53 increase was modest, the rise in p21 and PTEN, alongside suppression of MDM2, aligns with restored tumor suppressor activity and further enforces cell cycle arrest.

A marked reduction in EGFR, ERK, and SRC in all treatments, particularly in the combination group, underscores the effectiveness of AF as an EGFR inhibitor and highlights VC's potential as a sensitizer. This result is supported by studies showing that high-dose VC can act as a pro-oxidant in cancer cells, enhancing the efficacy of EGFR-targeted therapies [26]. Additionally, suppression of p85 and Akt suggests inhibition of the PI3K/Akt survival pathway, a critical axis in osteosarcoma growth and chemoresistance.

MEK1-4 levels were decreased, with combination of AF and VC expressed more pronounced inhibition. These proteins have been expressed in more progressive cancer; therefore, chemotherapeutic agent that targeted this pathway promising future [26-29].

The increase in Wnt/β-catenin signaling, vimentin and ROCK expression indicates a potential shift toward a mesenchymal phenotype, commonly associated with increased invasiveness. Although these changes were observed across all treatments, their functional implications require cautious interpretation. While EGFR inhibition typically suppresses epithelial–mesenchymal transition (EMT), oxidative stress has been reported to induce compensatory EMT-like responses in some models [28]. MnSOD upregulation, particularly in the VC group, may reflect mitochondrial antioxidant defense activation in response to ROS. Previous reports suggest that high MnSOD expressions may initially protect against ROS-induced damage, but sustained overexpression can lead to apoptosis via mitochondrial signaling [29]. VC also uniquely increased Smac/Diablo, a mitochondrial protein that promotes caspase activation by neutralizing IAPs [30].

MMP-2 and MMP-9, enzymes involved in extracellular matrix degradation and metastasis, were downregulated in all treatments, suggesting anti-invasive potential. The increase in vimentin, Wnt, ROCK, and β-catenin expression may indicate a compensatory activation of EMT or cytoskeletal remodeling, potentially as a stress response to treatment [30-31].

Future work should explore vivo validation using osteosarcoma animal models, detailed mechanistic studies on caspase-independent pathways, and whether this combination can sensitize drug-resistant osteosarcoma variants. Additionally, dose optimization, pharmacokinetics, and potential selective toxicity in normal osteoblasts versus tumor cells should be evaluated.

Conclusion

This study highlights combination of Afatinib and high-dose Vitamin C exerts synergistic cytotoxic effects in SaOS-2 osteosarcoma cells through enhanced ROS generation, mitochondrial dysfunction, suppression of survival signaling, and cell cycle arrest. While decreased caspase activity might seem contradictory to typical apoptosis, this has been observed under extreme oxidative condition where caspase-independent death prevails involving AIF and Smac/Diablo.

Key Findings

AF and VC act synergistically to reduce SaOS-2 cell viability by enhancing ROS generation, disrupting mitochondrial function, and suppressing oncogenic signaling. The combination increased Bax and reduced Bcl-2, supporting intrinsic apoptosis, but paradoxically decreased caspase activity, suggesting caspase-independent death involving Apaf-1 and Smac/Diablo. Cell cycle arrest was reinforced by reduced CDKs and cyclins with p21 and PTEN upregulation, while EGFR, ERK, SRC, PI3K/Akt, and MEK signaling were strongly suppressed. Although EMT-related markers (Wnt/β-catenin, vimentin, ROCK) increased, MMP-2 and MMP-9 declined, indicating potential anti-invasive effects alongside compensatory stress responses. Overall, AF and VC synergistically disrupt survival pathways and promote apoptosis in osteosarcoma cells, highlighting a promising therapeutic approach that warrants in vivo validation and further study of caspase-independent mechanisms.

Acknowledgments

The author thanks Union University for the source and support of research funding. The author also thanks colleagues and editing tools for assistance with improving the clarity of the manuscript.

References

[1] Xiang Y., Yang Y., Liu J., Yang X. Functional role of MicroRNA/p13K/AKT axis in osteosarcoma. *Frontiers Oncology* 2023; 10.3389/fonc.2023.1219211.

[2] Rothberg E.R., Ho X.D., Xu J., Wood D., Martson A., Maasalu K. Alternative splicing of leptin receptor overlapping transcript in osteosarcoma. *Exp Biol Med* (Maywood) 2020 ; 245 :1437–1443.

[3] Xu R., Feng F., Yu X., Liu Z., Lao L. LncRNA SNHG4 promotes tumor growth by sponging miR-224-3p and predicts poor survival and recurrence in human osteosarcoma. *Cell Proliferation* 2018 ; 51 : e12515.

[4] Izhakoff M.S., Bielack S.S., Meltzer P., Gorlick R. Osteosarcoma: current treatment and a collaborative pathway to success. *J Clin Oncol* 2015 ; 33 :3029–35.

[5] *https://seer.cancer.gov/statfacts/html/bones.htm*l. Access May 20, 2025.

[6] Mirabello L., Troisi R.J., Aavage S.A. International osteosarcoma incidence patterns in children and adolescent, middle ages and elderly persons. *Int J Cancer* 2009 ; 125 : 229-234.

[7] Amirhossein A., Goldin M., Awad M., Kulidjian A. Osteosarcoma: a comprehensive review. *Sicot J* 2018 ; 4 : 1-12.

[8] Hurvitz S.A., Shasky R., Harbeck N. Afatinib in the treatment of breast cancer. *Expert Opin Investing Drugs* 2014 ; 23 : 1039-1047.

[9] Molife L.R., Omlin O., Jones R.J., Karavasillis V., Bloomfield D., Lumsden G. Randomized Phase II trial of nintedanib, afatinib and sequential combination in castration-resistant prostate cancer. *Future Onc* 2014 ; 10 : 219-231.

[10] Seiwert T.Y., Fayette J., Cupissol D., Del Campo J.M., Clement P.M., Hitt R. A randomized phase II study of afatinib versus cetuximab in metastatic or recurrent squamous cell carcinoma of the head and neck. *Ann Oncol ESMO* 2014 ; 25 : 1813-1820.

[11] Wang S., Liu S., Zhao B., Yang F., Wang Y., Liang Q. Afatinib reverse multidrug resistance in ovarian cancer via dually inhibiting ATP binding cassette superfamily B member 1. *Oncotarget* 2015 ; 6 : 26142-26160.

[12] Li D., Ambrogio I., Shimamura T. BIBW2992, an irreversible EGFR/HER2 inhibitor highly effective in preclinical lung cancer models. *Oncogene* 2008 ; 27 : 4702-4711.

[13] Solca F., Dahl C., Zoephel A. Target binding properties and cellular activity of afatinib (BIBW 2992), an irreversible ErbB family blocker. *J Pharmacol Exp Ther* 2012 ; 343 : 342-350.

[14] Schoenfeld J.D., Sibenaller Z.A., Wagner B.A., Spitz D.R., Allen B.G. Redox active metals and H2O2 mediate the increased efficacy of pharmacological ascorbate in combination with gemcitabine or radiation in pre-clinical sarcoma models. *Redox Biology* 2018 ; 14 : 417-422.

[15] Du J., Martin S.M., Levine B.A., Wang S., Knudsen C.M., Cullen J.J. Mechanism of ascorbate-induced cytotoxicity in pancreatic cancer. *J Am.* Assoc. *Cancer Res* 2010 ; 16 :509-520.

[16] Chen Q., Espey M.G., Krishna M.C., Mitchell J.B., Corpe C.P., Buettner G.R., et al., Pharmacological ascorbic acid concentrations selectively kill cancer cells: action as a pro-drug to deliver hydrogen peroxide to tissues. *PNAS* 2005 ; 102 : 13604-13609.

[17] Chen Q., Espey M.G., Sun A.Y., Lee J.H., Buettner G.R., Levine M. Ascorbate in pharmacologic concentration selectively generate ascorbate radical and hydrogen peroxide in extracellular fluid *in vivo*. *PNAS* 2007 ; 104 : 8749-8754.

[18] Olney K.E., Du J., Van Erve T.J., Witmer J.R., Wagner B.A., Buettner G.R., et al., Inhibitors of hydroperoxide metabolism enhance ascorbate-induce cytotoxicity. *Free Radic Res* 2013 ; 47:154-163.

[19] Alam M., Shamsi A., Adnan M., Al-Soud W., Tippana A., Imtaiyaz H. Bax/Bcl2 cascade is regulated by the EGFR pathway: Therapeutic targeting of non-small cell lung cancer. *Front Oncol* 2022 ; 12 : 869672.

[20] Harris M.H., Thompson C.B. The role of the Bcl-2 family in the regulation of outer mitochondrial membrane permeability. *Cell Death & Differentiation* 2000 ; 7 : 1182 – 1191.

[21] Susin S.A., Lorenzo H.K., Zamzami N. Molecular characterization of mitochondrial apoptosis-inducing factor. *Nature* 1999 ; 397 (6718): 441.446.

[22] Guo X., Gu J., Shen L. High dose vitamin C inhibits the proliferation of osteosarcoma cells via downregulation of cyclins. *J Orthopedic Res* 2018 ; 36(5): 1353-1362.

[23] Pandey S.K., Shteinfer-Kuzmin A., Caspi V.C., Shoshan-Barmatz V. Non-apoptotic activity of the mitochondrial protein SMAC/Diablo in lung cancer: Novel target to disrupt survival, inflammation, and immunosuppression. Front Oncol 2022. 10.3389/fonc.2022.992260.

[24] Miljenko K., Davor J., Marija P., Maja G., Grahovac G., Gordana Z. EGFR and cyclin D1 in nodular melanoma: correlation with pathohistological parameters and overall survival. *Melanoma Research* 2014 ; 24(6) : 584-591.

[25] Il Na., Rho J.K., Choi J.C., Kim C.H., Park J., Koh J.S., et al. The survival outcomes of patients with resected non-small cell lung cancer differ according to EGFR mutations and the p21 expression. *Lung Cancer* 2007 ; 57 : 96-102.

[26] Mayo L.D., Donner D.B. The PTEN, Mdm2, p53 tumor suppressor–oncoprotein network. *Trends in Biochemical Sciences* 2002 ; 27 (9): 462-467.

[27] Li Y., Dong Q., Cui Y. Synergistic inhibition of MEK and reciprocal feedback networks for targeted intervention in malignancy. *Cancer Bio Med* 2019; 16: 415-434.

[28] Shimizy T., Kimura K., Sugihara E. MEK inhibition preferentially suppresses anchorage-independent growth in osteosarcoma cells and decreases tumors in vivo. *J Orthopaedic Res* 2021 ; 10.1002/jor 25023.

[29] Ruiz G.M., Maldonado V., Cancino G.C., Grajeda J.P.R., Zajgla J.M. Role of Smac/DIABLO in cancer progression. *J Exp Clin Cancer Res* 2008 27, 48.

[30] Loo S.Y., Hirpara J.L., Pandey V., Tan T.Z., Yap C.T., Lobie P.E., et al., Manganese superoxide dismutase expression regulates the switch between an epithelial and mesenchymal-like phenotype in breast cancer. *Antioxidant & Redox Signaling* 2016 ; 25 : 283-299.

[31] Wu K.J., Zhu G.D., Zhang L.L., Li L., Fan J.H., Wang X.Y., et al., Silibinin inhibits prostate cancer invasion, motility and migration by suppressing vimentin and MMP2 expression. *Acta Pharmacologica Sinica* 2009 ; 31 : 1162-1168.

Chapter 8

A Comparative Evaluation of Vitamin C and Etoposide Effects in SK-N-SH and SH-SY5Y Neuroblastoma Cells

Lunawati L. Bennett*, PhD, PharmD
Union University, College of Pharmacy, Jackson, Tennessee, USA

Abstract

Neuroblastoma is the most common extracranial malignancy in children which originates from the embryonic neural crest cell derivatives in the sympathetic nervous system. Based on the five-year-event-free survival, there are four subgroups' categories: very low risk, low risk, intermediate risk, and high risk. More than half of newly diagnosed neuroblastoma cases fall into very low or low risk categories. Current treatment regimen for high-risk neuroblastoma involved dose-intensive cycles of cisplatin and etoposide, alternating with Vincristine, doxorubicin, cyclophosphamide and topotecan. Modest clinical benefits, severe side effects, and frequent development of drug resistance are commonly encountered in neuroblastoma.

The goal of this study was to understand if high dose vitamin C (VC) addition into the current standard of etoposide (ET) has benefit effect. The study specifically investigates whether VC alone or in combination with a low dose of ET is more effective in treating neuroblastoma, utilizing SK-N-SH and SH-SY5Y as the models. Based on the results from sulforhodamine B assay, Rhodamine123, Hoechst 33342, and Western Blot assay, addition of VC to ET inhibits the growth of cancerous cells different signaling responses, reflecting distinct redox and differentiation states. These findings suggest that vitamin C potentiates the cytotoxic effects of etoposide through enhanced oxidative stress and mitochondrial-mediated apoptosis, supporting the potential therapeutic value of this combination.

Keywords: brain cancer, neuroblastoma, vitamin C, etoposide, SK-N-SH, SH-SY5Y

Abbreviations

ET	etoposide;
mTOR	mammalian target of rapamycin;

* Corresponding Author's Email: llbennett@uu.edu

MDM2	Mouse double minute 2 homolog;
MnSOD	Manganese superoxide dismutase;
MOMP	Mitochondrial outer membrane permeabilization;
p85	Phosphatidylinositol-3-kinase;
CDK-7	Cyclin dependent kinase 7;
Cyt C	Cytochrome C.

Introduction

Neuroblastoma is the most common extracranial cancer in children. It represents 8% of pediatric cancers that originate from the embryonic neural crest cell derivatives in the sympathetic nervous system. It has an insidious onset and rapid progression, accounting for 15% of childhood cancer deaths. The most common age of presentation is between 18 and 22 months with most cases being diagnosed before the age of 5. Older children are more likely to have aggressive cancers that are resistant to multimodal and cytotoxic therapies while infants less than 18 months can be successfully treated with surgery alone [1]. While a significant proportion of patients exhibit a favorable prognosis if the cancer is localized, approximately 50% of the diagnoses show a severe clinical course marked by widespread metastases to the bone and bone marrow. Despite intensive therapeutic modality, the survival rate remains below 35% [1-2].

Etoposide (ET) is a prototypical semi-synthetic epipodophyllotoxin derivative used for the treatment of cancers for more than 40 years. Both etoposide and its analogue teniposide derive from the precursor deoxy podophyllotoxin which is an aryl tetralin lignan commonly isolated from the roots and rhizomes of the medicinal plant *Sinopodophyllum hexandrum* (American May apple or mandrake, *Berberidaceae*), or from *Podophyllum peltatum* [3-5]. Since its approval by FDA in 1983, ET has been used for the treatment of testicular carcinoma, small cell lung cancer, lymphoma, sarcoma, neuroendocrine carcinoma, and acute lymphoblastic leukemia [6-8].

Pharmacological ascorbate, achieved through high-dose intravenous vitamin C (VC) to attain plasma levels of ≥ 20 mM, has recently emerged as a potential non-toxic adjuvant to standard care radio-chemotherapy-based cancer therapies across various disease sites [9-10]. The proposed anti-cancer mechanism of pharmacological VC involves redox-active metal-mediated or auto-oxidation of ascorbate, resulting in the formation of O_2 and H_2O_2 [10-12].

This study was designed to evaluate the chemo-enhancing potential of VC in combination with low-dose ET for treating neuroblastoma, utilizing SK-N-SH and SH-SY5Y cells as the models. The findings of this investigation reveal that the use of VC with ET demonstrated greater efficacy in the treatment of neuroblastoma. This marks a novel discovery in the field.

To evaluate the cytotoxic potential of high-dose VC, various antineoplastic agents - including paclitaxel, doxorubicin, etoposide, temsirolimus, bortezomib, afatinib, and sorafenib - were tested on human neuroblastoma using the model SK-N-SH and SH-SY5Y cell line. For combination studies, the lowest concentrations of each antineoplastic and high-dose VC that yielded a synergistic reduction in cell viability were selected. General experimental procedures followed the protocols outlined in Chapter 3 (Materials and Methods), while methodological details specific to this study are described below.

Rationale for Comparative Analysis

Given their shared neuroblastoma origin yet distinct phenotypic characteristics, the SH-SY5Y and SK-N-SH cell lines provide complementary models for evaluating redox-dependent cytotoxic mechanisms. SH-SY5Y represents a neuronally enriched and more differentiated phenotype, whereas SK-N-SH retains a heterogeneous population reflective of primary cancer diversity. Comparing their responses to VC, a redox-modulating agent, and ET, a DNA-damaging chemotherapeutic, allows for assessment of whether VC enhances or interferes with ET-induced apoptosis in neuroblastoma cells of differing differentiation states. This approach may provide insight into the role of oxidative stress and mitochondrial pathways in VC-mediated chemo sensitization within neural-derived cancers.

Cell Culture

1. The human neuroblastoma cell lines SK-N-SH (ATCC HTB-11) were cultured in EMEM media supplemented with 10% FBS and 1% streptomycin/penicillin, cultured and maintained in an incubator at 37°C in a 5% CO2 humidified environment. This cell is a product of J.L. Biedler's research, originated from the brain tissue of a 4-year-old female human patient diagnosed with neuroblastoma. This cell line exhibits distinctive genetic attributes, hyper diploidy and marker chromosomes 9q+ and 22q+. It consists of two major subtypes: neuroblastic (N-type) cells, which display small, rounded bodies with neurite-like processes, and substrate-adherent (S-type) cells, which are larger and more epithelial in appearance. This mixed phenotype reflects cancer's biological diversity and provides a useful system for investigating neuronal differentiation and tumor heterogeneity.
2. SH-SY5Y, a derivative from SK-N-SH line (ATCC CRL 2266), were cultured in 1:1 mixture of EMEM media and F12 Medium (GIBCO F12) with 15% FBS and 1% streptomycin/penicillin, cultured and maintained in an incubator at 37°C in a 5% CO2 humidified environment The cells exhibit a predominantly neuroblast-like morphology and possess the ability to differentiate into neuron-like cells when exposed to differentiation agents such as retinoic acid or brain-derived neurotrophic factor. SH-SY5Y cells express characteristic neuronal markers, including βIII-tubulin, MAP2, and tyrosine hydroxylase, consistent with dopaminergic and adrenergic features.

Results

Cell Viability and Selection of Doses

SK-N-SH cells treated with VC alone showed no significant change in viability at concentrations below 2.5 mM. Similarly, treatment with etoposide (ET) alone produced no marked cytotoxicity below 0.5 μM. Therefore, 2.5 mM VC and 0.5 μM ET were selected for combination treatment. The combined exposure resulted in a pronounced reduction in cell viability after 24, 48, and 72 h, indicating a synergistic cytotoxic effect in SK-N-SH cells. Comparable trends were observed in SH-SY5Y cells treated under the same conditions, confirming that the VC and ET combination effectively enhanced growth inhibition in both neuroblastoma cell lines.

The Chou–Talalay analysis revealed CI values below 1 for most combination points, confirming a synergistic interaction between ET and VC at lower VC concentrations (1.25–2.5 mM), while higher VC concentrations approached an additive effect (CI ≈ 1). This suggests that VC potentiates ET-induced cytotoxicity in SK-N-SH and SHSY5Y cells, especially within the sub-toxic range of VC. The observed synergy aligns with the hypothesis that redox modulation and mitochondrial stress contribute to enhanced susceptibility of neuroblastoma cells to low-dose ET in the presence of pharmacologic VC.

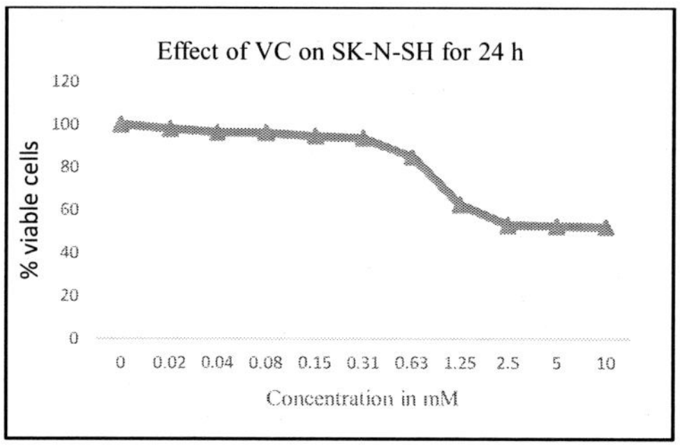

(a)

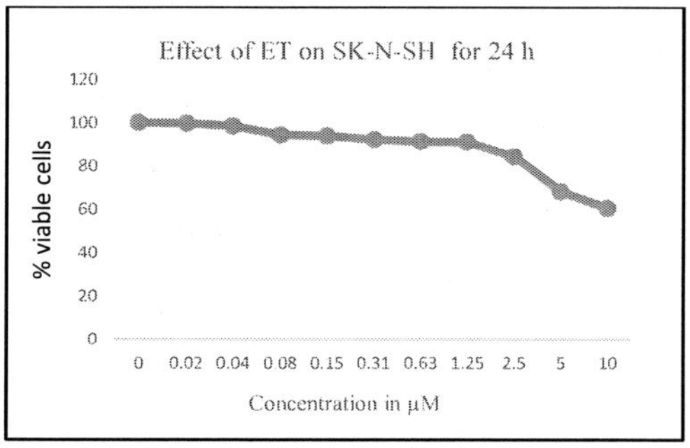

(b)

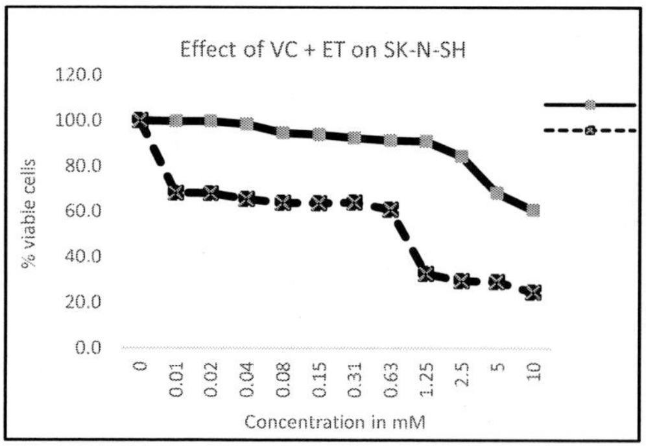

(c)

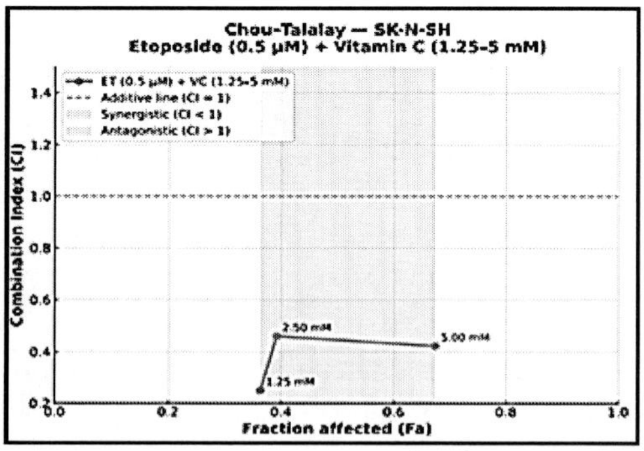

(d)

Figure 1. (Continued).

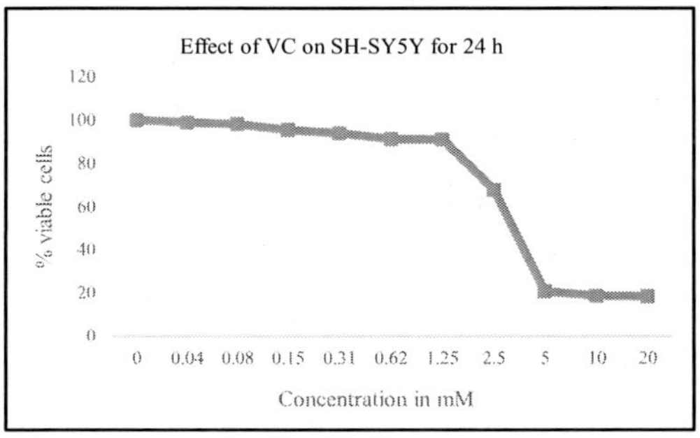

(e)

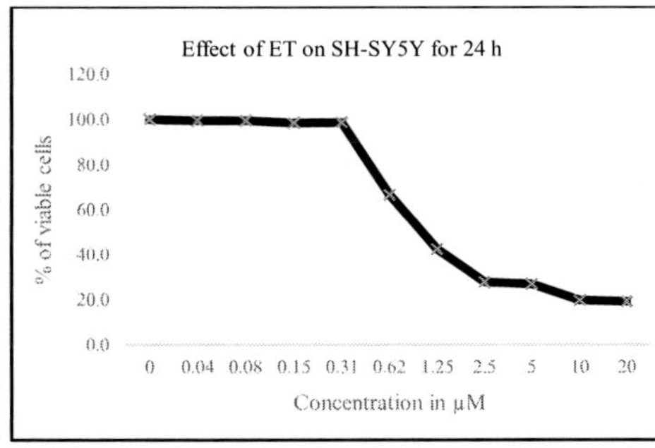

(f)

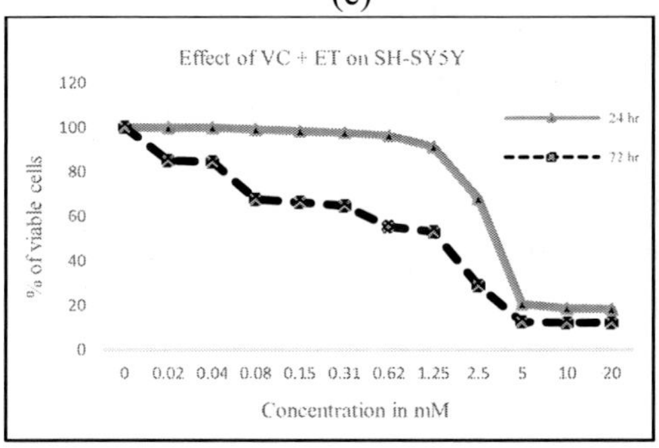

(g)

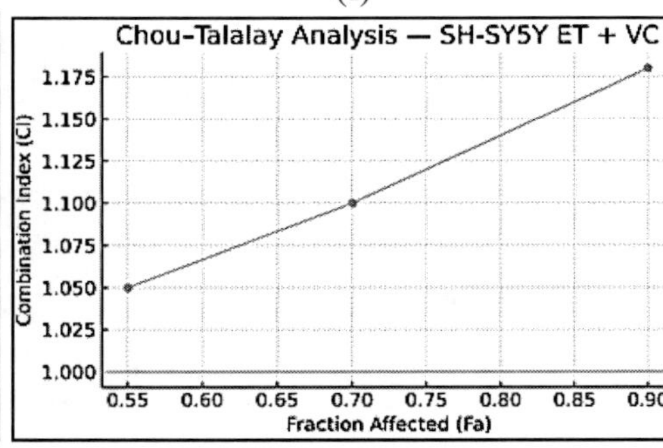

(h)

Figure 1. (a–d) SK-N-SH cells and (e–h) SH-SY5Y cells were treated with increasing concentrations of VC (0–20 mM) or ET (0–20 μM) for 24 h. Panels (a, e) show dose-dependent effects of VC alone, panels (b, f) depict ET alone, panels (c, g) illustrate the combined treatment of 2.5 mM VC + 0.5 μM ET at 24 and 72 h panel (d, h) show synergistic effect measure by Chou-Talalay method, showed synergistic effect for SKNSH (Fa = 0.43, CI 0.5) and for SHSY5Y (Fa = 0.72, CI = 0.95). Cell viability was determined by SRB assay and expressed as a percentage relative to untreated controls. Data represent mean ± SD of three independent experiments.

Changes Cells Morphology in SK-N-SH and SH-SY5Y

VC and ET induced marked morphological alterations in SK-N-SH and SH-SY5Y cells. In SK-N-SH cells, control cultures display healthy morphology with elongated processes and strong adherence after 24 h. Treatment with VC or ET alone resulted in reduced cell density, rounding, and partial detachment, indicating loss of viability. The combination of 2.5 mM VC and 0.5 μM ET produced the most pronounced effect, characterized by extensive cell shrinkage and detachment, with numerous cells appearing non-adherent or floating in the culture medium. Similar morphological trends were observed in SH-SY5Y cells, confirming that combined VC and ET treatment potentiated cytotoxicity and disrupted normal neuroblastoma cell morphology.

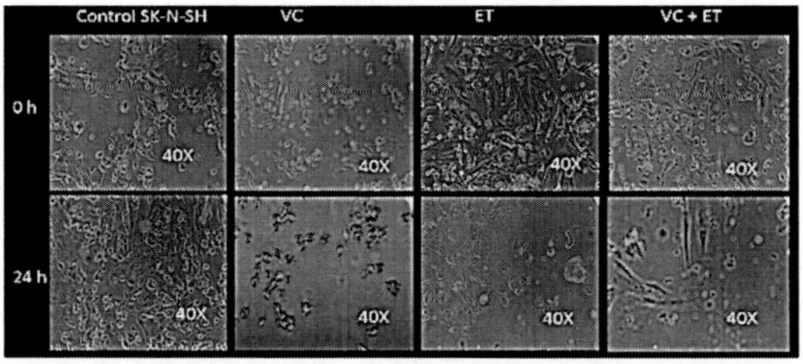

(a)

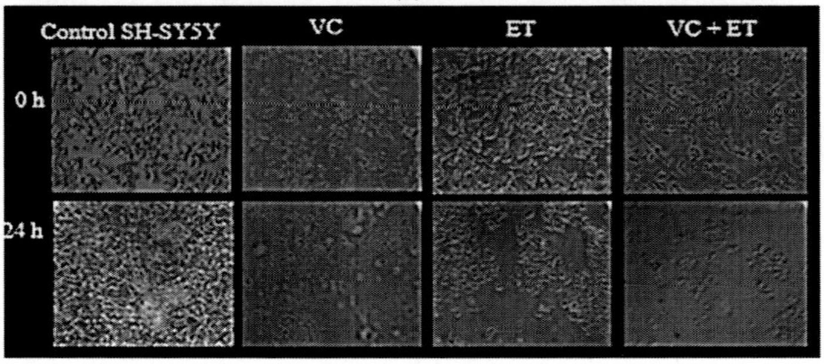

(b)

Figure 2. Representative phase-contrast micrographs show (a) SK-N-SH and (b) SH-SY5Y cells after 24 h of treatment with VC, ET), or their combination. Scale bar 40x using inverted microscope. Data are expressed as mean ± SD (n = 3).

Wound-Healing of SK-N-SH and SH-SY5Y

The migratory ability of neuroblastoma cells was markedly suppressed by the combined treatment of VC and ET. After 24 h, SK-N-SH cells treated with ET or the combination VC and ET exhibited significantly reduced migration, leaving a wider wound gap compared to cells treated with VC alone. In contrast, control cells migrated efficiently to close the wound area, indicating active motility and potential invasive capacity. Quantitative analysis confirmed a substantial increase in wound width under combination treatment relative to single-agent and control groups. Similar findings were observed in SH-SY5Y cells, where VC and ET treatment significantly impaired wound closure compared to control and single treatments (Figure 3c–d). These results suggest that VC enhances the anti-migratory effect of ET, thereby attenuating the invasive potential of neuroblastoma cells.

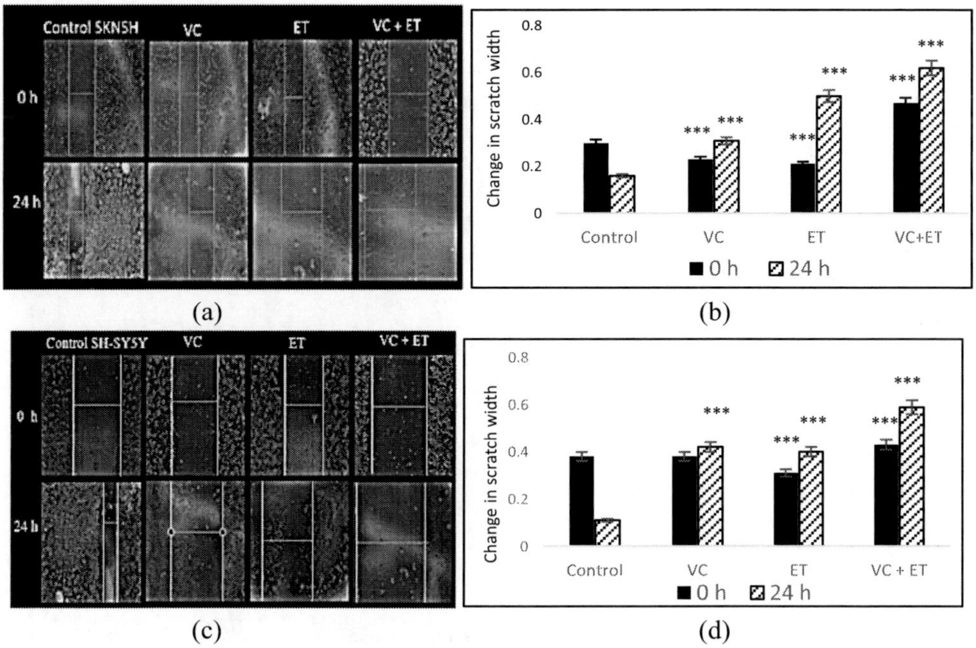

Figure 3. Representative wound-healing images of (a) SK-N-SH and (c) SH-SY5Y cells. Scale bar 40x using inverted microscope. Panels (b) and (d) show quantitative analysis of wound width, expressed as mean ± SD (n = 3), ***p < 0.001, according to the post hoc Newman-Keuls test.

Induction of Apoptosis in SK-N-SH and SH-SY5Y

Hoechst 33342 staining revealed increased nuclear condensation and fragmentation in both SK-N-SH and SH-SY5Y cells following combined VC and ET treatment, indicative of apoptosis. In SK-N-SH cells, control nuclei appeared uniformly round and faintly stained, whereas cells treated with VC or ET alone exhibited moderate chromatin condensation. The VC and ET combination markedly enhanced apoptotic morphology, with numerous brightly fluorescent, condensed, and fragmented nuclei. Quantitative analysis confirmed a significant increase in apoptotic cells under combination treatment compared to control and single-agent groups. A similar pattern was observed in SH-SY5Y cells, where VC and ET treatment led to a substantial rise in nuclear fragmentation and apoptotic index relative to controls. These results support that VC enhances ET-induced apoptosis in neuroblastoma cells.

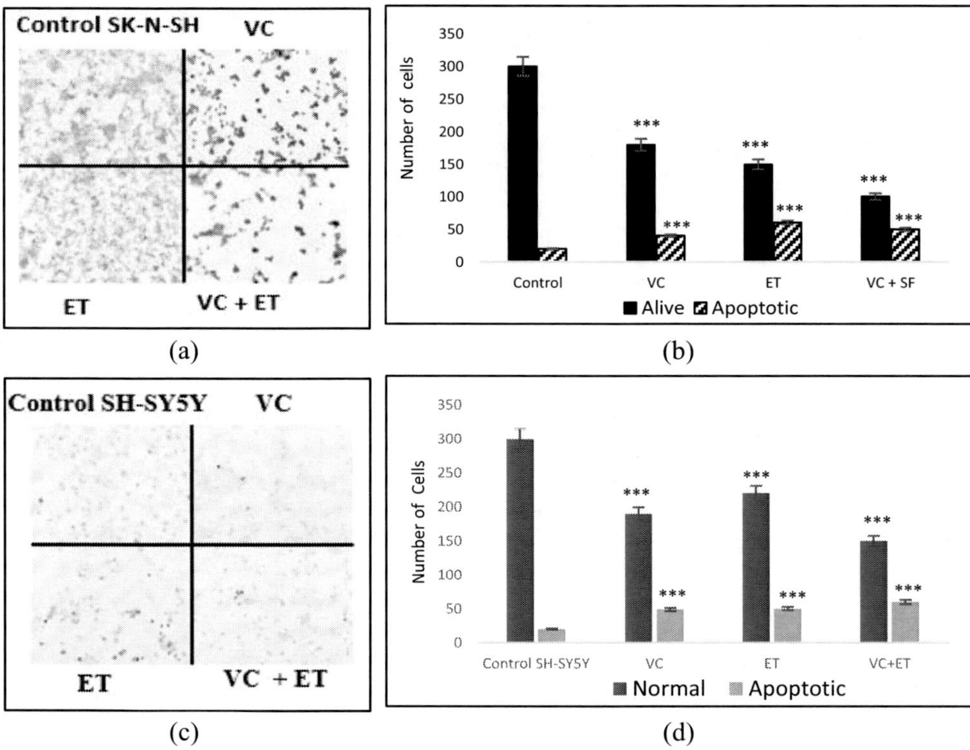

Figure 4. Representative fluorescence images of (a-b) SK-N-SH and (c-d) SH-SY5Y cells. Quantitative fluorescence intensity expressed as mean ± SD (n = 3). A significant increase in apoptotic cells was observed, with ***$p < 0.001$, as determined by the post hoc Newman-Keuls test.

Intracellular ROS in SK-N-SH and SY-SY5Y

ROS production was markedly increased in both SK-N-SH and SH-SY5Y cells following combined VC and ET treatment. In SK-N-SH cells, fluorescence intensity of H_2DCF-DA was modestly elevated after treatment with either VC or ET alone. The VC and ET combination, however, produced a strong green fluorescence signal, indicating a substantial rise in intracellular ROS levels. Quantitative analysis confirmed a significant increase in ROS intensity compared to single-agent and control groups. Similar results were observed in SH-SY5Y cells, suggesting that VC potentiates ET-induced oxidative stress, thereby contributing to enhanced cytotoxicity in neuroblastoma cells.

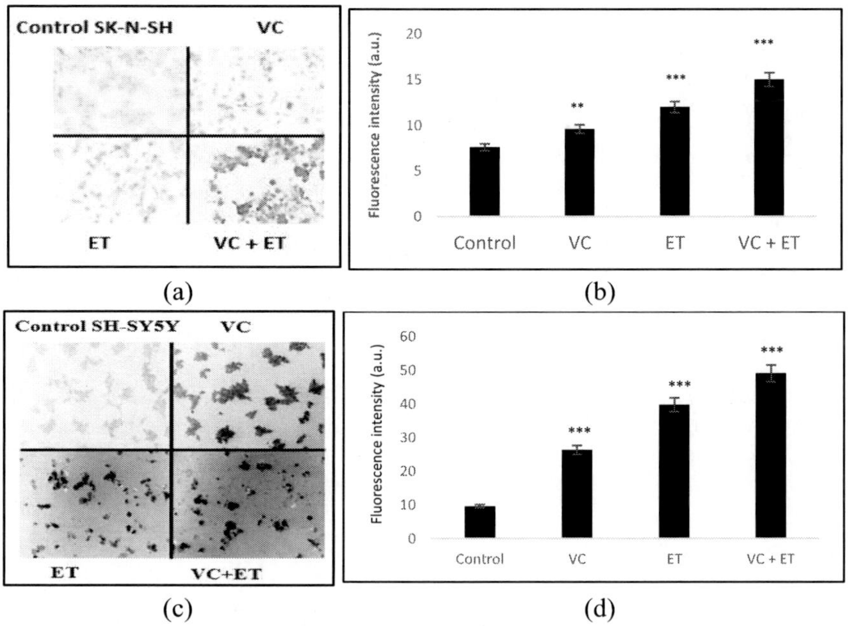

Figure 5. Representative fluorescence micrographs of (a-b) SK-N-SH and (c-d) SH-SY5Y cells. Quantitative fluorescence intensity expressed as mean ± SD (n = 3), indicated by $^{**}p < 0.01$, $^{***}p < 0.001$, according to the post hoc Newman-Keuls test.

Mitochondrial Membrane Potential in SK-N-SH and SH-SY5Y

Disruption of mitochondrial membrane potential ($\Delta\Psi m$) was evident after combined treatment with VC and ET. In SK-N-SH cells, control cultures exhibited strong Rhodamine 123 fluorescence, reflecting intact mitochondrial function. Treatment with VC or ET alone caused a moderate reduction in fluorescence intensity, while the combined treatment resulted in marked fluorescence loss, indicating mitochondrial depolarization. Quantitative data confirmed a significant decrease in $\Delta\Psi m$ in the combination group relative to control and single-agent treatments. Similar trends were detected in SH-SY5Y cells, further supporting that VC amplifies ET-induced mitochondrial dysfunction, consistent with ROS-mediated apoptotic signaling.

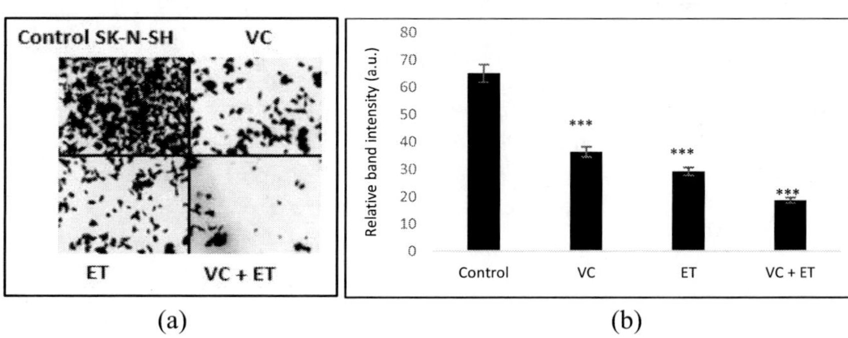

Figure 6. (Continued).

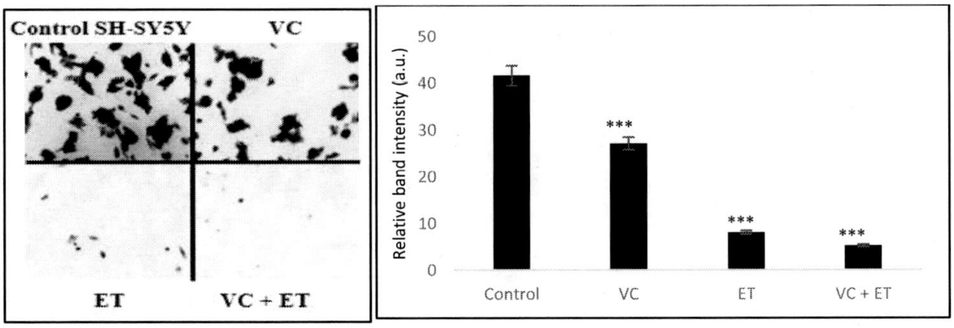

(c) (d)

Figure 6. Representative fluorescence images of (a-b) SK-N-SH and (c-d) SH-SY5Y cells. Quantitative fluorescence intensity data expressed as mean + SD (n = 3) indicated by ***p < 0.001, according to the post hoc Newman-Keuls test.

Modulation of Bax, Bcl2, AIF and Cyt C in SK-N-SH and SH-SY5Y

Western blot analysis revealed that the combination of VC and ET significantly modulated the expression of key apoptotic regulators in both SK-N-SH and SH-SY5Y cells. In SK-N-SH cells, treatment with VC or ET alone produced modest increases in cytochrome c and Bax expression with a reduction in Bcl-2. The combined VC and ET treatment markedly enhanced Cytochrome c release and Bax expression while further decreasing Bcl-2 levels, resulting in a pronounced increase in the Bax/Bcl-2 ratio as shown in the histogram. Similar expression patterns were observed in SH-SY5Y cells, supporting that VC amplifies ET-induced mitochondrial apoptosis through the intrinsic pathway. These findings are consistent with the observed ROS elevation and mitochondrial depolarization, indicating that VC synergistically enhances ET-mediated apoptotic signaling in neuroblastoma cells.

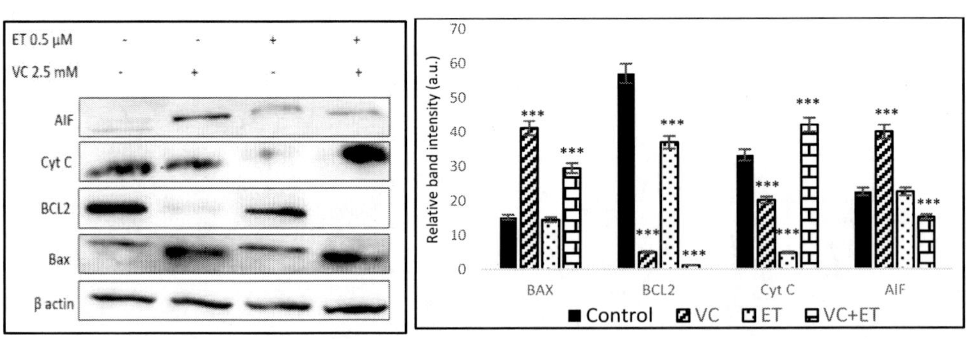

(a) (b)

Figure 7. (Continued).

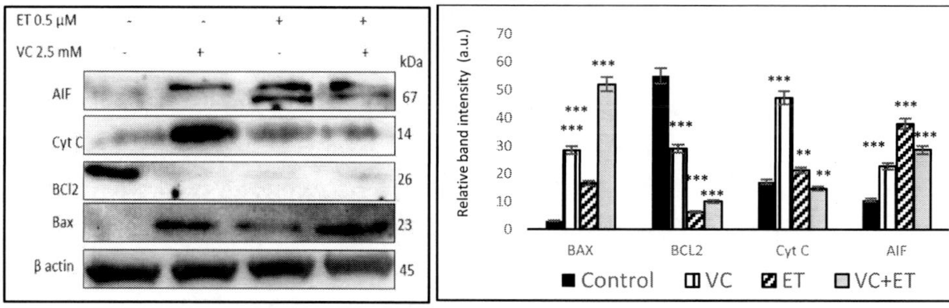

(c) (d)

Figure 7. Western blot analysis of Bax, BCl2, Cyt C, and AIF expression in SK-N-SH and SH-SY5Ycells following treatment with VC, ET or their combination. (a) Representative blots showing different proteins expressions in SK-N-SH. (c) Representative blots showing expression of proteins in SH-SY5Y. (b) Densitometric histogram compares relative protein levels normalized to β-actinin in SK-N-SH and (d) in SH-SY-5Y. Data are expressed as mean ± SD (n = 3). Statistical significance **p < 0.01 and ***p< 0.001 was determined using the Newman–Keuls post hoc test.

Modulation Mitochondrial Signaling in SK-N-SH and SH-SY5Y

The effects of VC, ET, and their combination on caspase activation were evaluated in SK-N-SH and SH-SY5Y cells. In SK-N-SH cells, VC treatment alone markedly increased the expression of initiator caspases (cas-8 and -9) and effector caspases (cas-3 and -7), as well as APAF-1. ET alone produced minimal or no change relative to the control. Interestingly, the VC and ET combination resulted in expression levels slightly lower than VC alone but still elevated compared to control, suggesting that excessive oxidative stress from the combination may trigger partial caspase suppression or post-apoptotic feedback regulation. In contrast, SH-SY5Y cells displayed a distinct pattern: VC or ET alone elicited minimal caspase activation, whereas the combination treatment led to a clear upregulation of caspase-3, -7, -8, -9, and APAF-1. These findings indicate that VC predominantly initiates caspase-mediated apoptosis in SK-N-SH cells, while in SH-SY5Y cells, VC synergizes with ET to activate the caspase cascade through both intrinsic and extrinsic pathways.

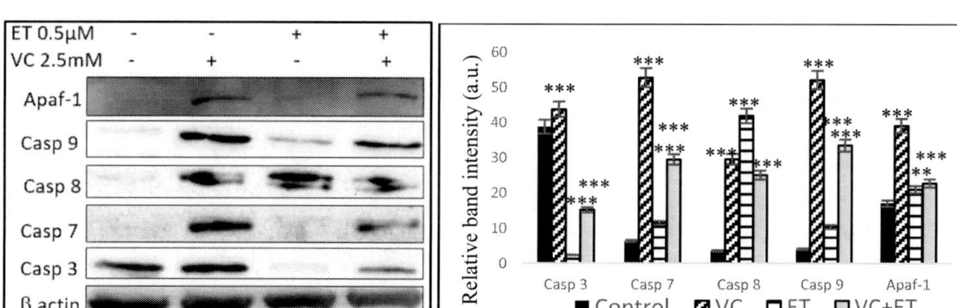

(a) (b)

Figure 8. (Continued).

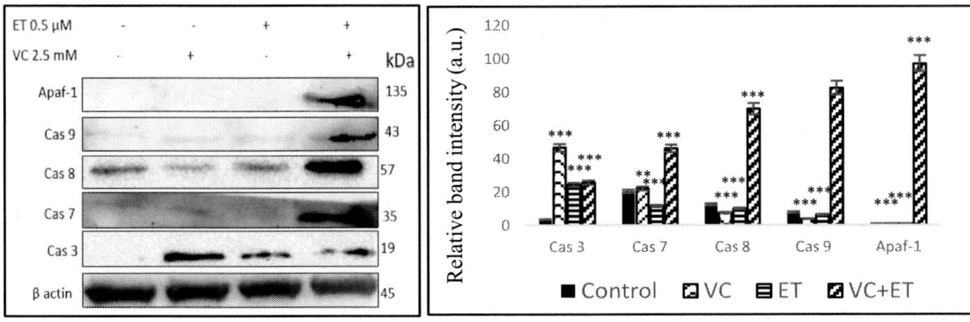

(c) (d)

Figure 8. Western blot analysis of expression caspase-3, -7, -8, -9, and APAF-1 protein in SK-N-SH and SH-SY5Ycells following treatment with VC, ET or their combination.
(a) Representative blots showing different proteins expressions in SK-N-SH. (c) Representative blots showing expression of proteins in SH-SY5Y. (b) Densitometric histogram compares relative protein levels normalized to β-actinin in SK-N-SH and (d) in SH-SY-5Y. Data are expressed as mean ± SD (n = 3). Statistical significance**p < 0.01 and ***p < 0.001 was determined using the Newman–Keuls post hoc test.

Modulation of MEK Kinase Pathway in SK-N-SH and SH-SY5Y

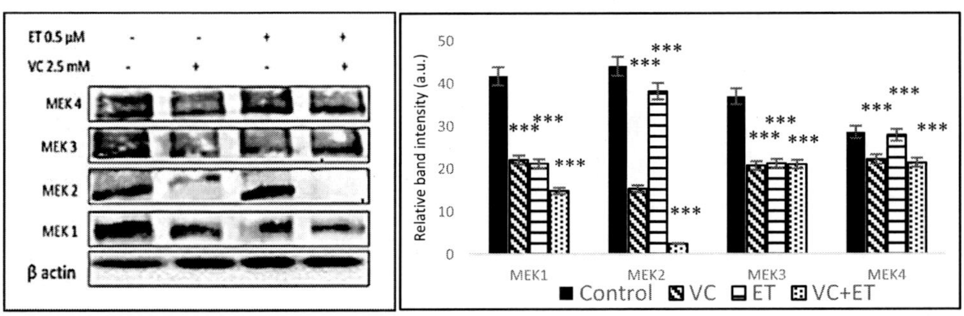

(a) (b)

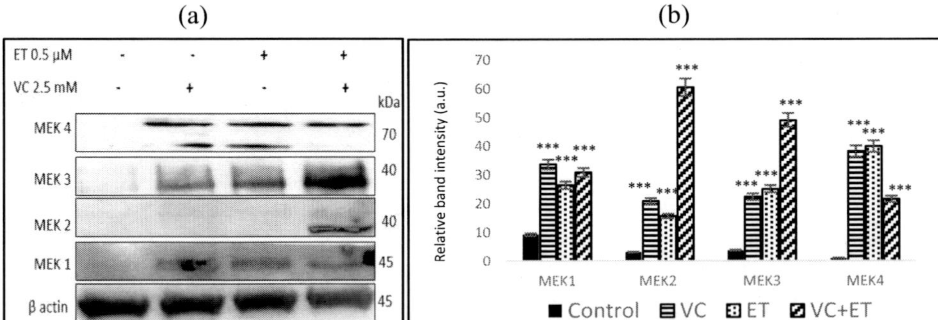

(c) (d)

Figure 9. Western blot analysis of expression MEK 1-4 proteins in SK-N-SH and SH-SY5Ycells following treatment with VC, ET or their combination. (a) Representative blots showing different proteins expressions in SK-N-SH. (c) Representative blots showing expression of proteins in SH-SY5Y. (b) Densitometric histogram compares relative protein levels normalized to β-actinin in SK-N-SH and (d) in SH-SY-5Y. Data are expressed as mean ± SD (n = 3). Statistical significance**p < 0.01 and ***p < 0.001 was determined using the Newman–Keuls post hoc test.

The expression of MEK isoforms (MEK1–4) was analyzed to determine whether VC, ET, or their combination affected MAPK pathway signaling in neuroblastoma cells. In SK-N-SH cells, all MEK isoforms showed reduced expression following treatment. VC and ET individually caused modest decreases, while the combination treatment led to the most pronounced suppression, particularly of MEK2, which exhibited minimal expression compared to the control. This downregulation suggests that the VC and ET combination inhibits the MEK-dependent survival signaling in SK-N-SH cells. In contrast, SH-SY5Y cells demonstrated a divergent response. VC alone markedly increased MEK1–3 expression and moderately elevated MEK4, indicating activation of compensatory signaling possibly linked to stress adaptation. ET alone or in combination with VC, however, decreased MEK4 expression and attenuated MEK1–3 levels relative to VC alone. These findings indicate that while VC and ET co-treatment suppresses MEK signaling in SK-N-SH cells, SH-SY5Y cells exhibit a mixed pattern - initial MEK activation by VC alone followed by inhibition under combined oxidative and genotoxic stress.

Modulation of Cell Cycle Regulatory in SK-N-SH and SH-SY5Y

To investigate whether VC, ET, or their combination affects the cell-cycle progression of neuroblastoma cells, the expression of cyclin-dependent kinases (CDK2, CDK7) and cyclins (cyclin B1, cyclin D1) was analyzed. In SK-N-SH cells, all tested proteins showed decreased expression following treatment, with the most pronounced reduction observed in the combination group. VC or ET alone caused moderate downregulation, whereas VC and ET led to further decrease in the expression of these proteins. In contrast, SH-SY5Y cells displayed an opposite pattern. While VC or ET alone caused mild decreases in CDK2, CDK7, and cyclin D1 expression relative to control, the combination treatment markedly increased all four proteins, particularly cyclin D1, CDK7, and CDK2, implying compensatory activation of cell-cycle regulators under combined redox and genotoxic stress. This biphasic response suggests that SK-N-SH cells undergo growth arrest and apoptotic commitment, whereas SH-SY5Y cells may activate transient survival signaling to counterbalance treatment-induced stress.

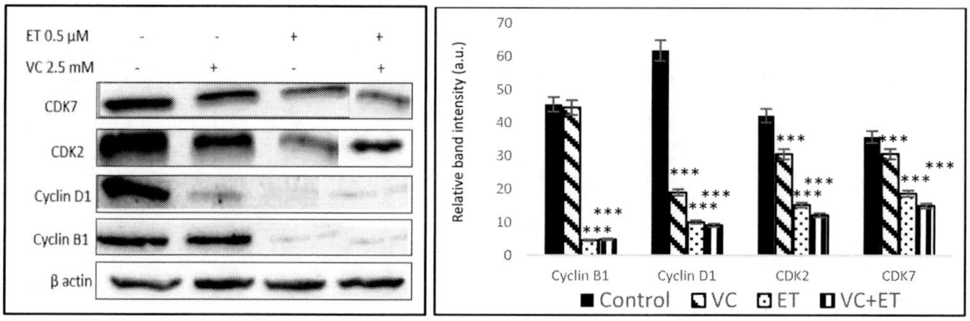

(a) (b)

Figure 10. (Continued).

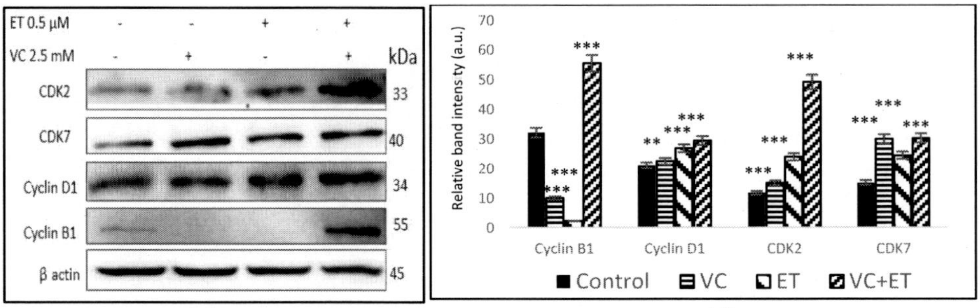

(c) (d)

Figure 10. Western blot analysis expression of cell cycle proteins in SK-N-SH and SH-SY5Ycells following treatment with VC, ET or their combination. (a) Representative blots showing different proteins exprcssions in SK-N-SII. (c) Representative blots showing expression of proteins in SH-SY5Y. (b) Densitometric histogram compares relative protein levels normalized to β-actinin in SK-N-SH and (d) in SH-SY-5Y. Data are expressed as mean ± SD (n = 3). Statistical significance**p < 0.01 and ***p < 0.001 was determined using the Newman–Keuls post hoc test.

Modulation of p21, p53, PTEN, and MDM2 in SK-N-SH and SH-SY5Y

To further delineate the molecular response of VC and ET, the expressions of PTEN, p53, p21, and MDM2, key regulators of cell survival and cell-cycle control were measured. In SK-N-SH cells, VC or ET alone resulted in reduced expression of PTEN and p53, and the combination treatment further suppressed both proteins. In contrast, p21 was consistently upregulated across all treatments, with the highest expression observed in the combination group, suggesting activation of cell-cycle checkpoint signaling despite diminished p53 levels. MDM2, a negative regulator of p53, was downregulated in all treatment groups, consistent with loss of the p53–MDM2 feedback loop. In SH-SY5Y cells, PTEN expression showed a slight increase following VC and ET treatment compared with control or single treatments, indicating partial restoration of tumor-suppressive signaling. Like SK-N-SH cells, p21 expression was markedly increased, while p53 and MDM2 decreased under all treatment conditions. These findings suggest that VC and ET modulate the PTEN–p53–p21–MDM2 regulatory axis in a cell-type–dependent manner: SK-N-SH cells exhibit pathway suppression with compensatory p21 induction, whereas SH-SY5Y cells retain partial PTEN activation alongside p21-mediated growth restraint (see Fig.11).

Modulation of Akt/p85/mTOR Pathway in SK-N-SH and SH-SY5Y

To assess the impact of VC, ET, and their combination on survival signaling, the expression of Akt, mTOR, and the PI3K regulatory subunit p85 were examined. In SK-N-SH cells, all three proteins showed reduced expression after treatment, with the most pronounced decrease observed in the VC and ET group. Both VC and ET alone caused moderate suppression of Akt and mTOR, while p85 expression was also diminished, indicating inhibition of the upstream PI3K/Akt/mTOR survival pathway. This downregulation suggests that VC enhances the cytotoxic effect of ET by attenuating pro-survival signaling cascades. In contrast, SH-SY5Y cells exhibited a distinct response. Treatment with VC or ET alone produced minor changes, but the combination markedly increased the expression of p85, Akt, and mTOR compared to control. This upregulation implies an adaptive activation of the PI3K/Akt/mTOR axis, possibly as a compensatory mechanism to counteract oxidative and genotoxic stress. Collectively, these findings indicate that while VC and ET synergistically suppress the Akt–mTOR pathway in SK-N-SH cells, it paradoxically activates the same signaling cascade in SH-SY5Y cells, highlighting intrinsic molecular heterogeneity between the two neuroblastoma subtypes (see fig.12).

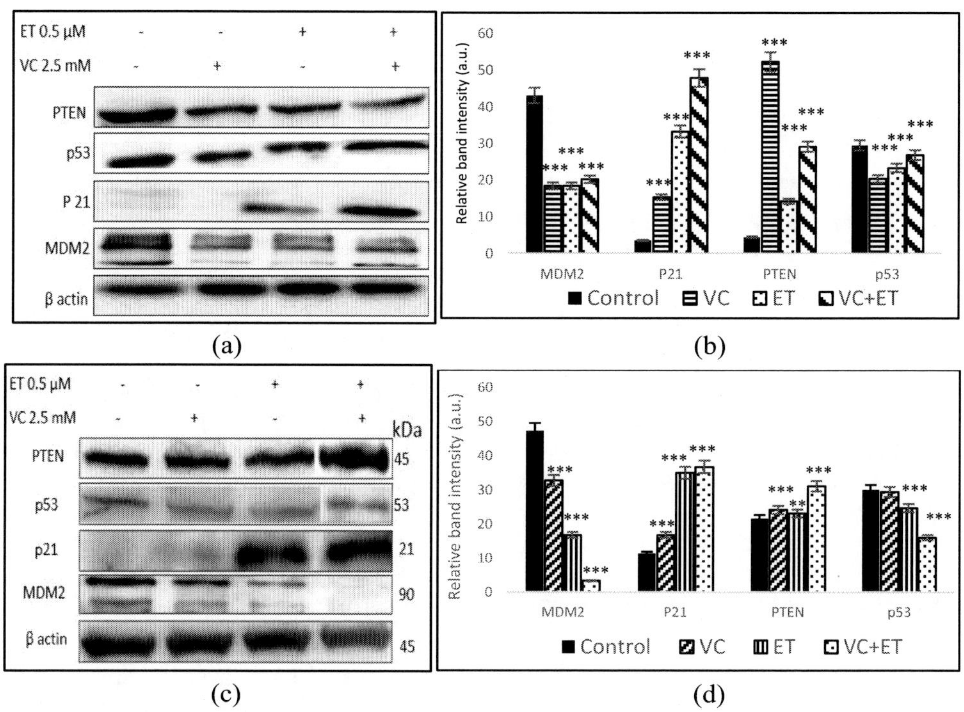

Figure 11. Western blot analysis expression of PTEN, p53, p21, and MDM2 in SK-N-SH and SH-SY5Ycells following treatment with VC, ET or their combination. (a) Representative blots showing different proteins expressions in SK-N-SH. (c) Representative blots showing expression of proteins in SH-SY5Y. (b) Densitometric histogram compares relative protein levels normalized to β-actinin in SK-N-SH and (d) in SH-SY-5Y. Data are expressed as mean ± SD ($n = 3$). Statistical significance $^{**}p < 0.01$ and $^{***}p < 0.001$ was determined using the Newman–Keuls post hoc test.

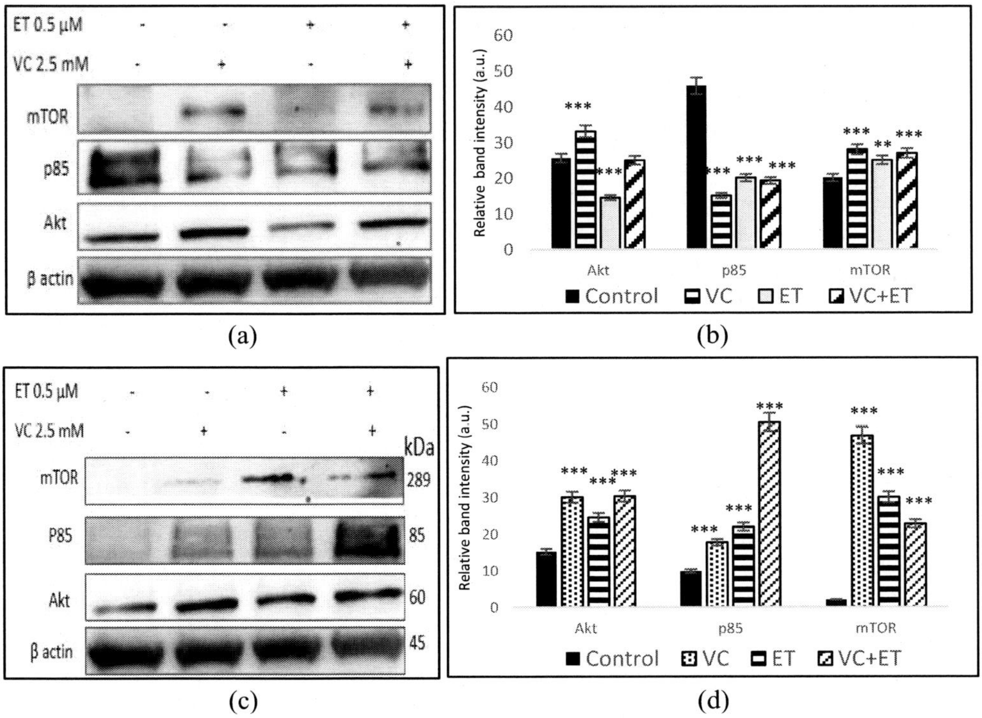

Figure 12. Western blot analysis expression of Akt, mTOR, and p85 in SK-N-SH and SH-SY5Ycells following treatment with VC, ET or their combination. (a) Representative blots showing different proteins expressions in SK-N-SH. (c) Representative blots showing expression of proteins in SH-SY5Y. (b) Densitometric histogram compares relative protein levels normalized to β-actinin in SK-N-SH and (d) in SH-SY-5Y. Data are expressed as mean ± SD ($n = 3$). Statistical significance**$p < 0.01$ and ***$p < 0.001$ was determined using the Newman–Keuls post hoc test.

Modulation of SAPK/JNK and p38 in SK-N-SH and SH-SY5Y

To further explore stress-responsive signaling mechanisms induced by VC and ET, the expression levels of p38 MAPK and SAPK/JNK were evaluated in both neuroblastoma cell lines. In SK-N-SH cells, treatment with VC or ET alone caused a reduction in p38 expression, while the combination further decreased p38 levels compared with control. In contrast, SAPK/JNK expression was markedly elevated in all treatment groups, with the strongest activation observed in the VC, suggesting enhanced stress signaling and pro-apoptotic response. A similar trend was observed in SH-SY5Y cells. While p38 expression decreased following VC, ET, or combination treatments, SAPK/JNK levels were significantly increased, especially under VC only. This consistent pattern across both cell lines indicates that VC and ET synergistically suppress p38-mediated survival signaling while concurrently activating the JNK pathway, a hallmark of stress-induced apoptosis.

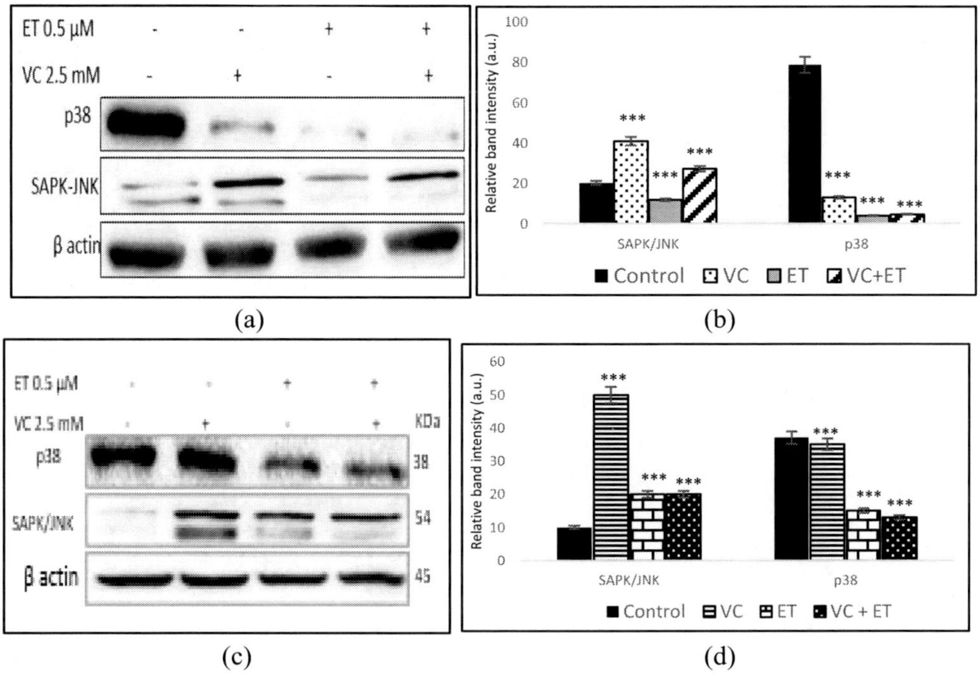

Figure 13. Western blot analysis expression of p38 and SAPK/JNK in SK-N-SH and SH-SY5Ycells following treatment with VC, ET or their combination. (a) Representative blots showing different proteins expressions in SK-N-SH. (c) Representative blots showing expression of proteins in SH-SY5Y. (b) Densitometric histogram compares relative protein levels normalized to β-actinin in SK-N-SH and (d) in SH-SY-5Y. Data are expressed as mean ± SD (n = 3). Statistical significance**p < 0.01 and ***p< 0.001 was determined using the Newman–Keuls post hoc test.

Modulation of ERK 1/2, Raf, and EGFR in SK-N-SH and SH-SY5Y

To delineate how VC and ET influence the upstream MAPK signaling cascade, the expression of EGFR, Raf, and ERK1/2 were analyzed in both SK-N-SH and SH-SY5Y cells. In SK-N-SH cells, VC or ET alone moderately reduced EGFR, Raf, and ERK1/2 expression, whereas the combination treatment produced a pronounced downregulation of all three proteins. The suppression of this signaling axis suggests effective inhibition of mitogenic and survival pathways, consistent with the observed apoptotic and growth-inhibitory responses in SK-N-SH cells. In contrast, SH-SY5Y cells exhibited the opposite pattern. VC or ET alone caused minor upregulation of EGFR, Raf, and ERK1/2, and the combination treatment further enhanced their expression levels compared with control. This coordinated activation indicates a compensatory engagement of the EGFR–Raf–ERK pathway, possibly reflecting a stress-adaptive response aimed at promoting survival signaling under combined redox and genotoxic stress. Together, these results highlight distinct regulatory dynamics between the two neuroblastoma subtypes - where SK-N-SH cells undergo suppression of MAPK-driven proliferation, while SH-SY5Y cells activate the same cascade as a protective mechanism.

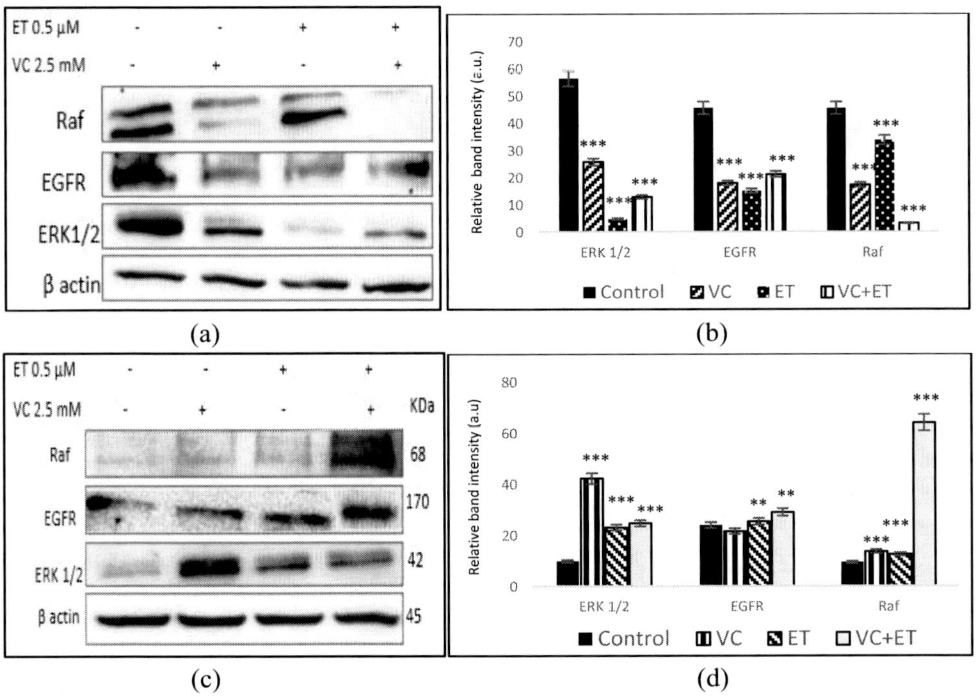

Figure 14. Western blot analysis expression of EGFR, Raf, and ERK1/2 in SK-N-SH and SH-SY5Ycells following treatment with VC, ET or their combination. (a) Representative blots showing different proteins expressions in SK-N-SH. (c) Representative blots showing expression of proteins in SH-SY5Y. (b) Densitometric histogram compares relative protein levels normalized to β-actinin in SK-N-SH and (d) in SH-SY-5Y. Data are expressed as mean ± SD (n = 3). Statistical significance $^{**}p < 0.01$ and $^{***}p < 0.001$ was determined using the Newman–Keuls post hoc test.

Modulation of Wnt, ROCK, and Vimentin in SK-N-SH and SH-SY5Y

Analysis of epithelial–mesenchymal and motility-associated markers revealed cell line–specific responses to VC, ET, and their combination. In SK-N-SH cells, ROCK and Wnt pathway protein levels were reduced following treatment, consistent with diminished ROCK-dependent contractility and suppression of canonical Wnt signaling. In contrast, vimentin - an intermediate filament and mesenchymal/EMT marker - was increased in SK-N-SH cells, with the highest expression observed in the ET-only group; VC alone and the VC and ET combination produced more moderate elevations relative to control. This pattern suggests that while upstream motility and Wnt signals are attenuated, ET alone may selectively promote mesenchymal marker expression in SK-N-SH cells. SH-SY5Y cells displayed an opposite trend: ROCK and Wnt expression were elevated in response to treatment, consistent with activation of motility and Wnt-linked survival pathways, whereas vimentin expression decreased across treatments. Together, these data indicate divergent regulation of EMT and motility programs between the two neuroblastoma lines - SK-N-SH showing increased mesenchymal marker expression (driven most strongly by ET) despite reduced ROCK/Wnt signaling, and SH-SY5Y showing activation of ROCK/Wnt with loss of vimentin. These opposing responses likely reflect intrinsic differences in cytoskeletal regulation and pathway crosstalk between the cell lines and may underline the distinct migration/invasion phenotypes observed earlier.

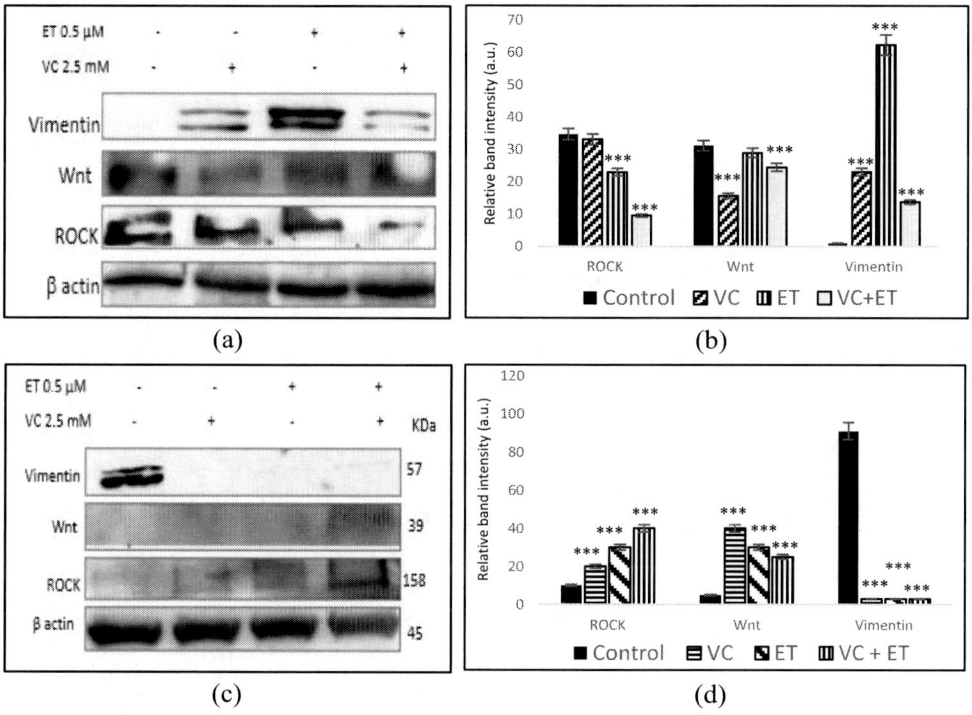

Figure 15. Western blot analysis expression of vimentin, Wnt, and ROCK in SK-N-SH and SH-SY5Ycells following treatment with VC, ET or their combination. (a) Representative blots showing different proteins expressions in SK-N-SH. (c) Representative blots showing expression of proteins in SH-SY5Y. (b) Densitometric histogram compares relative protein levels normalized to β-actinin in SK-N-SH and (d) in SH-SY-5Y. Data are expressed as mean ± SD (n = 3). Statistical significance ***$p < 0.001$ was determined using the Newman–Keuls post hoc test.

Modulation of MnSOD, Smac/Diablo, and Histone in SK-N-SH and SH- SY5Y

Analysis of mitochondrial (MnSOD, Smac/DIABLO) and chromatin-associated (core histone) proteins revealed opposing responses in the two neuroblastoma models. In SK-N-SH cells, core histone levels were generally reduced following treatment with VC or their combination but increased significantly in ET alone treatment. Smac/DIABLO was slightly elevated across treatment groups, consistent with partial release of mitochondrial pro-apoptotic factors, while MnSOD showed a small decrease, suggesting a modest reduction in antioxidant capacity. Collectively, these changes in SK-N-SH are concordant with enhanced mitochondrial apoptosis and reduced chromatin integrity under treatment, particularly when ET is present. By contrast, SH-SY5Y cells displayed a uniform upregulation of all three proteins: MnSOD, Smac/DIABLO, and core histone levels after VC, ET, and combination treatment. The MnSOD elevation implies an adaptive antioxidant response to oxidative stress; increased Smac/DIABLO may reflect mitochondrial priming for apoptosis that is not fully executed in this line; and higher histone levels could indicate altered chromatin remodeling or stress-related histone accumulation. Together, the SH-SY5Y profile suggests a stress-adaptive phenotype with concurrent mitochondrial signaling and chromatin changes that differ from the pro-apoptotic signature seen in SK-N-SH.

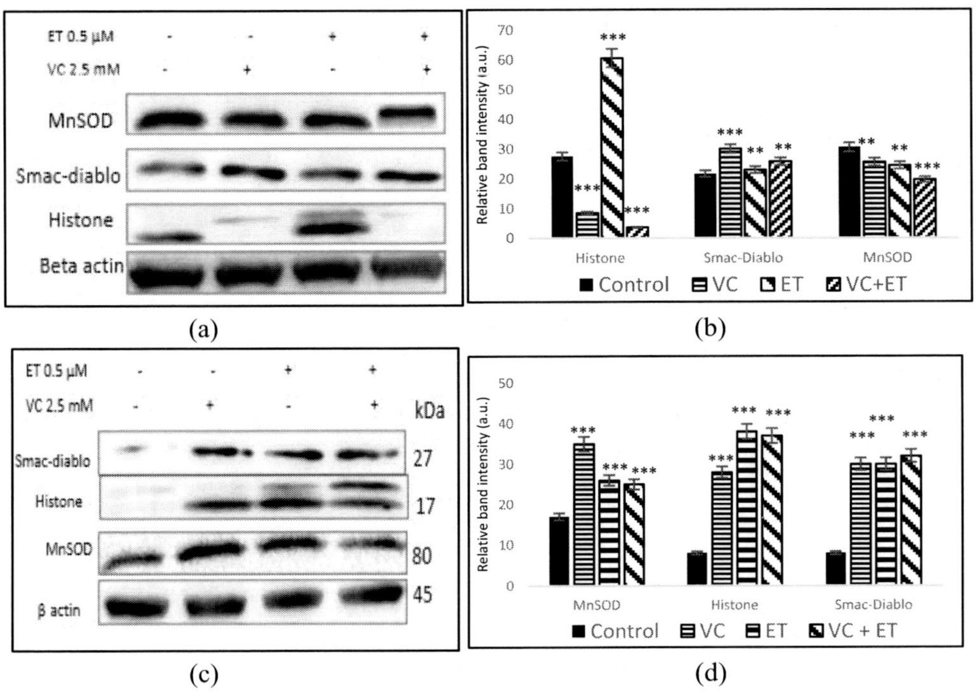

Figure 16. Western blot analysis expression of Histone, Smac/Diablo, and MnSOD in SK-N-SH and SH-SY5Ycells following treatment with VC, ET or their combination. (a) Representative blots showing different proteins expressions in SK-N-SH. (c) Representative blots showing expression of proteins in SH-SY5Y. (b) Densitometric histogram compares relative protein levels normalized to β-actinin in SK-N-SH and (d) in SH-SY-5Y. Data are expressed as mean ± SD (n = 3). Statistical significance$^{**}p < 0.01$ and $^{***}p < 0.001$ was determined using the Newman–Keuls post hoc test.

Modulation of MDR, PDL1 and PDK1 in SK-N-SH

Vitamin C and ET treatments led to coordinated downregulation of key proteins associated with immune evasion, drug resistance, and cellular metabolism. PD-L1 expression markedly decreased in all treatment groups, with the greatest reduction observed in ET only, suggesting suppression of immune checkpoint signaling. Similarly, PDK1 expression was reduced by VC and further suppressed by the combination, implying inhibition of glycolytic flux and mitochondrial reprogramming. MDR-ABC levels also declined slightly, consistent with reduced drug-efflux activity. The collective decrease in PD-L1, PDK1, and MDR-ABC indicates that VC, particularly in combination with ET, attenuates mechanisms of metabolic adaptation, immune escape, and chemoresistance, potentially sensitizing these neuroblastoma cells to apoptotic signaling (see Fig.17).

Modulation of MDR, BRCA1 and BRCA2 in SH-SY5Y

Vitamin C and ET elicited differential regulations of DNA repair and multidrug resistance markers. Both BRCA1 and BRCA2 exhibited notable reductions in expression across treatment groups, with the most pronounced decrease observed under combination treatment, indicating suppression of homologous recombination–mediated DNA repair pathways. In contrast, MDR-ABC expressions increased following VC or ET treatment alone, suggesting activation of drug-efflux and cytoprotective mechanisms. However, MDR-ABC levels declined under the combined VC and ET treatment, consistent with partial reversal of chemoresistance. Collectively, these findings suggest that while single-agent exposure triggers defensive responses in SH-SY5Y cells, the combination of VC and ET overcomes such adaptations, reducing both DNA repair and drug-efflux capacities, thereby enhancing cellular susceptibility to cytotoxic stress (see Fig. 18).

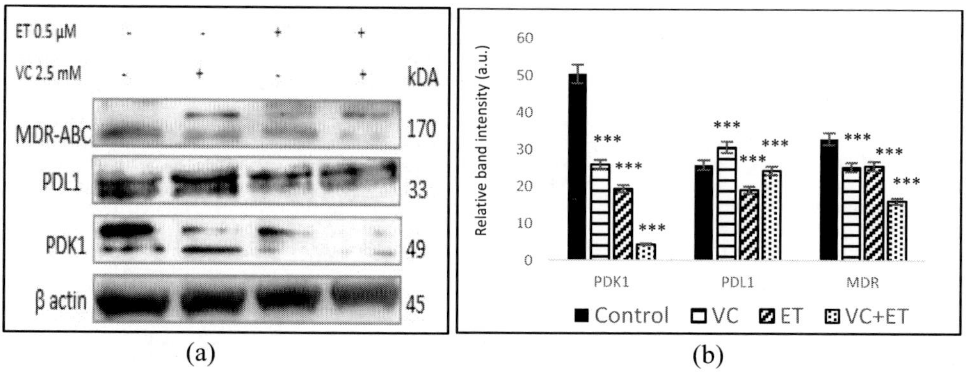

Figure 17. Western blot analysis of PDK1, PDL1, and MDR-ABC expressions in SK-N-SH following treatment with VC, ET, or their combination. (a) Representative blots showing differential expression of these proteins. (b) Densitometric histogram compares relative protein levels normalized to β-actin. Data represent mean ± SD (n = 3). Significant changes are marked as ***$p < 0.001$, according to the post hoc Newman-Keuls test.

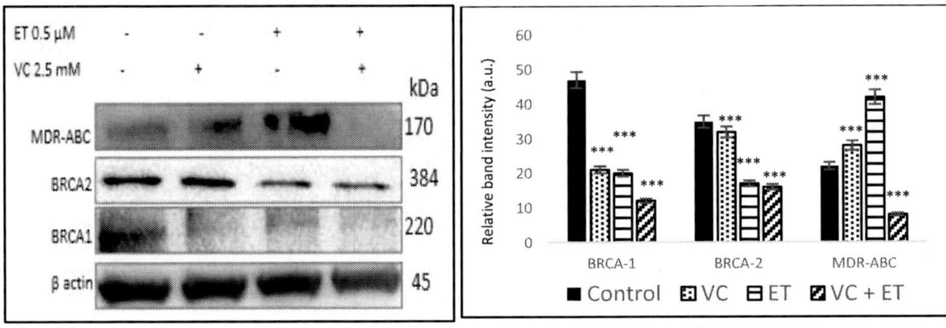

(a) (b)

Figure 18. Western blot analysis of BRCA1, BRCA2, and MDR-ABC expressions in SH-SY-5Y following treatment with VC, ET, or their combination. (a) Representative blots showing differential expression of these proteins. (b) Densitometric histogram compares relative protein levels normalized to β-actin. Data represent mean ± SD (n = 3). Significant changes are marked as ***p < 0.001, according to the post hoc Newman-Keuls test.

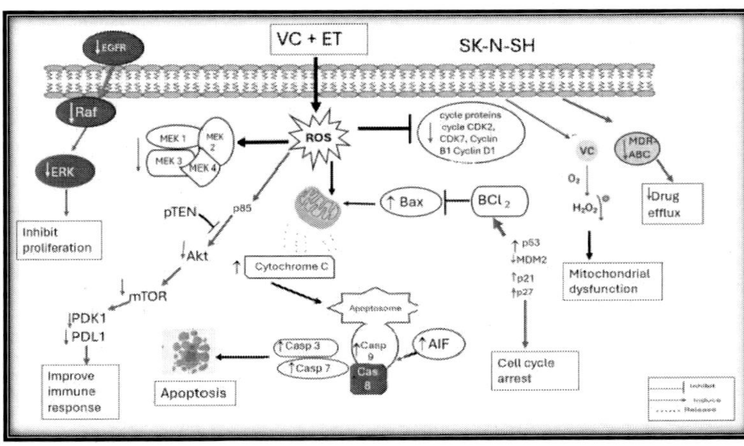

Figure 19. Proposed mechanistic model of VC and ET interaction in SK-N-SH.

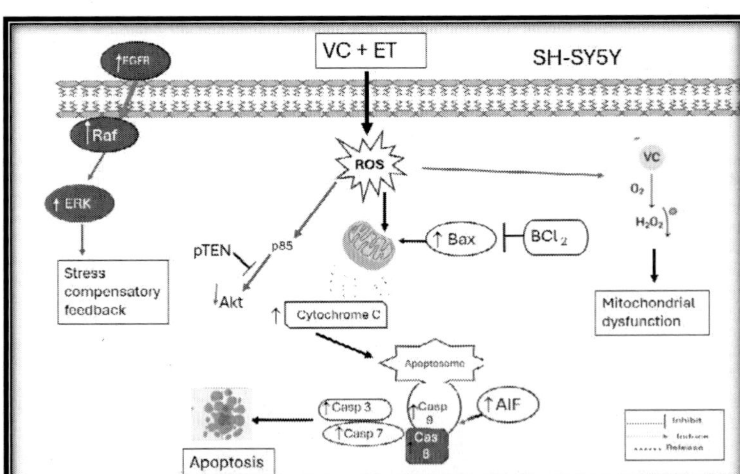

Figure 20. Proposed mechanistic model of VC and ET interaction in SH-SY5Y.

Discussion

As illustrated in Figures 19 and 20, the effects of VC, ET, and their combination on SK-N-SH and SH-SY5Y, caused different signaling pathways in cancer treatment. Both cell lines exhibited minimal sensitivity to sub-threshold doses of VC (<2.5 mM) or ET (<0.5 μM), consistent with prior reports indicating that low-dose VC or chemotherapeutic monotherapy often fails to induce substantial cytotoxicity in cancer cells [13-14]. However, the combination of VC and ET produced a robust synergistic reduction in cell viability over 24–72 h in both lines. Morphological assessment confirmed these results: SK-N-SH cells treated with the combination became rounded, detached, and fewer in number, while SH-SY5Y cells displayed milder morphological alterations, suggesting inherent differences in stress tolerance and adaptive capacity. Wound-healing assays further demonstrated impaired migratory ability under combination treatment, with SK-N-SH cells exhibiting the widest wound gaps, indicating stronger suppression of invasive potential.

At the molecular level, SK-N-SH cells underwent pronounced apoptosis in response to VC and ET, evidenced by increased Bax expression, cytochrome-c release, and downregulation of Bcl-2. Activation of both initiator (caspase-8, -9) and executioner caspases (caspase-3 and -7) along with Apaf-1 upregulation confirmed engagement of the intrinsic apoptotic pathway. Smac/DIABLO was modestly elevated, further supporting mitochondrial priming for apoptosis [15].

In contrast, SH-SY5Y cells displayed only limited apoptotic induction with VC or ET alone; significant caspase activation occurred predominantly under combination treatment, reflecting partial resistance and a requirement for dual redox and genotoxic stress to commit to cell death. Hoechst staining corroborated these findings, showing chromatin condensation and nuclear fragmentation in SK-N-SH, with milder nuclear changes in SH-SY5Y.

ROS generation and mitochondrial membrane depolarization were central to the observed cytotoxic effects. Both lines exhibited increased ROS (H2DCF-DA) and mitochondrial depolarization (Rhodamine 123), confirming that VC potentiates ET-induced oxidative stress and mitochondrial dysfunction. Notably, MnSOD levels were decreased in SK-N-SH but increased in SH-SY5Y, highlighting that SH-SY5Y cells are capable of partially buffering oxidative stress, which likely contributes to delayed apoptotic responses [16].

Analysis of survival and proliferative signaling revealed divergent responses. In SK-N-SH, VC and ET suppressed the PI3K/Akt/mTOR axis, MEK/ERK signaling, EGFR, and Raf expression, consistent with removal of key survival signals and sensitization to apoptosis. Conversely, SH-SY5Y exhibited upregulation of these pathways under combination treatment, indicating activation of compensatory survival mechanisms. Similarly, stress-responsive kinases showed differential regulation: p38 expression decreased while SAPK/JNK increased in both lines, aligning with oxidative stress-induced apoptotic signaling [17].

Cell-cycle regulators also reflected differential responses. SK-N-SH cells displayed decreased CDK2, CDK7, cyclin B1, and cyclin D1, coupled with p21 induction and suppression of MDM2 and PTEN. This pattern indicates G1/S and G2/M arrest, facilitating apoptosis. In SH-SY5Y, combination treatment led to increased CDK2, CDK7, cyclin B1, and cyclin D1, despite p21 upregulation, suggesting partial cell-cycle progression attempts and delayed apoptotic commitment [18].

DNA repair and drug-resistance pathways further distinguished the two lines. In SK-N-SH, PD-L1, PDK1, and MDR-ABC were reduced, indicating simultaneous suppression of immune evasion, metabolic adaptation, and efflux-mediated resistance [19] In SH-SY5Y, BRCA1 and BRCA2 decreased, while MDR-ABC was elevated with VC or ET alone but suppressed under combination treatment, highlighting that combined stress can overcome intrinsic resistance mechanisms in these cells [20].

Cytoskeletal and motility regulators exhibited cell-specific patterns. SK-N-SH cells demonstrated decreased ROCK and Wnt expression but increased vimentin, particularly under ET alone, consistent with transient EMT-like stress prior to apoptotic collapse. SH-SY5Y cells showed increased ROCK and Wnt but decreased vimentin, suggesting engagement of survival and repair pathways while migration remained impaired. These molecular signatures are aligned with wound-healing assays, confirming stronger inhibition of migration in SK-N-SH [21].

Finally, chromatin and mitochondrial priming indicators showed complementary trends. Histone levels decreased in SK-N-SH (except for modest ET-induced increase), whereas SH-SY5Y exhibited increased histone, MnSOD, and Smac/DIABLO, reflecting adaptive chromatin remodeling and enhanced mitochondrial defense. These findings support the notion that SK-N-SH cells are pushed toward irreversible apoptosis, while SH-SY5Y can transiently resist and adapt to oxidative and genotoxic stress [22].

Collectively, these results demonstrate that the VC and ET combination exerts multi-modal anticancer effects through ROS-mediated mitochondrial apoptosis, suppression of survival and proliferation signaling, impairment of DNA repair and drug-resistance pathways, and modulation of cell-cycle and cytoskeletal regulators. The differential responses between SK-N-SH and SH-SY5Y underscore the importance of intrinsic signaling plasticity and antioxidant capacity in determining sensitivity to redox-based combination therapy.

These observations are consistent with prior studies showing that pharmacological VC enhances chemotherapeutic efficacy via ROS generation, apoptosis induction, and inhibition of PI3K/Akt and MEK/ERK survival pathways [19-20]. At the same time, the adaptive responses observed in SH-SY5Y align with literature describing cell-type dependent buffering of oxidative stress and activation of compensatory survival signaling under pro-oxidant therapies [23].

Conclusion

This study reveals that VC, at pharmacological concentrations, synergizes with ET to induce cytotoxicity in neuroblastoma cells. However, the precise molecular routes differ markedly between SK-N-SH and SH-SY5Y. SK-N-SH follows a classical ROS-mitochondrial apoptotic pathway, supported by suppression of survival and cell-cycle signals and dismantling of resistance/immune markers. SH-SY5Y mounts stronger adaptive defenses (antioxidants, survival signaling, cell-cycle reprogramming) and requires dual redox and genotoxic stress to commit apoptosis. These divergent responses emphasize that VC–chemotherapy combinations must be tailored to cancer redox and signaling landscapes. Moving forward, rescue experiments (antioxidants, pathway inhibitors), time-course profiling, functional DNA-repair assays, and in vivo validation are essential to translate this mechanistic insight into predictive biomarkers and optimized therapeutic strategies.

Key Findings

The combination of pharmacological VC and ET exerts synergistic anticancer effects in neuroblastoma, but the underlying mechanisms are highly cell-context dependent. In SK-N-SH cells, the combination drives a decisive apoptotic program characterized by oxidative stress, mitochondrial dysfunction, caspase activation, and suppression of PI3K/Akt/mTOR and MEK/ERK survival pathways - ultimately dismantling cell-cycle control and resistance markers such as PD-L1, PDK1, and MDR-ABC. In contrast, SH-SY5Y cells exhibit a more adaptive phenotype, initially activating antioxidant MnSOD and pro-survival PI3K/Akt, MEK/ERK responses before succumbing to combined oxidative and genotoxic stress. These contrasting outcomes highlight that VC's redox activity can either reinforce or overwhelm cancer cell defenses depending on intrinsic signaling plasticity.

Acknowledgments

The author thanks Union University for the source and support of research funding as well as colleagues and editing tools for assistance with improving the clarity of the manuscript.

References

[1] Newman E.A., Abdessalam S., Aldrink J.H., Austin M., Heaton T.E., Bruny J., et al., APSA Cancer committee. Update on neuroblastoma. *J Pediatric Surg.* 2019 ;54(3) :383-389.

[2] Mercaldo F., Brunese L., Martinelli F., Santone A., Cesarelli M. Explainable convolutional neural networks for brain cancer detection and localization. *Sensors* 2023 ; 23 : 7614.

[3] Bailly C. Etoposide: a rider on the cytokine storm. *Cytokine* 2023 ; 168 : 156234.

[4] Shah Z., Gohar U.F., Jamshed I., Mushtaq A., Mukhtar H., Manea R., et al., Podophyllotoxin: history, recent advances and prospects. *Biomolecules* 2021 ; 11(4) : 603.

[5] Schultz B.J., Kim S.Y., Lau W., Sattely E.S. Total biosynthesis for milligram-scale production of etoposide intermediates in a plant chassis. *J Am Chem Soc* 2019 ; 141 : 19231-19235.

[6] Montecucco A., Zanetta F., Biamonti G. Molecular mechanisms of etoposide. *ECCLI J* 2015;14: 95-108.

[7] Fan H.Y., Zhu Z.L., Xian H.C., Wang H.F., Chen B.J., Tang Y.J., et al., Insight into the molecular mechanism of podophyllotoxin derivatives as anticancer drugs. *Fron Cell Dev Biol* 2021 ; T9 : 709075.

[8] Li X., Ma Q., Chang C., Li H., Cao D. First-line treatment of ocrelizumab with chemotherapy in advanced gastro enter pancreatic neuroendocrine carcinoma: Study protocol for a prospective, multicenter, phase II study. *Front Oncol* 2022 ; 12: 958905.

[9] Du J., Martin S.M., Levine B.A., Wang S., Knudsen C.M., Cullen J.J. Mechanism of ascorbate-induced cytotoxicity in pancreatic cancer. *J Am. Assoc. Cancer Res*. 2010 ; 16 :509-520.

[10] Chen Q., Espey M.G., Krishna M.C., Mitchell J.B., Corpe C.P., Buettner G.R., et al., Pharmacological ascorbic acid concentrations selectively kill cancer cells : action as a pro-drug to deliver hydrogen peroxide to tissues. *PNAS* 205 ; 102 : 13604-13609.

[11] Chen Q., Espey M.G., Sun A.Y., Lee J.H., Buettner G.R., Levine M. Ascorbate in pharmacologic concentration selectively generate ascorbate radical and hydrogen peroxide in extracellular fluid *in vivo*. *PNAS* 2007 ; 104 : 8749-8754.

[12] Olney K.E., Du J., Van Erve T.J., Witmer J.R., Wagner B.A, Buettner G.R., et al., Inhibitors of hydroperoxide metabolism enhance ascorbate-induce cytotoxicity. *Free Radic Res* 2013 ; 47 :154-163.

[13] Szarka A., Kapuy O., Lorincz T., Banhegyi G. Vitamin C and Cell death. *Antioxidants and Redox* signaling 2021 ; 34 ,11.

[14] Szarka A., Lorincz T., Hajdinak P. Friend or foe: the relativity of (anti)oxidative agents and pathways. Int *J Mol Sci* 2022 ; 23 (9), 5188.

[15] Mussa A., Hamid M., Hajissa K., Murtadha A.H. Pharmacological vitamin C-induced high H2O2 generation mediates apoptotic cell death by caspases 3/7 activation in breast cancer tumor spheroids. *J of Translational Med* 2025 ; 23, 31.

[16] Cao X., Yi Y., Ji M., Liu Y., Wang D., Zhu H. The dual role of vitamin C in cancer: from antioxidant prevention to prooxidant therapeutic applications. *Sec Precision Medicine* 2025, 12.

[17] Hayes J.D., Kostova A.D., Tew K.D. Oxidative stress in cancer. *Cancer Cell* 2020 ; 38 : 167-197.

[18] Matthews H.K., Bertoli C., de Bruin R.A.M. Cell cycle control in cancer. *Nature Rev Mol Cell Biol* 2022; 23: 74-88.

[19] Jiang Y., Chen M., Nie H., Yuan Y. PD-1 and PD-L1 in cancer immunotherapy: clinical implications and future considerations. *Human Vaccines & Immunotherapeutics* 2019 ; 15(5) : 1111-1122.

[20] Li S., Silvestri V., Leslie G., Rebbeck T.R., Neuhausen S.L., Hopper J.L., et al., Cancer risks associated with BRCA1 and BRCA2 pathogenic variants. *J Clin Oncol* 2022 ; 40, 14.

[21] Xue W., Yang L., Chen C., Ashrafizadeh M., Tian Y., Sun R. Wnt/β-catenin-driven EMT regulation in human cancer. *Cellular & Mol Life Sci* 2024 ; 81, 79.

[22] Brabson J.P., Leesang T., Mohammad S., Cimmino L. Epigenetic regulation of genomic stability by vitamin C. *Sec Nutrigenomics* 2021 ; 12.

[23] Landriscina M., Maddalena F., Laudiero G., Esposito F. Adaptation to oxidative stress, chemoresistance, and cell survival. *Antioxidants & Redox Signaling* 2009 ; 11, 11.

Chapter 9

The Synergistic Anticancer Effects of Vitamin C and Bortezomib via Modulation of Apoptotic and Cell Cycle Pathways in Colorectal Cancer

Lunawati L. Bennett*, **PhD, PharmD**
Union University, College of Pharmacy, Jackson, Tennessee, USA

Abstract

Colorectal cancer globally ranks the third most common cancer in men and the second most common in women. While colorectal incidence is relatively low before the age of 50, a significant increase is observed with advancing age. In developed countries, the median age at diagnosis is around 70 years. Survival rates for individuals diagnosed with metastatic colorectal cancer indicate that approximately 70% to 75% survive beyond one year, 30% to 35% beyond three years, and fewer than 20% beyond five years from diagnosis.

The goal of this study was to understand if vitamin C has a benefit effect on colorectal cancer treatment. The study specifically investigates whether vitamin C alone or in combination with a low dose of bortezomib is more effective, utilizing Caco2 as the model. Based on the results from SRB assay, Rhodamine123, Hoechst 33342, and Western Blot assay, addition of vitamin C to bortezomib inhibits the growth of cancerous cells by suppressing Akt, p85, MDM2 and Bcl2, cell cycle proteins, MEK 1-4, and increasing p21, Bax, p53, and PTEN expressions. Together, these findings indicate that vitamin C enhances the cytotoxic and pro-apoptotic effects of bortezomib by disrupting survival signaling and cell cycle progression, suggesting a promising therapeutic strategy for improving cancer treatment outcomes.

Keywords: gastrointestinal cancer, colorectal cancer, vitamin C, bortezomib, caco2

Abbreviations

APAF	Apoptotic peptidase activating factor;
Bax	Bcl2 Associated X-protein;
Bcl2	B cell lymphoma 2;
Cas	Caspase;

* Corresponding Author's Email: llbennett@uu.edu

CDK7	Cyclin dependent kinase 7;
Cyt C	Cytochrome C;
ROCK	Rho-associated kinase;
ROS	Reactive oxygen species;
SAPK/JNK	Stress-activated protein kinase/c-Jun N-terminal kinase;
MAPKs	Mitogen-activated protein kinases;
MEKs	Mitogen-activated protein kinase kinases;
MDM2	Mouse double minute 2 homolog.

Introduction

Colorectal cancer (CRC) holds a significant place among the 'big four' cancer types in the United States, standing alongside breast, lung, and prostate cancer. Globally, it ranks as the third most common cancer in men and the second most common in women. While CRC incidence is relatively low before the age of 50, a significant increase is observed with advancing age. In developed countries, the median age at diagnosis hovers around 70 years [1-2]. Beyond demographics, additional risk factors of CRC include family history, inflammatory bowel disease, smoking, excessive alcohol consumption, high intake of red and processed meat, obesity, and diabetes. Recent studies have also introduced the potential role of infectious agents, such as Helicobacter pylori, Fusobacterium, and others, which are currently under investigation [3].

Colorectal cancer has a significant global impact, affecting over 1.85 million individuals annually and resulting in more than 850,000 deaths. Survival rates for individuals diagnosed with metastatic colorectal cancer indicate that approximately 70% to 75% survive beyond one year, 30% to 35% beyond three years, and fewer than 20% beyond five years from diagnosis [4]. However, it's important to note that the five-year relative survival rate is more favorable in high-income countries such as Australia, Canada, the USA, and various European nations. The stage at which the cancer is diagnosed is identified as the most crucial prognostic factor, significantly influencing survival outcomes [3].

Research has extensively focused on key tumor suppressor genes like p53 and recurrent cytogenetic aberrations, particularly 18q loss of heterozygosity. These genes play a crucial role in the malignant transformation of colon epithelial cells, exerting specific effects on cell behavior [5]. Additionally, common mutations in CRC involve APC, CTNNB1, KRAS, BRAF, SMAD4, TGFBR2, and PIK3CA, influencing key signaling pathways like Wnt, β-catenin, EGFR, MAPK, p85, and TGFβ, as well as genes regulating critical cellular behaviors such as DNA repair and proliferation. Detecting these mutations provides insights into CRC progression, enabling early diagnosis and facilitating early treatment [6].

Bortezomib (BZ) is a dipeptidyl boronic acid that selectively and reversibly inhibits the ubiquitin 26S proteasome pathway which plays a role in the degradation of many intracellular proteins involves in cell-cycle regulation, transcription factor activation, and apoptosis [7-8]. The FDA approved BZ (Velcade®) in 2003 for the treatment of multiple myeloma and mantle cell lymphoma [7].

Pharmacological achieved through high-dose intravenous vitamin C (IVC) to attain plasma levels of $\geq$ 20 mM, has recently emerged as a potential non-toxic adjuvant to standard care radio-chemotherapy-based cancer therapies across various disease sites [9-10]. The proposed anti-cancer mechanism of pharmacological VC involves redox-active metal-mediated or auto-oxidation of ascorbate, resulting in the formation of O_2 and H_2O_2 [10-12].

This study was designed to evaluate the chemo-enhancing potential of VC in combination with low-dose BZ for treating colorectal cancer, utilizing Caco2 cells as the model. The findings of this investigation reveal that the use of VC with BZ demonstrated greater efficacy in the treatment of colorectal cancer. This marks a novel discovery in the field.

To evaluate the cytotoxic potential of high-dose VC, various antineoplastic agents - including paclitaxel, doxorubicin, etoposide, temsirolimus, bortezomib, afatinib, and sorafenib - were tested on human colorectal cancer using the model CaCo2 cell line. For combination studies, the lowest concentrations of each antineoplastic and high-dose VC that yielded a synergistic reduction in cell viability were selected. General experimental procedures followed the protocols outlined in Chapter 3 (Materials and Methods), while methodological details specific to this study are described below.

Cell Culture

The colorectal adenocarcinoma cell line Caco2 (ATCC HTB-37) was cultures in EMEM media supplemented with 20% FBS and 1% streptomycin/penicillin. This epithelial cell was isolated from colon tissue derived from a 72-year-old, white male with colorectal adenocarcinoma. The cells were cultured in T75 dishes and maintained in an incubator at 37°C in a 5% CO_2 humidified environment.s

Results

Cell Viability and Selection of Doses

Cells treated with vitamin C (VC) alone showed no significant change in viability at concentrations below 5 mM. Treatment with bortezomib (BZ) alone resulted in only a slight reduction in cell viability at concentrations below 500 nM, with a noticeable decrease beginning at 62.5 nM. Therefore, 62.5 nM BZ was selected for subsequent combination treatments with VC to assess potential synergistic effects. The combination of VC and BZ significantly reduced Caco-2 cell viability compared to either agent alone after 24 or 48 h of exposure. Based on the results, 5 mM VC, 62.5 nM BZ, and their combination were chosen for further experiments.

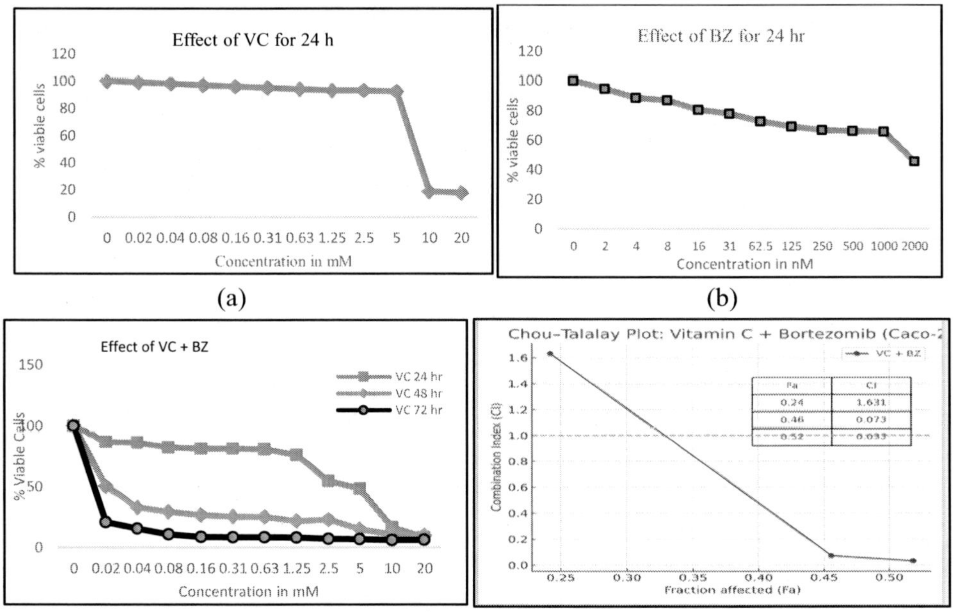

(c) (d)

Figure 1. Effects of VC and BZ on Caco-2 cell viability. (a) Dose-dependent effects of VC (0–20 mM) on cell viability after 24 and 48 h of treatment. (b) Effects of increasing BZ concentrations (0–500 nM) on cell viability at 24 h.(c) Synergistic reduction in cell viability following combined treatment with 5 mM VC and 62.5 nM BZ for 24, 48 and 72 h, compared to either agent alone. (d) Chou-Talalay data showed strong synergistic at Fa = 0.46, CI 0.073. Data represents SD from at least three independent experiments.

Changes in Cell Morphology

Treatment of Caco2 cells with VC and BZ showed alteration in cell morphologies in all groups compared to the control. While control cells remained healthy, showing increased numbers and adherence after 24 h, cells treated with VC or BZ alone exhibited reduced viability and morphological changes. The combination of VC and BZ led to even greater of cell death, with many cells appearing floating in the culture dish.

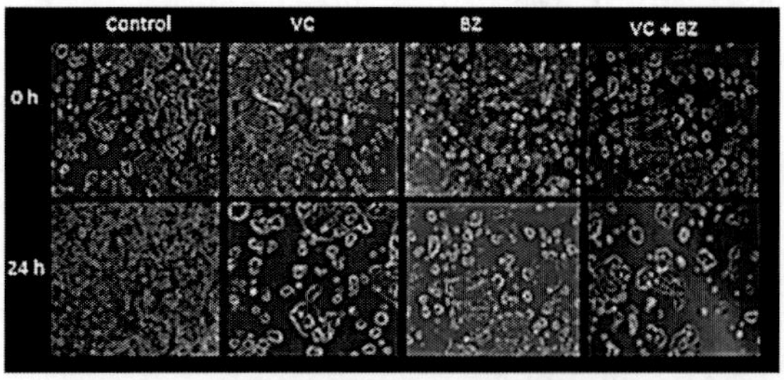

Figure 2. Results from inverted microscopic images of Caco2 cells (40x) after 24 h of treatment with VC, BZ, or their combination. Cells treated with VC or BZ alone exhibited some morphological changes. In the combination treatment, most cells became detached from the dish, with only a few remaining attached.

Wound-Healing

After 24 h of treatment, the combination of VC and BZ led to significantly reduced migration of Caco2 cells, resulting in a wider wound gap compared to treatments with VC or BZ alone. In contrast, control cells migrated closer together indicating early signs of invasion and potential cancer metastasis, with histogram comparing the wound widths across control, VC, BZ, and combination treatments.

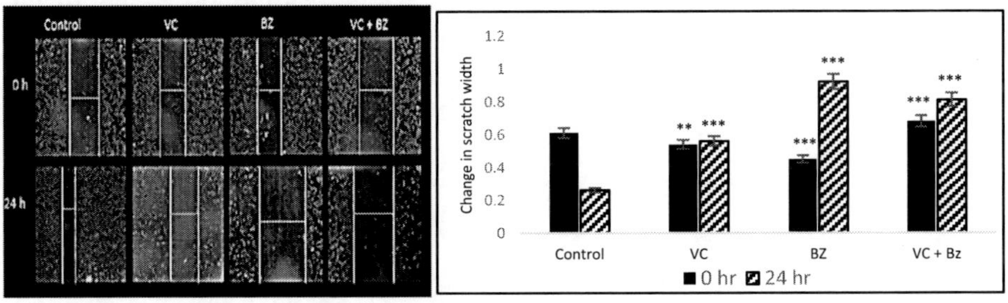

(a) (b)

Figure 3. Wound healing assay of Caco2 cells. (a) Representative images at 0 and 24 h for control, VC, BZ, and combination treatments. (b) Histogram comparing wound width across treatment groups after 24 h. Data are expressed as mean ± SD; significant differences are indicated by $^{**}p < 0.01$, $^{***}p < 0.001$ (post hoc Newman–Keuls test).

Induction of Apoptosis

The combination of VC and BZ resulted in a lower rate of apoptosis in Caco2 cells compared to treatment with VC or BZ alone. This finding, confirmed by Hoechst 33342 staining and observed in fluorescence microscopy images reveals that control cells had lower fluorescence intensity, indicating normal, healthy nuclei. In contrast, apoptotic cells exhibited bright blue fluorescence due to nuclear condensation and fragmentation. Quantitative analysis confirms a significantly lower percentage of viable cells in those treated with VC, BZ, or the combination compared to the control.

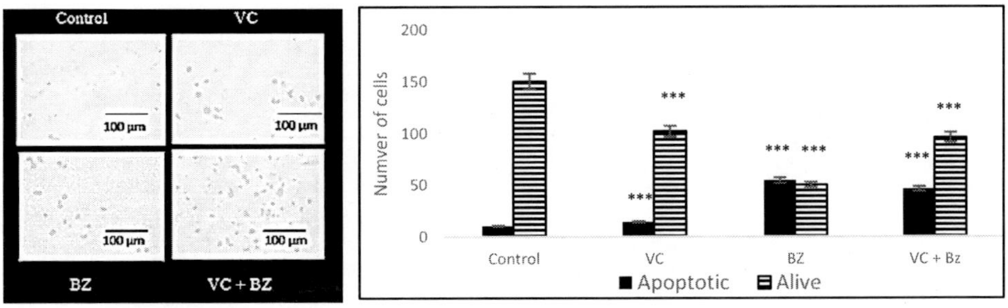

(a) (b)

Figure 4. (a) shows fluorescence microscopic images of Caco2 cells treated for 24 h with VC, BZ, or their combination. The scale bar represents 100 µm. Figure 4(b) presents a histogram of the percentage of apoptotic cells relative to non-apoptotic cells. Data is expressed as mean ± SD (n = 3). A significant increase in apoptotic cells was observed, with $^{***}p < 0.001$, as determined by the post hoc Newman-Keuls test.

Intracellular ROS Generation

The generation of intracellular ROS was assessed in Caco2 cells following treatment with VC, BZ, or their combination, using H2DCFDA staining. Variations in fluorescence intensity through microscopic images, with higher ROS generation indicated by increased fluorescence intensity. Significant ROS generation was observed in response to VC, BZ, and the combination treatments compared to the control, with darker colors indicating lower ROS generation. Histogram of fluorescence intensity corresponding to the VC, BZ, and combined treatments.

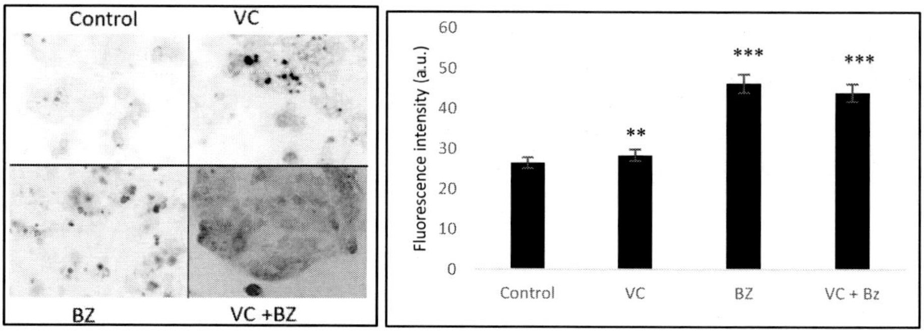

(a) (b)

Figure 5. Intracellular ROS generation in Caco2 cells after 24 h treatment. (a) Representative fluorescence microscopy images following H2DCF staining. Scale bar indicating 100 μm. (b) Histogram of fluorescence intensity corresponding to treatments with VC, BZ, or their combination versus the control. Data are expressed as mean ± SD (n = 3); significant change in ROS levels was observed, indicated by ** $p < 0.01$ and ***$p < 0.001$, according to the post hoc Newman-Keuls test.

Mitochondrial Membrane Potential (Ψ_m)

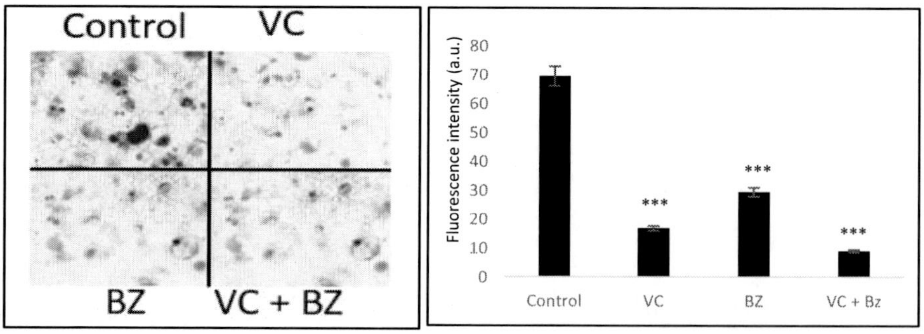

(a) (b)

Figure 6. (a) shows the results of fluorescence microscopic examination depicting changes in mitochondrial membrane depolarization in treated Caco2 cells compared to control cells. The scale bar represents 100 μm. (b) Histogram illustrating the fluorescence intensity corresponding to the control, VC, BZ, or combination treatments, with a significant decrease indicated by ***$p < 0.001$, according to the post hoc Newman-Keuls test.

The generation of reactive oxygen species (ROS) in Caco2 cells indicated cell death attributed to the depletion of mitochondrial membrane potential, as detected with Rhodamine 123 staining. Treatments with VC, BZ, or the combination of VC and BZ induced cell death. Control cells exhibited higher fluorescence intensity, indicating healthy mitochondria, compared to treated cells, as illustrated in the histogram.

Modulation of Bax, Bcl2, Cytochrome C, and AIF

In apoptotic cells, the intracellular generation of ROS is linked to alterations in the expressions of Bax and Bcl2 proteins. Increase in Bax and decrease in Bcl2 expressions in Caco2 cells treated with a combination of VC and BZ. ROS generation also led to a reduction in mitochondrial membrane potential, resulting in an increased release of cytochrome C into the cytosol, which further induced apoptosis. A decrease in the expression of apoptosis-inducing factor (AIF) was observed in all cells except control.

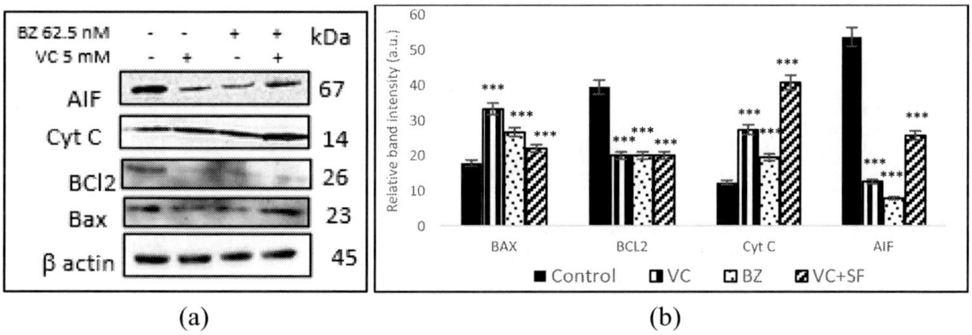

Figure 7. Western blot analysis of Bax, BCl2, cyt C, and AIF following treatment with VC, BZ, or their combination. (a) Representative blots showing expression of these proteins. (b) Densitometric histogram compares relative protein levels normalized to β-actin. Data are expressed as mean ± SD (n = 3). Statistical significance was determined using the Newman–Keuls post hoc test (**p < 0.001).

Modulation Mitochondrial Signaling Proteins

Mitochondrial apoptosis, triggered by a loss of membrane potential, involves several key proteins, including caspases -3, -7, -8, and -9 in VC alone while BZ alone caused only a slight elevation of these caspases. Notably, the combination of VC and BZ led to a decrease in caspases -3 and -7, while caspases -8 and -9 were elevated. Histograms indicate modulation of these caspases compared to the control.

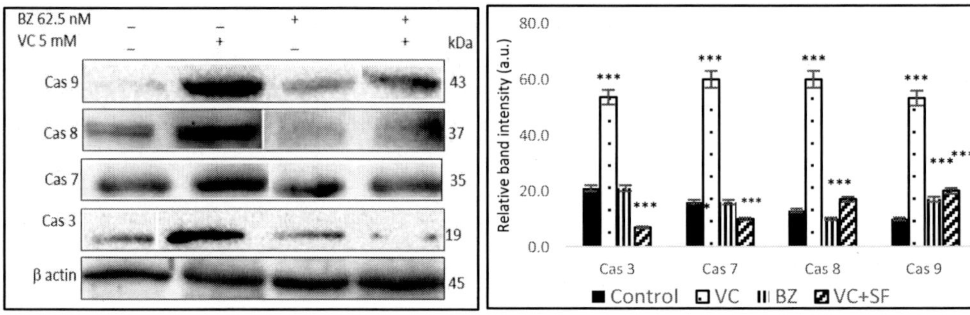

(a) (b)

Figure 8. Western blot analysis of expressions of cas -3, -7, -8, and -9. in Caco2 cells following treatment with VC, BZ, or their combination. (a) Representative blots showing expression of these proteins. (b) Densitometric histogram compares relative protein levels normalized to β-actin. Data are expressed as mean ± SD (n = 3). Statistical significance was determined using the Newman–Keuls post hoc test (**p < 0.001).

Modulation of MEK Kinase Pathway

To investigate the potential mechanism of VC, BZ, or their combination in modulating aberrant cell signaling of mitogen-activated protein kinases (MAPKs), the expression of MEK isoforms was examined in Caco-2 cells. Significant decreases in MEK-1, -2, -3, and -4 expression levels were observed across all treatment groups, indicating that both VC and BZ effectively suppress upstream MAPK activation. Since MEK kinases serve as key regulatory nodes that relay proliferative and survival signals from receptor tyrosine kinases to ERK-dependent transcriptional programs, the downregulation of multiple MEK isoforms suggests a broad inhibition of growth-promoting pathways. These findings support a role for VC and BZ in attenuating MAPK-driven oncogenic signaling, with combination treatment producing the most pronounced inhibitory effect.

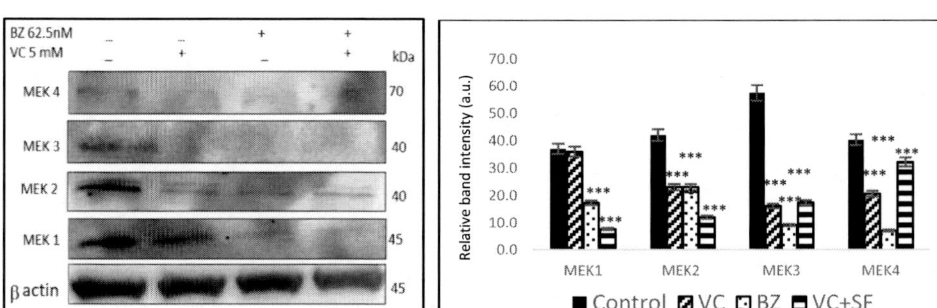

(a) (b)

Figure 9. Western blot analysis of MEK -1, -2, -3 and -4 expression in Caco2 cells following treatment with VC, BZ, or their combinations. (a) Representative blots showing expression of these proteins. (b) Densitometric histogram compares relative protein levels normalized to β-actin. Data are expressed as mean ± SD (n = 3). Statistical significance was determined using the Newman–Keuls post hoc test (***p < 0.001).

Modulation of Cell Cycle Regulatory Proteins

The inhibition of cell cycle progression is recognized as a key strategy in managing colorectal cancer. Treatment of Caco-2 cells with VC, BZ, or their combination resulted in decreased levels of key cell cycle regulatory proteins, including CDK7, CDK2, cyclin B1, and cyclin D1. An exception was observed in cells treated with BZ alone, which showed an increase in CDK7 expression.

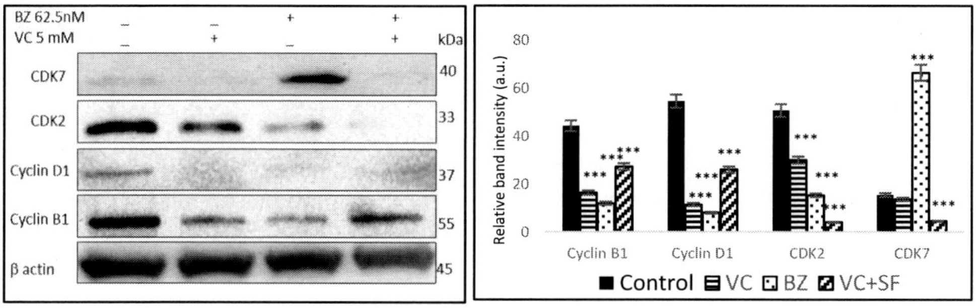

(a) (b)

Figure 10. Western blot analysis of Cyclin B1, DI and CDK2 and 7 expressions in Caco2 cells following treatment with VC, BZ, or their combination. (a) Representative blots showing expression of these proteins. (b) Densitometric histogram compares relative protein levels normalized to β-actin. Data are expressed as mean ± SD (n = 3). Statistical significance was determined using the Newman–Keuls post hoc test (***$p < 0.001$).

Modulation of p21, PTEN, and MDM2

The impact of VC, BZ, and their combination on the expression of key regulatory proteins, including p21, PTEN, and MDM2, was assessed in Caco2 cells. There was a significant increase in the expression levels of p21 and PTEN after BZ alone or its combination with VC, indicative of a positive regulatory effect on cell tumor suppression. The expression of MDM2 decreased, suggesting an inhibitory effect of VC, BZ or their combination (see Fig.11).

Modulation of Akt/p85/mTOR

The effect of VC, BZ, and their combination on Akt, p85 (a regulatory subunit of P13K), and mammalian target of rapamycin (mTOR) proteins was assessed. Decreases in Akt, mTOR, and p85 expressions were observed in all treatments, except mTOR expressions increase in BZ only treatment. These findings suggest that VC when used alone or in combination may exert greater inhibitory effects on p13k/Akt/mTOR pathway. Histogram represents the modulation of Akt, p85 and mTOR in Caco2 (see Fig. 12).

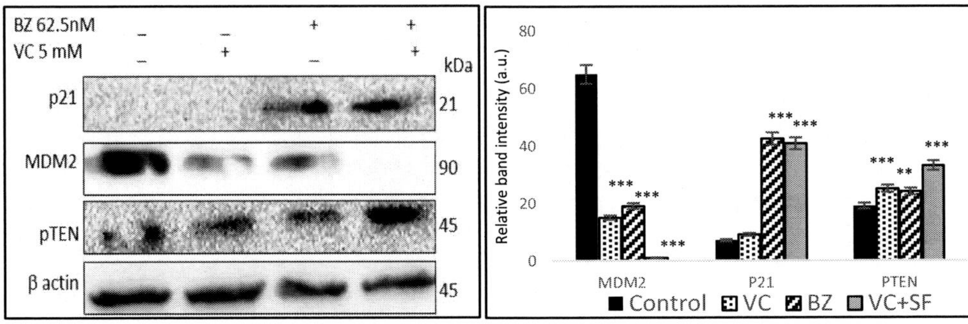

(a) (b)

Figure 11. Western blot analysis of PTEN, p21, MDM2 expressions in Caco2 cells following treatment with VC, BZ, or their combination. (a) Representative blots showing expression of these proteins. (b) Densitometric histogram compares relative protein levels normalized to β-actin. Data are expressed as mean ± SD (n = 3). Statistical significance was determined using the Newman–Keuls post hoc test (**p < 0.001, ***p < 0.001).

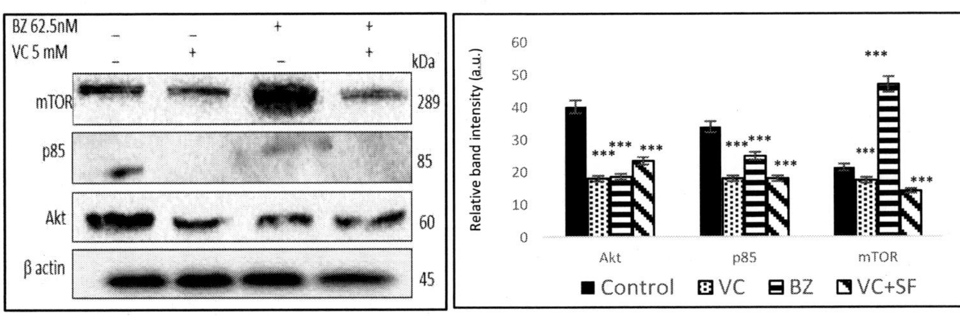

(a) (b)

Figure 12. Western blot analysis data showing the modulation of Akt, p85, and mTOR expressions after treatment of Caco2 cells with VC, BZ, or their combination.
(b) Densitometric histogram compares relative protein levels normalized to β-actin. Data are expressed as mean ± SD (n = 3). Statistical significance was determined using the Newman–Keuls post hoc test (***p < 0.001).

Modulation of SAPK/JNK and p38

The impact of VC, BZ, and their combined treatment on SAPK/JNK and p38 proteins was evaluated in Caco2 cells. VC, BZ, or their combination caused decreased the expression of SAPK/JNK and p38, with slight decrease of p38 in the combinational treatment.

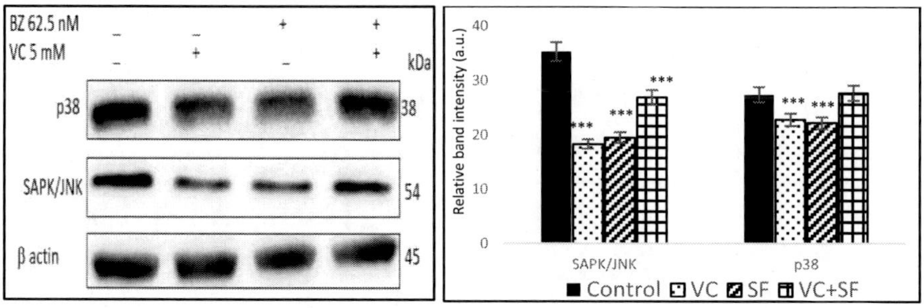

(a) (b)

Figure 13. Western blot analysis of SAPK/JNK and p38 expressions after treatment of Caco2 cells with VC, BZ, or their combination. (a) Representative blots showing expression of these proteins. (b) Densitometric histogram compares relative protein levels normalized to β-actin. Data are expressed as mean ± SD (n = 3). Statistical significance was determined using the Newman–Keuls post hoc test (***p < 0.001).

Modulation of ERK 1/2 AND EGFR

The impact of VC, BZ, and their combined treatment on ERK and EGFR proteins was assessed in Caco2 cells. Decreased expressions of ERK and EGFR in VC, BZ, or their combination indicate a favorable effect in causing decrease cancer progression.

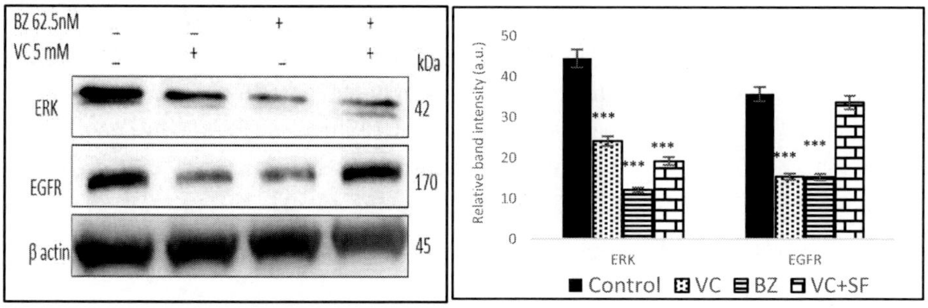

(a) (b)

Figure 14. Western blot analysis expressions of ERK 1/2 and EGFR in Caco2 cells following treatment with VC, BZ, or their combination. (a) Representative blots showing expression of these proteins. (b) Densitometric histogram compares relative protein levels normalized to β-actin. Data are expressed as mean ± SD (n=3). Statistical significance was determined using the Newman–Keuls post hoc test (***p < 0.001).

Modulation of β-catenin, Wnt, and ROCK

The effects of VC, BZ, and their combination on β-catenin, Wnt, and ROCK protein expression were examined in Caco-2 cells. Treatment with VC or BZ alone resulted in decreased expression of β-catenin and ROCK, suggesting a potential inhibitory effect on cancer progression pathways. Interestingly, the combination of VC and BZ led to an increase in β-catenin and ROCK expression compared to either agent alone. In contrast, Wnt expression was consistently reduced across all treatment groups.

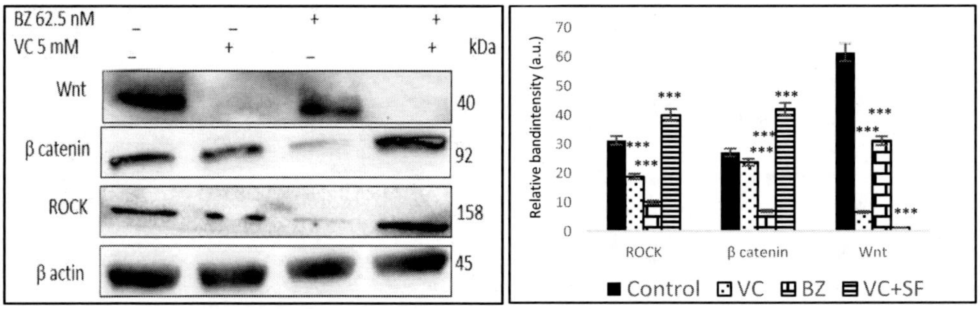

(a) (b)

Figure 15. Western blot analysis data of ROCK, β catenin and Wnt expressions in Caco2 cells following treatment with VC, BZ, or their combination. (a) Representative blots showing expression of these proteins. (b) Densitometric histogram compares relative protein levels normalized to β-actin. Data are expressed as mean ± SD (n = 3). Statistical significance was determined using the Newman–Keuls post hoc test (***p < 0.001).

Modulation of MnSOD, Smac/Diablo, E-cadherin, and Vimentin

The effects of VC, BZ, and their combination on the expression of MnSOD, Smac/Diablo, E-cadherin, and Vimentin were evaluated in Caco2 cells. An increase in Smac/Diablo expression following combined VC and BZ treatment suggests a synergistic pro-apoptotic effect, which was not observed with either agent alone. Conversely, increased Vimentin expression in all treatment groups - VC, BZ, and their combination - indicates a potential enhancement of cancer cell invasiveness. E-cadherin expression decreased with individual treatments but increased with the combination, suggesting partial reversal of epithelial-mesenchymal transition (EMT). MnSOD levels were elevated in the VC and combination groups.

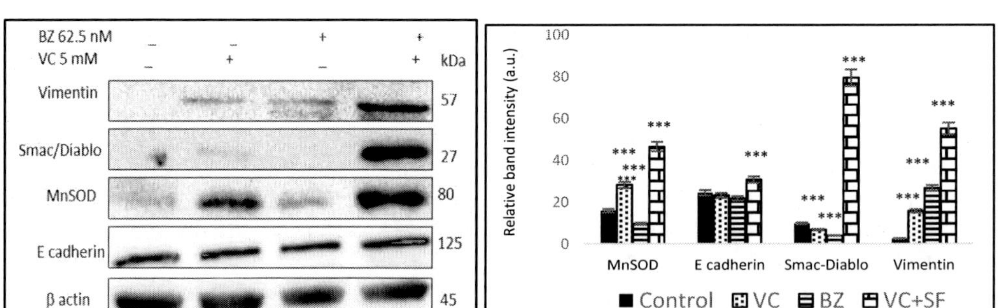

(a) (b)

Figure 16. Western blot analysis data showing the modulation of MnSOD, Smac/Diablo, Vimentin, and E cadherin expressions after treatment of Caco2 cells with VC, BZ, or their combination. (a) Representative blots showing expression of these proteins. (b) Densitometric histogram compares relative protein levels normalized to β-actin. Data are expressed as mean ± SD (n = 3). Statistical significance was determined using the Newman–Keuls post hoc test (***p < 0.001).

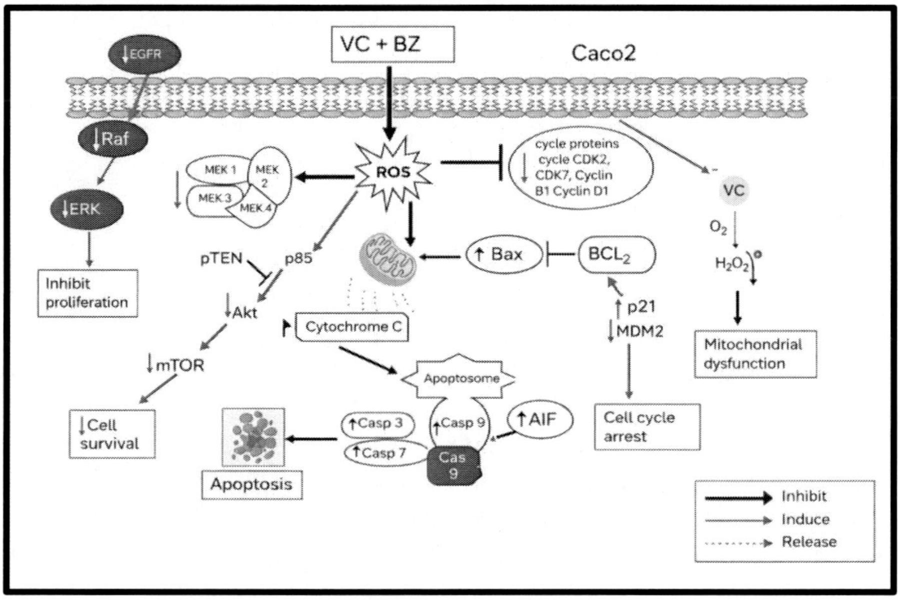

Figure 17. Proposed mechanistic model of VC and BZ in colorectal cancer.

Discussion

As illustrated in Figure 17, the molecular impact of VC, BZ, and their combination on colorectal adenocarcinoma Caco2 cells revealed broad alterations in key signaling pathways, cell cycle arrests, and decrease in invasion/metastasis-related proteins, highlighting the multifaceted nature of the treatment response. Combination treatment with VC and BZ resulted in a significant increase in Bax and cytochrome c levels, accompanied by a consistent decrease in Bcl-2. These changes strongly indicate the activation of the intrinsic mitochondria-mediated apoptotic pathway, a hallmark of effective chemotherapeutic intervention [13-14].

Bortezomib treatment alone resulted in only a modest increase in the expression of caspases -3, -7, -8, and -9, suggesting a limited ability to trigger apoptosis via either the intrinsic or extrinsic pathways. This limited pro-apoptotic effect is further supported by the minimal changes observed in mitochondrial apoptotic regulators such as Bax, cytochrome c, and Bcl-2 under BZ-only conditions. In contrast, VC treatment led to a marked increase in all four caspases, particularly caspase-9 and caspase-3, which are central to the intrinsic mitochondrial apoptotic pathway. This aligns with the observed elevation of Bax and cytochrome c and the suppression of Bcl-2, indicating that VC more effectively initiates mitochondrial outer membrane permeabilization (MOMP), leading to downstream caspase activation [15].

The relative inefficacy of BZ may stem from its primary mechanism of action, which might not strongly engage the apoptotic machinery directly but instead targets other cellular processes such as microtubule stabilization, oxidative stress modulation, or anti-inflammatory pathways [16]. Unlike VC, which directly promotes ROS generation and mitochondrial dysfunction, BZ may lack sufficient mitochondrial disruption capacity on its own to activate caspase cascades robustly. Interestingly, when VC and BZ were combined, a differential caspase response was observed: caspase-3 and -7 levels decreased, while caspase-8 and -9 levels increased. This shift could suggest a complex interaction where VC's pro-apoptotic mitochondrial effects dominate, but BZ modifies the downstream signaling - possibly enhancing initiator caspase-8/9 expression while modulating effector caspase-3/7 degradation or inhibition. The selective upregulation of Smac/Diablo in the combination group further supports this synergistic effect, as Smac antagonizes IAPs, thereby facilitating caspase activation that might otherwise be suppressed.

Cell cycle analysis revealed a marked reduction in cyclin B1, cyclin D1, CDK2, and CDK7 across all treatments, except for CDK7, which was specifically downregulated in the BZ-only group. This suggests that both VC and BZ can arrest the cell cycle at multiple checkpoints (G1 and G2/M), with BZ exerting stronger transcriptional regulatory effects via CDK7 suppression [17]. These alterations align with known effects of proteasome inhibition in halting cancer cell proliferation [16].

The PI3K/AKT/mTOR pathway was broadly downregulated, as seen by the decrease in AKT and p85 across all groups, and a reduction in mTOR in VC and combination treatments. Interestingly, BZ alone led to increased mTOR expression, which may reflect compensatory survival signaling in response to proteasome stress, as previously documented in cancer cells adapting to BZ exposure [18].

Notably, tumor suppressors p21 and PTEN were upregulated in all treatment groups, accompanied by a decrease in MDM2. This profile supports the reactivation of the p53 signaling axis, which promotes growth arrest and apoptosis in response to DNA damage and oncogenic stress [19].

MAPK signaling was also suppressed, as shown by reduced levels of SAPK/JNK, p38, and ERK. This broad inhibition may contribute to reduced proliferation and survival of Caco-2 cells, given the importance of these pathways in colorectal cancer pathogenesis [20]. Furthermore, EGFR expression was consistently downregulated, aligning with prior studies reporting the suppressive effects of VC and BZ on EGFR-mediated growth signals [21].

Wnt signaling and its downstream effectors (e.g., β-catenin) were reduced by VC and BZ individually, but the combination unexpectedly increased β-catenin and ROCK expression. While β-catenin is typically associated with tumor proliferation and stemness, the dual increase with ROCK suggests enhanced cytoskeletal reorganization and possible metastatic potential in some contexts [22]. This underscores a need for caution in interpreting the invasiveness-related consequences of combination therapy.

The observed increase in Vimentin and decrease in E-cadherin in individual treatments further supports the potential promotion of epithelial-mesenchymal transition (EMT), a process linked to metastasis. However, the combination therapy partially reversed this pattern - restoring E-cadherin expression while still maintaining high Vimentin - suggesting an incomplete or transitional EMT state [23]. These findings echo recent reports that proteasome inhibitors can produce mixed EMT profiles depending on cellular context.

Finally, the elevation of MnSOD in VC and combination groups may reflect increased oxidative stress buffering capacity. While MnSOD is generally cytoprotective, its role in modulating redox sensitive signaling can also influence cell survival, mitochondrial function, and resistance to apoptosis [24].

Conclusion

The results suggest that VC and BZ, particularly in combination, have potent antiproliferative and pro-apoptotic effects in Caco2 cells. However, the upregulation of certain metastasis-related markers such as ROCK and β-catenin under combination treatment highlights the complexity of therapeutic responses and warrants further in vivo validation. These findings contribute to the growing evidence for combining redox-active compounds and proteasome inhibitors in colorectal cancer treatment but also emphasize the importance of context-specific pathway modulation.

Key Findings

VC and BZ exert complementary anticancer effects on Caco-2 cells through the modulation of multiple molecular pathways. VC strongly activated the mitochondrial apoptotic cascade marked by increased Bax, cytochrome and decreased BCl2, whereas BZ alone showed modest apoptotic activity. When combined, VC and BZ enhanced intrinsic apoptosis and upregulated Smac/Diablo, suggesting synergistic crosstalk between redox stress and proteosome inhibition. Both agents suppressed P13k/AKT/mTOR and MAPK signaling and reduced cyclin and CDK expression, consistent with growth arrest and inhibition of proliferation. Upregulation of p21 and PTEN with concurrent downregulation of MDM2 supports reactivation of p53-dependent stress responses. Individual treatments downregulated β-catenin and ROCK, the combination increased their expression, indicating possible cytoskeletal or migratory adaptations. VC enhances apoptotic and antiproliferative responses of BZ in colorectal cancer.

Acknowledgments

The author thanks Union University for the source and support of research funding and thanks colleagues and editing tools for assistance with improving the clarity of the manuscript.

References

[1] Ferlay J., Soerjomataram I., Dikshit R., Eser S., Mathers C., Rebelo M., et al., Cancer incidence and mortality worldwide: sources, methods and major patterns in GLOBOCAN 2012. *Int J Cancer* 2015 ; 136(5) : E359-386.

[2] Rahib L., Smith B.D., Aizenberg R., Rosenzweig A.B., Fleshman J.M., Matrisian L.M. Projecting cancer incidence and deaths to 2030: the unexpected burden of thyroid, liver, and pancreas cancers in the United States. *Cancer Res* 2014 ; 74(11) :2913-2921.

[3] Biller L.H., Schrag D. Diagnosis and Treatment of Metastatic Colorectal Cancer: A Review. *JAMA* 2021 ; 325(7) :669-685.

[4] Brenner H., Kloor M., Pox C.P. Colorectal cancer. *Lancet* 2014 ;383(9927) :1490-1502.

[5] Grady W.M., Pritchard C.C. Molecular alterations and biomarkers in colorectal cancer. *Toxicol Patho* 2014 ; 42(1):124-139.

[6] Wu Z., Li Y., Zhang Y., Hu H., Wu T., Liu S., et al., Colorectal Screening Methods and Molecular Markers for Early Detection. *Technol Cancer Res Treat* 2020 ; 19 :1533033820980426.

[7] Yamamoto S., Egashira N. Pathological mechanisms of bortezomib-induced peripheral neuropathy. *Int J Mol Sci* 2021; 22(2):888.

[8] Meuser B., Hirsch C., Jarosch E., Sommer T. ERAD: the long road to destruction. *Nat Cell Biol* 2005 ; 7 :766–772.

[9] Voorhees P.M., Orlowski R.Z. The proteasome and proteasome inhibitors in cancer therapy. *Annu Rev Pharmacol Toxicol* 2006 ; 46 :189–213.

[10] Chen Q., Espey M.G., Krishna M.C., Mitchell J.B., Corpe C.P., Buettner G.R., et al., Pharmacological ascorbic acid concentrations selectively kill cancer cells: action as a pro-drug to deliver hydrogen peroxide to tissues. *PNAS* 2005 ; 102 : 13604-13609.

[11] Chen Q., Espey M.G., Sun A.Y., Lee J.H., Buettner G.R., Levine M. Ascorbate in pharmacologic concentration selectively generate ascorbate radical and hydrogen peroxide in extracellular fluid *in vivo*. *PNAS* 2007 ; 104 : 8749-8754.

[12] Olney K.E., Du J., Van Erve T.J., Witmer J.R., Wagner B.A., Buettner G.R., et al., Inhibitors of hydroperoxide metabolism enhance ascorbate-induce cytotoxicity. *Free Radic Res* 2013 ; 47 :154-163.

[13] Engur S., Dikmen M. The evaluation of the anti-cancer activity of ixazomib on Caco2 colon solid tumor cells, comparison with bortezomib. *Int J Clin Lab Med* 2017 ; 6 : 391-398.

[14] Fahy B.N., Schlieman M.G., Mortenson M.M., Virudachalam S., Bold R.J. Targeting BCL-2 overexpression in various human malignancies through NF-kB inhibition by the proteosome inhibitor bortezomib. Cancer *Chemother Pharmacol* 2005 ; 56 : 46-54.

[15] Szarka A., Kapuy O., Lorincz T., Banhegyi G. Vitamin C and cell death. *Antioxidants & Redox Signaling* 2021 ; 34, 11.

[16] Mujtaba T., Dou Q.P. Advances in the understanding of mechanisms and therapeutic use of bortezomib. *Discov Med* 2011 ; 12(67) : 471-480.

[17] Dutta R.P., Kumar R., Tembhare P.R., Bagal B. Targeting transcriptional kinase of CDK7 halts proliferation of multiple myeloma cells by modulating the function of canonical NF-kB pathway and cell cycle Regulatory proteins. *Trans Oncol* 2023 ; 35, 101729. 2016.

[18] Kralian S., Carr B.I. *Molecular pathways. Diagnosis and Treatment.* Third Edition. Springer 2016.

[19] Shamloo B., Usluer S. p21 in cancer research. *Cancers* 2019 ; 11(8), 1178.

[20] Pranteda A., Piastra V., Stramucci L., Fratantonio D., Bossi G. The p38 MAPK signaling activation in colorectal cancer upon therapeutic treatments. *Int J Mol Sci* 2020 ; 21(8) : 2773.

[21] Wagner E.F., Nebreda A.R. Signal integration by JNK and p38 MAPK pathways in cancer development. Nat. Rev. *Cancer* 2009 ; 9 :537–549.

[22] Shi W., Xu C., Gong Y., Yan Z., Mei L., Tang C., et al., RhoA/Rock activation represents a new mechanism for inactivating Wnt/β-catenin signaling in the aging-associated bone loss. *Cell Regen* 2021 ; 3 : 10, 8.

[23] Zhou J., Cheng H., Wang Z., Chen H. Bortezomib attenuates renal interstitial fibrosis in kidney transplantation via regulating the EMT induced by TNF-Smurf1-AkT-mTOR-p70S6K pathway. *J Cellular Mol Med* 2019; 23:5390-5402.

[24] Robbins D., Zhao Y. Manganese superoxide dismutase in cancer prevention. *Antioxidants & Redox Signaling* 2014 ; 20 : 10.

Chapter 10

Vitamin C and Doxorubicin in Pancreatic Cancer -Mechanistic Insights into Apoptosis, Oxidative Stress, and Signaling Pathway

Lunawati L. Bennett* **PhD, PharmD**
Union University, College of Pharmacy, Jackson, Tennessee, USA

Abstract

Pancreatic cancer is a leading cause of cancer-related death worldwide, and its global burden has more than doubled over the past 25 years. Approximately 90% of pancreatic cancers are pancreatic ductal adenocarcinoma with a 5-year survival rate of 11%. The combination regimens using leucovorin, 5-fluorouracil, irinotecan and oxaliplatin known as FOLFIRINOX or gemcitabine plus nab-paclitaxel have prolonged the median overall survival of the patients to 8.5–13 months, but with a significant toxic burden. Numerous attempts have been made to improve systemic therapies, but they have either failed to improve efficacy or have added significant toxic side effects.

The goal of this study was to understand if high dose vitamin C added into chemotherapy has a benefit effect in treating pancreatic cancer, utilizing BxPC-3 epithelial pancreas adenocarcinoma as the model. Based on the results from SRB assay, Rhodamine123, Hoechst 33342, and Western Blot assay, VC inhibits expressions of p38, EGFR, ERK, Akt and induction of tumor suppressor p21 and PTEN marked novel therapeutic in the treatment of pancreatic cancer. Collectively, these findings suggest that high-dose vitamin C exerts potent antitumor activity by suppressing proliferative and survival pathways while activating intrinsic tumor-suppressive mechanisms, supporting its potential as a promising adjunct in pancreatic cancer therapy.

Keywords: pancreatic cancer, doxorubicin, vitamin C, pancreatic ductal adenocarcinoma

* Corresponding Author's Email: llbennett@uu.edu

Abbreviations

AIF	Apoptosis inducing factor;
Bax	Bcl2 Associated X-protein;
Bcl2	B cell lymphoma 2;
Cas	Caspase;
CDK7	Cyclin dependent kinase 7;
Cyt C	Cytochrome C;
EGFR	Epidermal growth factor receptor;
ERK	Extracellular signal-regulated kinase;
PTEN	Phosphatase and tensin homolog;
ROCK	Rho-associated kinase.

Introduction

Over the past 25 years, pancreatic cancer incidence and global burden have more than doubled [1]. Approximately 90% of pancreatic cancers are pancreatic ductal adenocarcinoma (PDAC) with most affected individuals (80%) present with advanced-stage PDAC and usually have a 5-year survival rate of only 11%. The highest incidence rates of PDAC are observed in Blacks, followed by White, Hispanic, and Asian populations [2-4]. PDAC is more prevalent in men than in women and is rarely diagnosed before the age of 55. It predominantly affects elderly populations, with the highest incidence observed in people over 70 years old [1, 5]. In advanced disease, this cancer can metastasize to liver, peritoneal, or lung showing as hepatomegaly, ascites, abdominal distension, cough, dyspnea, or chest pain. Gastrointestinal bleeding, venous thromboembolism and back pain or other neurological symptoms are associated with vascular and nerve invasion [6-7].

The potential for curing pancreatic cancer lies in a combination of thorough resection and systemic multi-agent chemotherapy. Despite this approach, the overall recurrence rate remains high, ranging from 70-80%. For patients diagnosed with locally advanced or metastatic PDAC, the condition is generally deemed non-curative, and the focus shifts to palliative management. Numerous trials have demonstrated that systemic chemotherapy known as FOLFIRINOX utilizing a combination of 5-Fluorouracil, irinotecan, and oxaliplatin, can enhance overall survival in advanced PDAC cases with the median overall survival to 8.5–13 months [8].

Doxorubicin (DX) has anticancer properties against leukemia, lymphoma, breast, thyroid and osteosarcoma and has been used widely in many chemotherapy regimens [9-10]. As an anthracycline, DX is isolated from the pigment of fungus *Streptomyces peucetius* var. *Caesius*. In 1950, the antitumor activity of DX was first revealed, and its application as an antitumor compound was approved in 1963 [10-11].

Pharmacological VC achieved through high-dose intravenous (IVC) to attain plasma levels of $\geq$ 20 mM, has recently emerged as a potential non-toxic adjuvant to standard care radio-chemotherapy-based cancer therapies across various disease sites

[12-13]. The proposed anti-cancer mechanism of pharmacological VC involves redox-active metal-mediated or auto-oxidation of ascorbate, resulting in the formation of O_2 and H_2O_2 [13-15]. A phase I/IIa study investigating the pharmacokinetic interaction between intravenous VC and gemcitabine showed that pharmacological ascorbate induced cell death in pancreatic cancer cells with diverse mutational backgrounds [16].

This study was designed to evaluate the chemo-enhancing potential of VC in combination with low-dose of DX for treating PDAC using BxPC-3 epithelial pancreas adenocarcinoma as the model. The findings of this investigation reveal that the use of VC with DX demonstrated greater efficacy in the treatment of neuroblastoma. This marks a novel discovery in the field.

To evaluate the cytotoxic potential of high-dose VC, various antineoplastic agents - including paclitaxel, doxorubicin, etoposide, temsirolimus, bortezomib, afatinib, and sorafenib - were tested on human pancreatic cancer using the model BxPC-3 cell line. For combination studies, the lowest concentrations of each antineoplastic and high-dose VC that yielded a synergistic reduction in cell viability were selected. General experimental procedures followed the protocols outlined in Chapter 3 (Materials and Methods), while methodological details specific to this study are described below.

Cell Culture

BxPC-3 (ATCC CRL-1687), is a cell line exhibiting epithelial morphology that was isolated from the pancreas tissue of a 61-year-old, female patient with adenocarcinoma, were cultured in RPMI 1640 media supplemented with 10% FBS and 1% streptomycin/penicillin. The cells were cultured in T75 dishes and maintained in an incubator at 37°C in a 5% CO2 humidified environment.

Results

Cell Viability and Selection of Doses

VC treatment BxPC-3 alone reduced cell viability in a dose-dependent manner, while DX alone produced a pronounced cytotoxic effect, with ~50% reduction at mid-range concentrations. The combination of VC and DX produced a synergistic decrease in cell viability, and these conditions were selected for subsequent experiments The combination of VC and DX at the tested doses shows consistent synergy across all tested effect levels (Fa $\approx$ 0.7), with observed cytotoxicity ($\approx$72–73% cell death) is greater than expected if VC and DX acted independently.

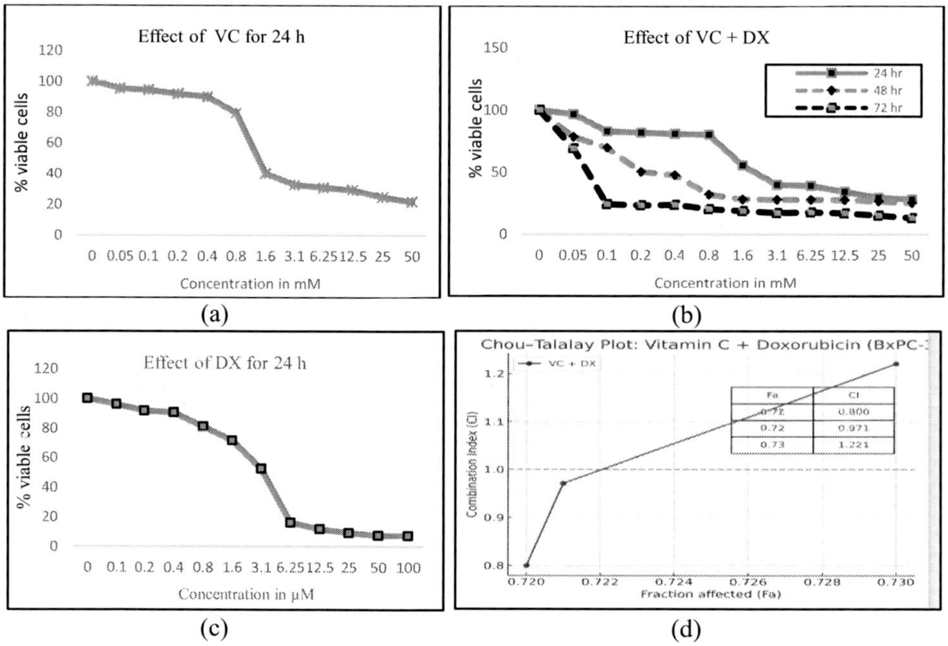

Figure 1. SRB assay results for BxPC-3 cells treated for 24 h with (a) VC (0 to 50 mM) showing decreased viability at 3 mM after 24 h; (b) combination treatment of 3 mM VC and 3μM DX at 24, 48 and 72 h, highlighting a combined effect of VC and DX; (c) DX (0-100 3μM) with 50% reduction in cells at 3 μM. (d) Using the combination of VC 3 mM and DX 3 μM, Chou-Talalay graph showed synergistic effect with Fa = 0.72 with CI < 1.

Changes in Cells Morphology

The morphological changes in BXPC-3 cells after 24 h treatment were observed with VC, DX, or their combination. Control cells exhibited healthy morphology with increased cell numbers and adherence to the culture dish. In contrast, cells treated with VC or DX alone showed reduced cell viability and altered morphology. The combination treatment with VC and DX resulted in further cell death, as indicated by the presence of floating cells on the culture dish.

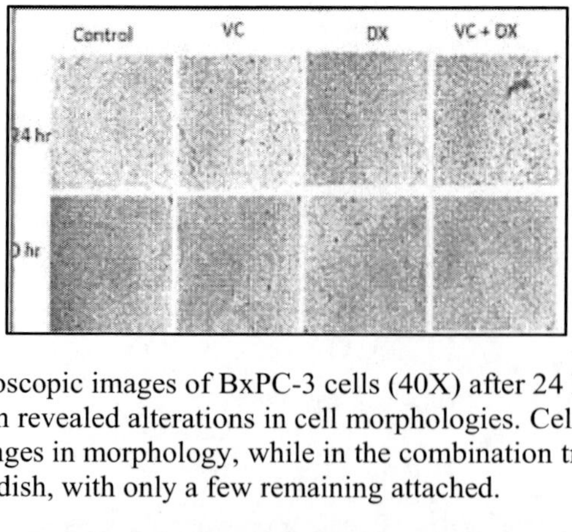

Figure 2. Inverted microscopic images of BxPC-3 cells (40X) after 24 h treatment with VC, DX, or their combination revealed alterations in cell morphologies. Cells treated with VC or DX exhibited some changes in morphology, while in the combination treatment, most cells were detached from the dish, with only a few remaining attached.

Wound-Healing

After 24 h of treatment, the combination of VC and DX led to significantly reduced migration of BxPC-3 cells, resulting in a wider wound gap compared to treatments with VC or DX alone. In contrast, control cells migrated closer together, indicating early signs of invasion and potential cancer metastasis. Quantitative analysis comparing the wound widths across control, VC, DX, and combination treatments.

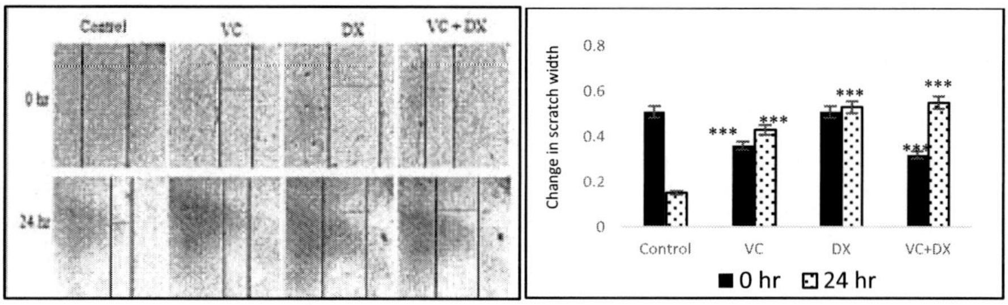

(a) (b)

Figure 3. Wound healing assay of BxPC-3 cells. (a) Representative images at 0 and 24 h for control, VC, DX, and combination treatments. (b) Histogram comparing wound width across treatment groups after 24 h. Data are expressed as mean ± SD; significant differences are indicated by ***p < 0.001 (post hoc Newman–Keuls test).

Induction of Apoptosis

Hoechst 33342 staining revealed that apoptosis was most pronounced in BxPC-3 cells treated with VC alone, whereas DX or the combination of VC and DX induced relatively fewer apoptotic events. Control cells maintained normal nuclear morphology with low fluorescence intensity, while apoptotic cells showed condensed and fragmented bright blue nuclei. Quantitative analysis confirmed a significantly lower percentage of viable cells in the VC-treated group compared to DX or combination treatments.

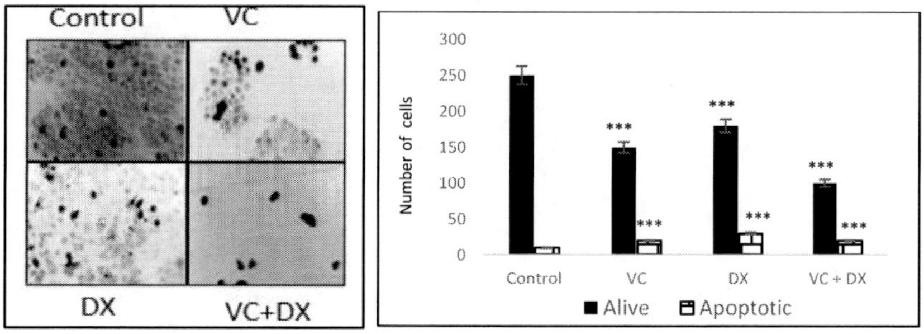

(a) (b)

Figure 4. Apoptosis analysis in BxPC-3 cells after 24 h. of treatment. (a) Representative fluorescence microscopy images of control, VC, DX, and combination groups stained with Hoechst 33342. Scale bar = 100 μm. (b) Histogram shows the percentage of apoptotic versus viable cells across treatment groups. Data are presented as mean ± SD (n = 3); ***p < 0.001 vs control (post hoc Newman–Keuls test).

Intracellular ROS Generation

ROS analysis demonstrated that all treatments induced a marked increase in intracellular ROS generation compared to control cells. This was evident from enhanced fluorescence intensity in VC, DX, and combination-treated groups, indicating elevated oxidative stress in BxPC-3 cells.

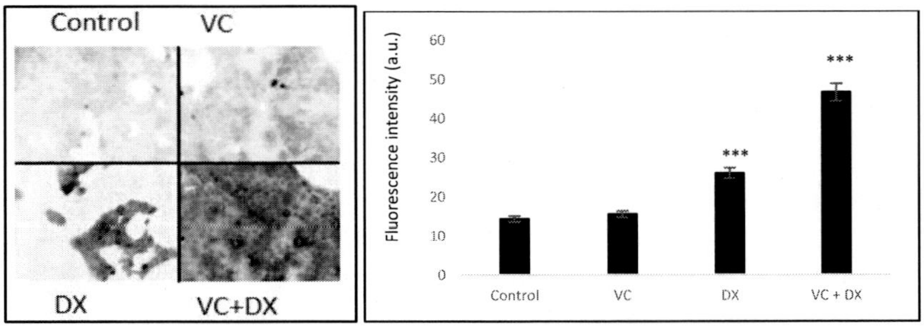

(a) (b)

Figure 5. Intracellular ROS generation in BxPC-3 cells after 24 h of treatment. (a) Representative fluorescence microscopy images following H2DCFDA staining. Increased fluorescence intensity corresponds to higher ROS levels. Scale bar = 100 µm. (b) Histogram of fluorescence intensity comparing control, VC, DX, and combination treatments. Data are expressed as mean ± SD (n = 3); ***$p < 0.001$ vs control (post hoc Newman–Keuls test).

Mitochondrial Membrane Potential (Ψ_m)

Assessment of mitochondrial membrane potential using Rhodamine 123 revealed a marked loss of fluorescence intensity in VC, DX, and combination-treated BxPC-3 cells compared to controls, consistent with mitochondrial depolarization and treatment-induced cell death. The results suggest that treatment disrupts mitochondrial ΔΨ_m, impairing mitochondrial function and triggering downstream apoptotic/necrotic pathways.

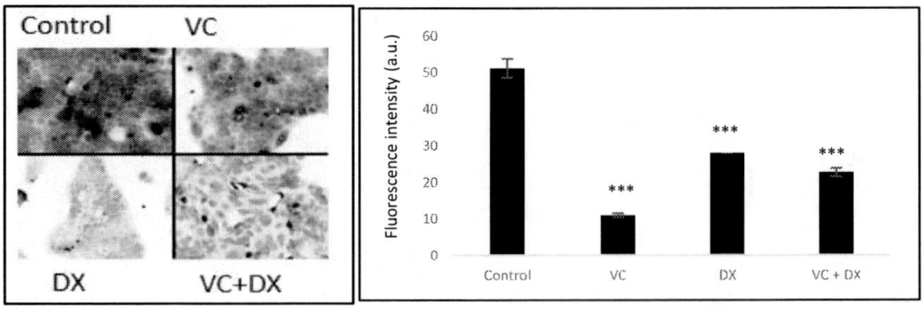

(a) (b)

Figure 6. Mitochondrial membrane potential in BxPC-3 cells after 24 h of treatment. (a) Representative fluorescence microscopy images stained with Rhodamine 123, showing reduced fluorescence intensity in VC, DX, and combination groups relative to control. Scale bar = 100 µm. (b) Histogram of fluorescence intensity quantifying mitochondrial depolarization across groups. Data are expressed as mean ± SD (n = 3); ***$p < 0.001$ vs control (post hoc Newman–Keuls test).

Modulation of Bax, Bcl2, and Cytochrome C

ROS generation was associated with modulation of mitochondrial apoptosis regulators. Combination treatment with VC and PX increased Bax expression and decreased BCl2 favoring a pro-apoptotic shift. In parallel, cytochrome c release was enhanced across treatments, consistent with mitochondrial membrane depolarization.

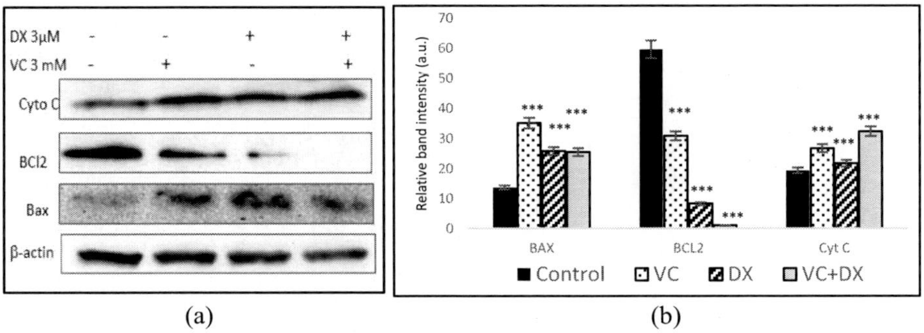

Figure 7. Western blot analysis of apoptosis-related proteins in BxPC-3 cells after 24 h of treatment. (a) Representative blots showing expression of Bax, Bcl-2 and cytochrome c in control, VC, DX, and combination groups. (b) Band intensity histogram quantifying protein expression relative to control. Data are presented as mean ± SD (n = 3); ***p < 0.001 vs control (post hoc Newman–Keuls test).

Modulation of Mitochondrial Signaling Proteins

Mitochondrial apoptosis markers were modulated following treatment with VC, DX, or their combination. Western blot analysis showed that combined VC and DX treatment markedly increased AIF-1 expression, while single treatments elevated Cas-8 and cleaved Cas-9, but caused decrease in Cas-3 and Cas-7. Densitometric quantification confirmed significant upregulation of Cas-8, cleaved Cas-9, and AIF-1 across treatment groups.

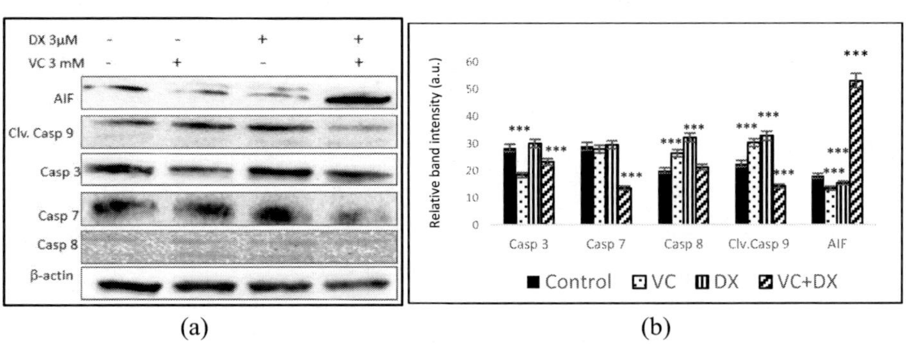

Figure 8. Western blot analysis of cas -3, -7, -8, -9, and AIF expressions in BxPC-3 cells following treatment with VC, DX, or their combination. (a) Representative blots showing expression of these proteins. (b) Densitometric histogram compares relative protein levels normalized to β-actin. Data are presented as mean ± SD (n = 3); ***p < 0.001 vs control (post hoc Newman–Keuls test).

Modulation of MEK Kinase Pathway

To explore the role of MAPK signaling, Western blot analysis was performed to evaluate phosphorylated MEK isoforms in BxPC-3 cells treated with VC, DX, or their combination. All treatments caused a significant decrease in MEK-2, indicating a potential favorable effect. In contrast, MEK-1, MEK-3, and MEK-4 levels were consistently increased across treatment groups, suggesting an unfavorable regulatory response.

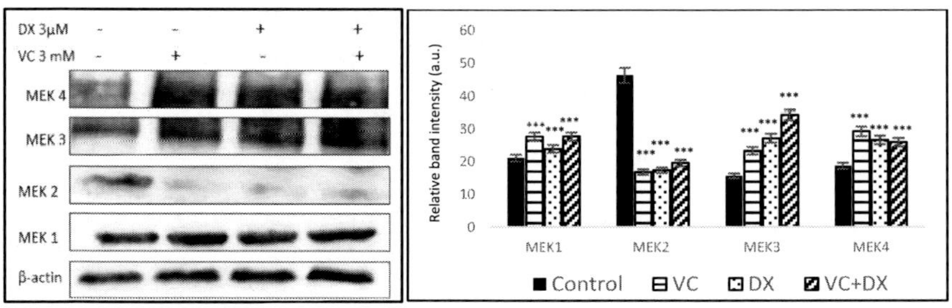

(a) (b)

Figure 9. Western blot analysis expressions of MEK-1, -2, -3, and -4 in BxPC-3 cells following treatment with VC, DX, or their combination. (a) Representative blots showing expression of these proteins. (b) Densitometric histogram compares relative protein levels normalized to β-actin. Data are expressed as mean ± SD (n = 3). Significant change indicated by ***$p < 0.001$, according to the post hoc Newman-Keuls test.

Modulation of Cell Cycle Regulatory Proteins

To evaluate the impact of VC, DX, and their combination on cell cycle progression in BxPC-3 cells, Western blot analysis of key regulatory proteins was performed. Combined VC and DX treatment resulted in a marked increase in CDK7, CDK2, cyclin B1, and cyclin D1 compared to control reflect un unfavorable effect of VC and DX in pancreatic cancer cells.

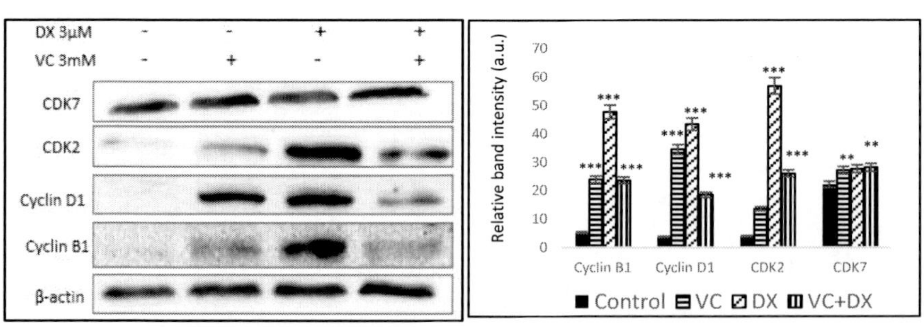

(a) (b)

Figure 10. Western blot analysis expressions of CDK7, CDK2, cyclin B1, and cyclin D1 in BxPC-3 cells following treatment with VC, DX, or their combination. (a) Representative blots showing expression of these proteins. (b) Densitometric histogram compares relative protein levels normalized to β-actin. Data are expressed as mean ± SD (n = 3). Significant change indicated by ** $p < 0.01$ and ***$p < 0.001$, according to the post hoc Newman-Keuls test.

Modulation of p21, PTEN, and MDM2

The effects of VC, DX, and their combination on key regulatory proteins were examined in BxPC-3 cells. Western blot analysis showed no detectable expression of p53 in this cell line. Treatment with VC significantly increased p21 expression, indicating a favorable role in cell cycle regulation and tumor suppression. PTEN expressions were also elevated following treatment with VC, DX, or their combination, further suggesting a beneficial effect on tumor suppressor pathways.

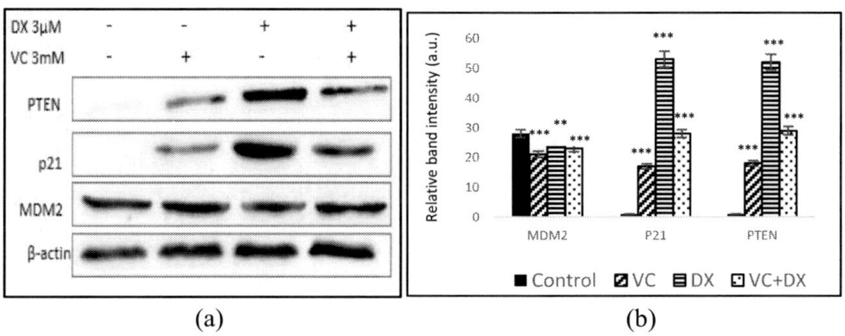

Figure 11. Western blot analysis expressions of p21, PTEN, and MDM2 in BxPC-3 cells following treatment with VC, DX, or their combination. (a) Representative blots showing expression of these proteins. (b) Densitometric quantification of protein expression. Significant changes are marked as **p < 0.01 and ***p < 0.001, according to the post hoc Newman-Keuls test.

Modulation of Akt/P13K

The effects of VC, DX, and their combination on the PI3K/Akt pathway were examined in BxPC-3 cells. Western blot analysis revealed a significant increase in PI3K expression across all treatment groups, indicating an unfavorable regulatory effect. Akt expression showed decrease expression suggesting a positive impact on this pathway. Given the close interconnection of PI3K and Akt, these changes highlight potential feedback interactions within the signaling cascade.

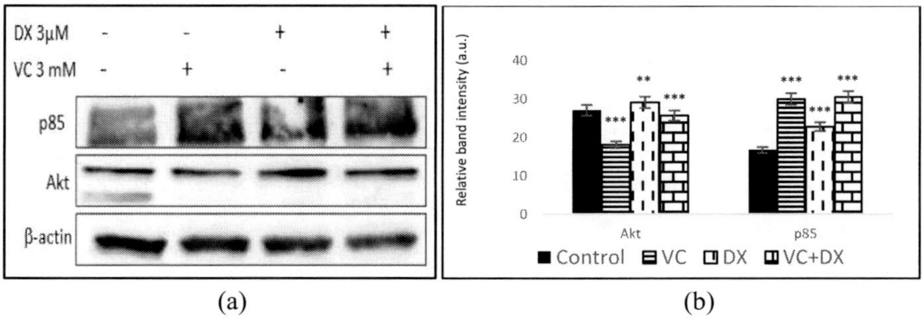

Figure 12. Western blot analysis expressions of PI3K and Akt in BxPC-3 cells following treatment with VC, DX, or their combination. (a) Representative blots showing expression of these proteins. (b) Densitometric histogram compares relative protein levels normalized to β-actin. Data are expressed as mean ± SD (n = 3). Statistical significance was determined using the Newman–Keuls post hoc test (***p < 0.001).

Modulation of SAPK/JNK and p38

The effects of VC, DX, and their combination on SAPK/JNK and p38 were assessed in BxPC-3 cells. Western blot analysis showed that p38 expression was consistently reduced across all treatment groups, with the most pronounced decrease observed in the VC–DX combination. In contrast, SAPK/JNK expression increased significantly with DX alone. Densitometric quantification confirmed these patterns, indicating opposing regulatory effects on SAPK/JNK and p38 signaling.

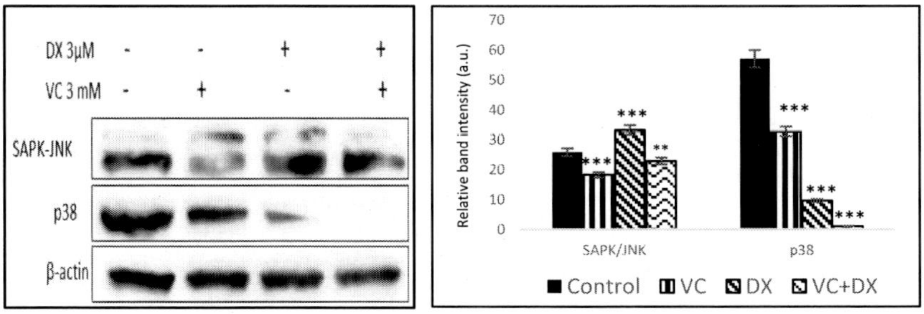

(a) (b)

Figure 13. Western blot analysis of SAPK/JNK and p38 proteins in BxPC-3 cells following treatment with VC, DX, or their combination. (a) Representative blots showing expression of these proteins. (b) Densitometric histogram compares relative protein levels normalized to β-actin. Data are expressed as mean ± SD (n = 3). Statistical significance was determined using the Newman–Keuls post hoc test (***$p < 0.001$).

Modulation of ERK, EGFR and SRC

The effects of VC, DX, and their combination of ERK, EGFR, and SRC were evaluated in BxPC-3 cells. Western blot analysis revealed a marked decrease in EGFR expression across all treatment groups, suggesting a favorable effect of VC and DX. In contrast, ERK1/2 and SRC expressions were increased and showed unfavorable effect of combination of VC and DX.

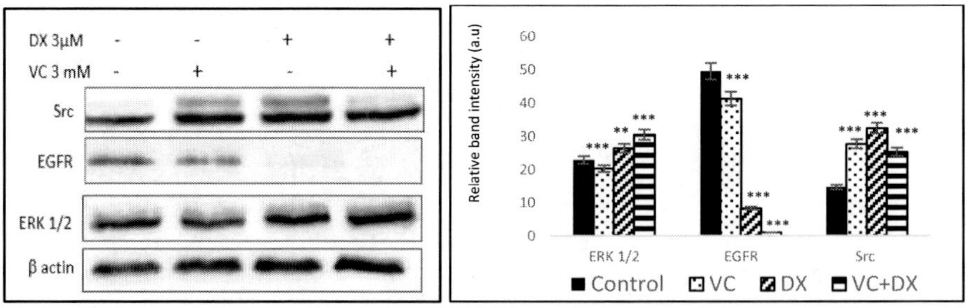

(a) (b)

Figure 14. Western blot analysis of ERK, EGFR and SCR in BxPC-3 cells following treatment with VC, DX, or their combination. (a) Representative blot analysis of these protein expressions. (b) Densitometric histogram compares relative protein levels normalized to β-actin. Data are expressed as mean ± SD (n = 3). Significant changes are marked as ** $p < 0.01$, ***$p < 0.001$, according to the post hoc Newman-Keuls test.

Modulation of Wnt, β Catenin, and ROCK

The effects of VC, DX, and their combination on Wnt, ROCK, β-catenin, and histone proteins were examined in BxPC-3 cells. Western blot analysis showed that Wnt, ROCK, and β-catenin expression levels were significantly increased across all treatment groups, indicating an unfavorable regulatory effect of VC, DX, or their combination of these signaling proteins. Densitometric quantification confirmed these findings (see Fig 15).

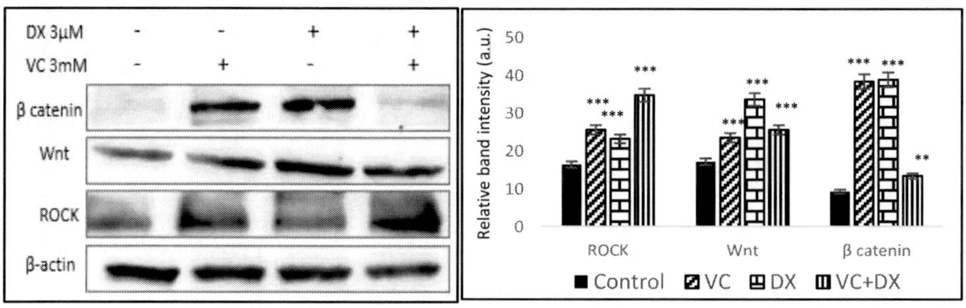

(a) (b)

Figure 15. Western blot analysis expressions of Wnt, ROCK, β-catenin, and histone in BxPC-3 cells following treatment with VC, DX, or their combination. (a) Representative blots showing expression of these proteins. (b) Densitometric histogram compares relative protein levels normalized to β-actin. Data are expressed as mean ± SD (n = 3). Significant changes are marked as ** $p < 0.01$ and ***$p < 0.001$, according to the post hoc Newman-Keuls test.

Modulation of MnSOD, Smac/Diablo, and E-cadherin

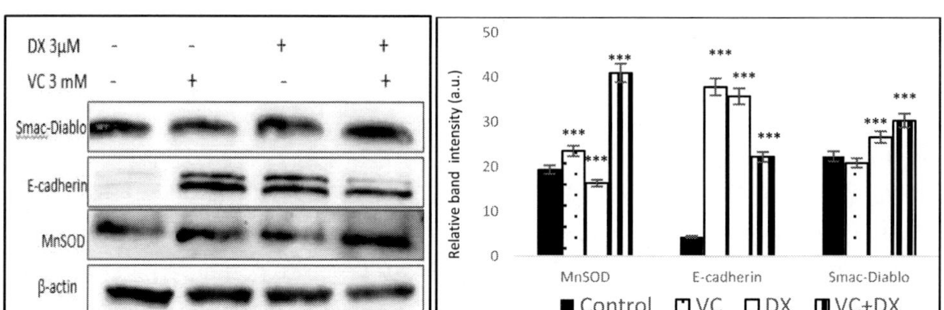

(a) (b)

Figure 16. Western blot analysis of MnSOD, E-cadherin, and Smac/DIABLO expression in BxPC-3 cells following treatment with VC, DX, or their combination. (a) Representative blots showing expression of these proteins. (b) Densitometric histogram compares relative protein levels normalized to β-actin. Data are expressed as mean ± SD (n = 3). Significant changes are marked as ***$p < 0.001$, according to the post hoc Newman-Keuls test.

The effects of VC, DX, and their combination on MnSOD, Smac/Diablo, and E-cadherin expression were examined in BxPC-3 cells. Western blot analysis revealed a modest increase in Smac/Diablo levels across all treatment groups suggesting a favorable pro-apoptotic effect. In contrast, E-cadherin expression was elevated following VC, DX, and their combination, which may indicate an unfavorable effect by promoting invasive potential. MnSOD levels were variably modulated but did not show a consistent directional change compared with control (see Fig.16).

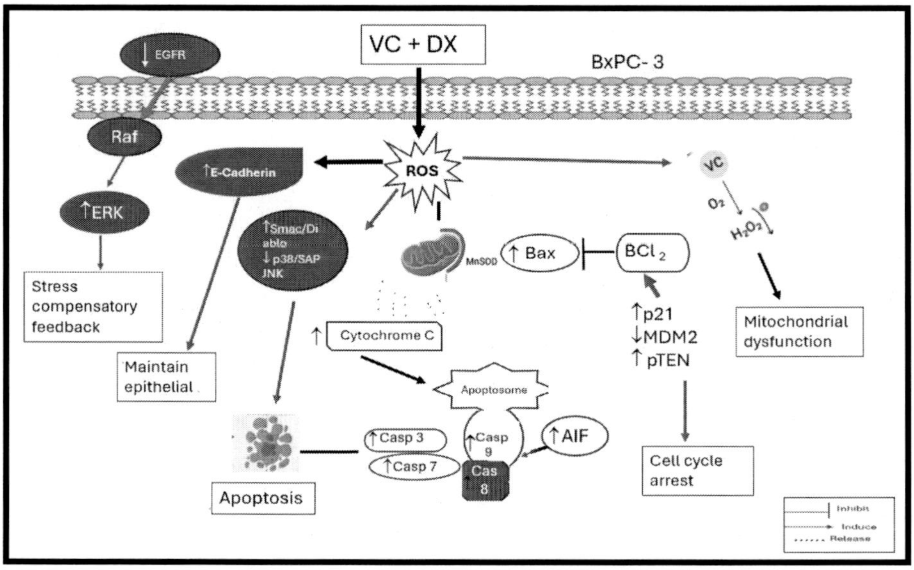

Figure 17. Proposed mechanistic model of VC and DX in pancreatic cancer.

Discussion

As illustrated in Figure 17, VC, DX and the combination enhance therapeutic efficacy in pancreatic cancer BxPC-3 cells by inducing significant alterations in cell morphology, viability, apoptosis, oxidative stress, mitochondrial function, and various signaling pathways. These effects suggest a complex interplay between VC and DX, warranting further exploration.

Treatment with VC, DX, and their combination led to reduced cell viability and altered morphology in BxPC-3 cells. The combination treatment resulted in further cell death, as indicated by the presence of floating cells, suggesting enhanced cytotoxicity. These observations align with previous studies indicating that high-dose VC can sensitize cancer cells to chemotherapeutic agents by generating H_2O_2, which induces oxidative stress in cells [12-15].

Microscopic staining revealed pronounced apoptosis in VC-treated cells, while DX and the combination induced relatively fewer apoptotic events. This discrepancy may be attributed to the different mechanisms of action of VC and DX. VC has been widely reported to induce apoptosis primarily through the generation of ROS, which can disrupt mitochondrial homeostasis, cause depolarization of the mitochondrial membrane, and trigger the release of pro-apoptotic factors leading to cell death [17]. This mitochondrial-centered stress response explains why VC-treated cells displayed robust apoptotic features. DX, on the other hand, is classically known to act through direct DNA damage by intercalates into DNA strands and inhibits topoisomerase II, resulting in double-strand breaks and replication stress [18]. While this also leads to apoptosis, the visible apoptotic changes may be less pronounced at the same treatment window compared with the rapid mitochondrial disruption triggered by VC. All treatments induced a marked increase in intracellular ROS generation, as evidenced by enhanced fluorescence intensity. This elevation in ROS levels was associated with a loss of mitochondrial membrane potential, indicating mitochondrial depolarization and treatment-induced cell death. These findings are consistent with studies demonstrating that VC can enhance lipid peroxidation and ROS production in cancer cells, contributing to cell death [19-20].

Western blot analysis provided additional insight into the apoptotic signaling events. The VC–DX combination markedly increased AIF-1, a protein released from mitochondria that promotes caspase-independent apoptosis. In contrast, the single treatments elevated caspase-8 and cleaved caspase-9 levels, both hallmarks of caspase-dependent apoptosis. However, levels of executioner caspases -3 and -7, were reduced in the combination group compared with single treatments. This suggests that VC and DX do not simply converge on the same apoptotic pathway but instead activate parallel, and perhaps competing, routes to cell death. VC's effect is more closely tied to mitochondrial disruption and AIF-1–mediated apoptosis [17], whereas DX primarily triggers the classical caspase cascade [18]. When combined, the treatments appear to engage both mitochondrial and caspase-dependent pathways, producing a broader but more complex apoptotic profile.

Combined VC and DX treatment resulted in a marked increase in CDK7, CDK2, cyclin B1, and cyclin D1 expression compared with control. These alterations suggest differential modulation of cell cycle regulators across treatment groups. The upregulation of these proteins may indicate a compensatory mechanism in response to DNA damage induced by VC and DX, promoting cell cycle progression and survival.

Additionally, VC, DX, and their combination affected MAPK signaling pathway. All treatments caused a significant decrease in MEK-2, indicating a potential favorable effect, while MEK-1, MEK-3, and MEK-4 levels were consistently increased, suggesting an unfavorable regulatory response. These findings are in line with studies indicating that VC can modulate MAPK signaling pathways, influencing cell survival and proliferation Additionally, the combination treatment led to increased PI3K expression, indicating an unfavorable regulatory effect. Akt expression showed decreased expression, suggesting a positive impact on this pathway. Given the close interconnection of PI3K and Akt, these changes highlight potential feedback interactions within the signaling cascade [20].

The molecular pattern produced by VC and DX points to a concurrent activation of intrinsic apoptosis and a pro-invasive/partial-EMT pathway - a duality increasingly recognized in cancer cells exposed to severe stress. Mechanistically, the apoptosis signature is consistent with mitochondrial (intrinsic) pathway activation i.e., mitochondrial damage and outer membrane permeabilization release proteins such as Smac/Diablo and cytochrome-c, and allowance of initiator Cas-9 to assemble the apoptosome and activate effector Cas-3 and -7. Smac/DIABLO both sensitizes cells to classical chemotherapeutics and synergizes with agents that trigger mitochondrial outer membrane permeabilization

Upregulation of MnSOD and evidence of increased MAPK, ERK1/2 signaling and β-catenin/Wnt/ROCK axis activation are coherent with a stress-response network driven by elevated ROS produced by both pharmacologic VC and DX. DX is well documented to increase mitochondrial ROS and thereby engage redox-sensitive responses. MnSOD upregulation is a canonical mitochondrial antioxidant response to increased superoxide and is commonly seen after DX exposure as a cell attempts to buffer oxidative damage representing an adaptive antioxidant program, which can transiently protect mitochondria from ROS but, if ROS generation exceeds buffering capacity, the same mitochondria will release apoptogenic factors (Smac/DIABLO and cytochrome-c) - explaining as why both MnSOD induction and caspase activation in parallel.

Reactive oxygen species and DNA damage signaling can crosstalk with the canonical Wnt/β-catenin pathway, via phosphorylation events that alter β-catenin stability/localization and with RhoA/ROCK signaling that controls cytoskeletal contractility and migration. Activation of Wnt/β-catenin and ROCK is frequently associated with increased motility, matrix remodeling and EMT-like behaviors that promote invasion and metastasis. Importantly, these pathways can be triggered as adaptive responses to chemotherapeutic stress and can promote survival of subpopulations that evade death - a plausible molecular explanation for why apoptosis markers and invasion-promoting signals are co-present [21-23].

ERK activation further complicates the picture because ERK can be pro-apoptotic or pro-survival depending on intensity, duration and subcellular localization. ROS and stress kinases commonly lead to transient ERK activation; sustained ERK signaling, however, tends to drive transcriptional programs that support survival, migration and cytoskeletal rearrangements. In the presence of strong mitochondrial damage and Smac release, some cell subpopulations proceed to apoptotic death (caspase activation), while others may engage ERK-mediated survival and motility programs that favor persistence and invasion.

Future studies should focus on elucidating the molecular mechanisms by which VC and DX modulate signaling pathways and contribute to drug resistance. Investigating the effects of VC and DX in vivo will provide insights into their therapeutic potential and safety profiles. Additionally, exploring the combination of VC and DX with other therapeutic agents may enhance treatment efficacy and overcome resistance mechanisms.

Conclusion

The combination of VC and DX exhibits complex effects on BxPC-3 cells, inducing apoptosis, modulating cell cycle progression, and affecting various signaling pathways. While the combination treatment enhances cytotoxicity and apoptosis, it also induces changes that may promote invasiveness and resistance. These findings underscore the need for a comprehensive understanding of the molecular mechanisms underlying the effects of VC and DX in pancreatic cancer treatment.

Key Findings

VC, DX, and their combination reduced BxPC-3 cell viability, with the combination showing the strongest cytotoxic effect. VC increased tumor suppressors p21 and PTEN, while MDM2 and cell cycle proteins (CDK2, CDK7, cyclins) were variably modulated. MAPK, PI3K/Akt, Wnt/β-catenin, and EMT-related proteins were differentially regulated, reflecting both favorable (e.g., EGFR downregulation, p38 decrease) and unfavorable (e.g., β-catenin, E-cadherin) effects. Overall, VC enhances DX cytotoxicity but also activates pro-survival and invasive pathways, suggesting the need for combinatorial strategies to maximize therapeutic efficacy.

Acknowledgments

The author thanks Union University for the source and support of research funding. The author thanks colleagues and editing tools for assistance with improving the clarity of the manuscript.

References

[1] Siegel R., Miller K.D., Jemal A. Cancer statistics. *Cancer Journal for Clinicians* 2023 ; 73(1) : 17-48.

[2] Stoffel E.M., Brand R.E., Goggins M. Pancreatic cancer: changing epidemiology and new approaches to risk assessment, early detection, and prevention. *Gastroenterology* 2023 ; 164 (5) : 752-765.

[3] National Cancer Institute. Surveillance, Epidemiology and End Results Program. *www.seer.cancer.gov*. Accessed September 10, 2024.

[4] Klein A.P. Pancreatic cancer epidemiology: understanding the role of lifestyle and inherited risk factors. *Nat Rev Gastroenterol Hepatol* 2021 ; 18 :493–502.

[5] Rawla P., Sunkara T., Gaduputi V. Epidemiology of Pancreatic Cancer: Global Trends, Etiology and Risk Factors. *World J Oncol* 2019 ; 10(1) :10-27.

[6] Kisiel J.B., Taylor W.R. Diagnostic approaches in pancreatic cancer: From imaging to biomarkers. *J of Gastrointestinal Oncology* 2024 ; 15(4) : 1012-1023.

[7] Yoshida K., Nakamura Y. Advances in biomarker discovery and imaging techniques for pancreatic cancer. *J of Translational Medicine* 2023 ; 21(1), 298.

[8] Hochster C.M.R., Ko M.A.M.Z., Ross H.A.M., Jones D.G.S., Williams T.L., Tempero W.S., et al., Erlotinib plus gemcitabine compared with gemcitabine alone in patients with advanced pancreatic cancer : a phase III trial of the National Cancer Institute of Canada Clinical Trials Group. *J Clin Oncol* 2007 ; 25 :1960–1966.

[9] Almajidi Y.Q., Kadhim M.M., Jalil A.T., Sayyid N.H., Jawhar Z.H., Gupta J., et al., Doxorubicin loaded micelles in tumor cell-specific chemotherapy. *Environmental Res* 2023 ; 227 : 115722.

[10] Mohajeri M., Sahekabar A. Protective effect of curcumin against doxorubicin-induced toxicity and resistance. *Review* 2018 ; 122 : 30-51.

[11] Morabito A., Gattuso D., Stani S.C., Fanelli M., Castallena M.A. Safety and activity of the combination of pegylated liposomal doxorubicin and weekly docetaxel in advanced breast cancer. *Breast Cancer* 2004 ; 86 (3) : 249-258.

[12] Du J., Martin S.M., Levine B.A., Wang S., Knudsen C.M., Cullen J.J. Mechanism of ascorbate-induced cytotoxicity in pancreatic cancer. *J Am Assoc Cancer Res* 2010 ; 16 :509-520.

[13] Chen Q., Espey M.G., Krishna M.C., Mitchell J.B., Corpe C.P., Buettner G.R., et al., Pharmacological ascorbic acid concentrations selectively kill cancer cells : action as a pro-drug to deliver hydrogen peroxide to tissues. *PNAS* 2005 ; 102 : 13604-13609.

[14] Chen Q., Espey M.G., Sun A.Y., Lee J.H., Buettner G.R., Levine M. Ascorbate in pharmacologic concentration selectively generate ascorbate radical and hydrogen peroxide in extracellular fluid *in vivo*. *PNAS* 2007 ; 104 : 8749-8754.

[15] Olney K.E., Du J., Van Erve T.J., Witmer J.R., Wagner B.A., Buettner G.R., et al., Inhibitors of hydroperoxide metabolism enhance ascorbate-induce cytotoxicity. *Free Radic Res* 2013 ; 47 :154-163.

[16] Polireddy K., Dong R., Reed G., Chen P., Williamson S., Pessetto Z., et al., High dose parenteral ascorbate inhibited pancreatic cancer growth and metastasis: mechanisms and a phase I/IIa study. *Sci Rep* 2017 ; 7 : 17188.

[17] Liu Y., Huang P., Li Z., Xu C., Wang H., Jia B., et al., Vitamin C sensitizes pancreatic cancer cells to erastin-induced ferroptosis. *Oxidative Med Cell Longevity* 2022 ;298(1) :101-113.

[18] Zhang M., Harashima N., Moritani T., Huang W., Harada M. The roles of ROS and caspases in TRAIL-induced apoptosis in pancreatic cancer cells. *PLoS One* 2015 ;10(6) : e0127386.

[19] Bedhiafi T., Inchakalody V.P., Fernandes Q. The potential role of vitamin C in empowering cancer immunotherapy. *Biomed & Pharmacotherapy* 2022 ; 112553.

[20] Fan D., Liu X., Shen Z., Wu P., Zhong L., Lin F. Cell signaling pathways based on vitamin C and their implications in cancer therapy. *Biomed Pharmacother* 2023 ; 156 :113883.

[21] Zhou Q., Zhou Y., Liu X., Shen Y. GDC-0449 improves the antitumor activity of nano-doxorubicin in a fibroblast-enriched microenvironment in pancreatic cancer. *Sci Rep* 2017 ;7(1) :13869.

[22] Rebelo R., Polonia B., Santos L.L., Vasconcelos MH, Xavier CPR. Drug repurposing opportunities in pancreatic ductal adenocarcinoma. *Pharmaceuticals* 2021 ;14(3) :280.

[23] Aslan M., Shahbazi R., Ulu Bayram K., Ozpolat B. Targeted therapies for pancreatic cancer and hurdles in their clinical application. *Anticancer Res* 2018 ;38(12) :6591-6598.

Chapter 11

How a Combined Vitamin C and Sorafenib Treatment Targets HER2–BRCA–ERα Axis and Promotes Mitochondrial Apoptosis in Luminal Breast Cancer Cells

Lunawati L. Bennett*, PhD, PharmD
Union University, College of Pharmacy, Jackson, Tennessee, USA

Abstract

Breast cancer is the most common cancer among women worldwide and can be classified into four subtypes based on the presence or absence of specific receptors as estrogen receptor-positive, progesterone receptor-positive, human epidermal growth factor receptor 2-positive, or triple-negative breast cancer. Treatment options for breast cancer include surgery, radiation therapy, chemotherapy, hormone therapy, immunotherapy, and targeted drug therapies. However, these treatments often result in significant side effects, including cardiotoxicity and bone marrow neoplasia.

The aim of this study was to evaluate whether the addition of vitamin C to the current standard chemotherapy regimen provides additional therapeutic benefits. Specifically, the study investigates whether vitamin C alone or in combination with a low dose of the chemotherapeutic agent sorafenib is more effective in treating invasive ductal luminal breast cancer, using the MCF-7 cell line (ER+, PR+, HER2-) as a model. Results from SRB assays, Rhodamine 123, Hoechst 33342 staining, and Western blot analysis showed that the addition of vitamin C to sorafenib inhibits cancer cell growth by inducing Bax, increasing caspases, suppressing matrix metalloproteinase -9 and -2, Bcl-2, cell cycle proteins, p38, SAP/JNK, Akt, Vimentin, EGFR and ERK genes.

Keywords: breast cancer, vitamin C, MCF-7, estrogen positive, progesterone positive

---

* Corresponding Author's Email: llbennett@uu.edu

Abbreviations

Bax	Bcl2 Associated X-protein;
Bcl2	B cell lymphoma 2;
Cas	Caspase;
CDK7	Cyclin dependent kinase 7;
Cyt C	Cytochrome C;
EGFR	Epidermal growth factor receptor;
ERK	Extracellular signal-regulated kinase;
MAPKs	Mitogen-activated protein kinases;
MEKs	Mitogen-activated protein kinase kinases;
MDM2	Mouse double minute 2 homolog;
MnSOD	Manganese superoxide dismutase.

Introduction

Breast cancer is a highly heterogeneous neoplasm that has a distinct molecular subtype identified through gene expression analysis. These subtypes are categorized based on the immunohistochemical presence of hormone receptors: ER^+, PR^+, $HER2^+$, and triple-negative breast cancer (ER-, PR-, $HER2^-$) [1].

Invasive ductal carcinoma (IDC) is the most common type of breast cancer, accounting for approximately 70-80% of all breast cancer cases. It originates in the milk ducts of the breast and invades the surrounding tissue. The "luminal" subtype refers to ER^+ and/or PR^+. This subtype is further classified into two main categories: luminal A and luminal B, with Luminal A generally being more responsive to hormone therapy and having a better prognosis compared to luminal B [2-4].

The exact cause of IDC, like many cancers, is multifactorial. Several risk factors contribute to its development, including genetic mutations, particularly in the BRCA1 and BRCA2 genes, family history, age, and lifestyle factors such as alcohol consumption and hormone replacement therapy. Hormonal imbalances and prolonged exposure to estrogen, either naturally or *via* external sources, are significant contributors. Other factors include early onset of menstruation, late menopause, and obesity, especially after menopause, which increases estrogen levels due to fat tissue.

Survival rates for IDC vary depending on the stage of diagnosis, cancer grade, and hormone receptor status. The five-year survival rate for localized IDC (cancer confined to the breast) is around 99%. When the cancer has spread to nearby lymph nodes (regional stage), the five-year survival rate drops to about 86%, and if distant metastasis occurs, it reduces to approximately 30%. Luminal A cancers, which tend to grow more slowly and have a better prognosis, often have higher survival rates compared to Luminal B, which are more aggressive and may involve HER2. IDC is curable, especially when detected early. Treatment options typically include surgery (lumpectomy or mastectomy), radiation therapy, chemotherapy, hormone therapy (for hormone receptor-positive cancers), and targeted therapies such as trastuzumab for

HER2+. Hormone receptor-positive cancers, particularly luminal A, often respond well to hormone therapies such as tamoxifen or aromatase inhibitors. The curability of IDC depends heavily on early detection, as well as the tumor's receptor status and stage at diagnosis [4-7].

Sorafenib (SF) has been used for the treatment of hepatocellular carcinoma, renal -cell carcinoma and thyroid cancer [8-10]. It works by inhibiting several key kinases involved in cancer growth and angiogenesis. It targets serine/threonine kinases in the RAF/MEK/ERK pathway, particularly RAF-1 and BRAF, that regulate cell proliferation and inhibit cancer growth [11].

Pharmacological achieved through high-dose intravenous vitamin C (IVC) to attain plasma levels of ≥20 mM, has recently emerged as a potential non-toxic adjuvant to standard care radio-chemotherapy-based cancer therapies across various disease sites [12-13]. The proposed anti-cancer mechanism of pharmacological VC involves redox-active metal-mediated or auto-oxidation of ascorbate, resulting in the formation of O_2 and H_2O_2 [13-14].

This study was designed to evaluate the chemo-enhancing potential of VC in combination with low-dose sorafenib for treating breast cancer, utilizing MCF-7 cells as the model. The findings of this investigation reveal that the use of VC with SF demonstrated greater efficacy in the treatment of breast cancer. This marks a novel discovery in the field.

To evaluate the cytotoxic potential of high-dose VC, various antineoplastic agents - including paclitaxel, doxorubicin, etoposide, temsirolimus, bortezomib, afatinib, and sorafenib - were tested on human breast cancer using the MCF-7 cell line. For combination studies, the lowest concentrations of each antineoplastic and high-dose VC that yielded a synergistic reduction in cell viability were selected. General experimental procedures followed the protocols outlined in Chapter 3 (Materials and Methods), while methodological details specific to this study are described below.

Cell Culture

Human breast cancer cell line MCF7 (ATCC HTB-22), was first isolated in 1970 from the pleural effusion of a 69-year-old Caucasian female patient with metastatic mammary carcinoma. It is the first hormone-responding breast cancer cell line with ER+, PR+, and glucocorticoid receptors (GR+) that serve as a valuable *in vitro* model [15-16]. It was cultured in Eagle's Minimum Essential Medium (EMEM) supplemented with 10% fetal bovine serum (FBS), 1% streptomycin/penicillin, and human recombinant insulin and zinc solution. The cells were cultured in T75 dishes and maintained in an incubator at 37°C in a 5% CO_2 humidified environment.

Results

Cell Viability and Selection of Doses

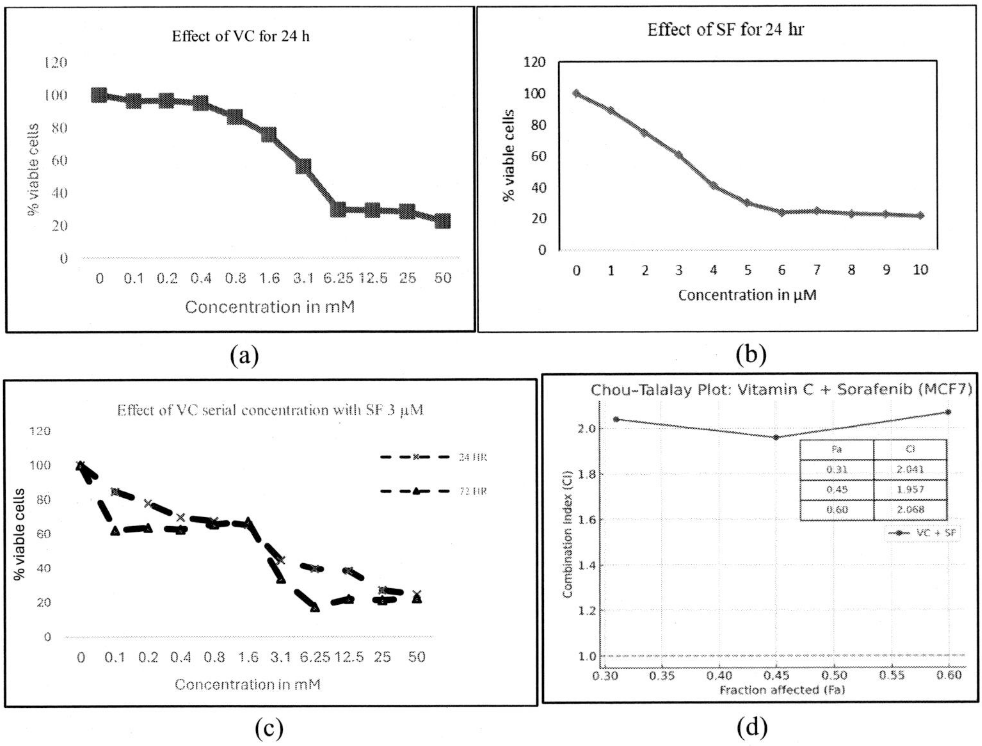

Figure 1. (a) shows that MCF7 cell viability decreased with increasing VC concentrations (0 to 50 mM) after 24 h. Figure 1(b) indicates a reduction in cell viability starting at 3 μM SF, and Figure 1(c) demonstrates a further decrease in viability with a 24 h, 48 h, and 72 h treatment of 3 mM VC and 3 μM SF, highlighting a combined effect.(d) the combination of VC and SF showed synergistic effect with Fa = 0.6, CI 0.77 according to Chou-Talalay calculation.

Cells treated with VC alone showed no significant change in viability at dosages lower than 3 mM (Figure 1a). Similarly, cells treated with SF alone exhibited no change in viability below 3 μM. A concentration of 3 μM SF was selected for serial VC treatment to determine if the combination treatment could further decrease the viability of MCF7 cells. The combination of VC and SF showed a synergistic effect after 24, 48, and 72 h. Based on the SRB assay results, 3 μM SF, 3 mM VC, and their combination were chosen for further experiments (see Fig.1 above).

Changes in Cells Morphology

MCF7 cell morphology was altered in all treatment groups compared to the control. While control cells remained healthy, showing increased numbers and adherence after 24 h, cells treated with VC or SF alone exhibited reduced viability and morphological changes. The combination of VC and SF led to even greater cell death, with many cells appearing floating in the culture dish.

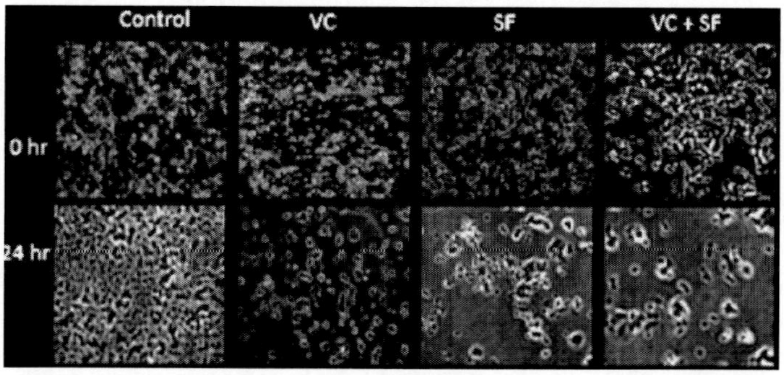

Figure 2. Inverted microscopic images of MCF7 cells (40X) after 24 h treatment with VC, SF, or a combination revealed alterations in cell morphologies.

Wound Healing

After 24 h of treatment, the combination of VC and SF led to significantly reduced migration of MCF7 cells, resulting in a wider wound gap compared to treatments with VC or SF alone. In contrast, control cells migrated closer together, indicating early signs of invasion and potential cancer metastasis. Histogram comparing the wound widths across all treatments.

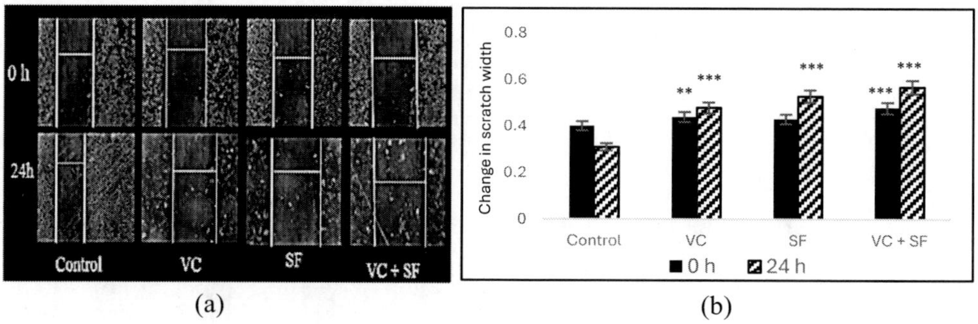

Figure 3. (a) results of the wound healing assay in MCF7 cells treated with VC, SF, or their combination, compared to the control at 0 and 24 h. Figure 3(b) shows a histogram comparing wound widths across different treatment groups. Data are expressed as mean ± SD of three experiments. $^{**}p < 0.01$ and $^{***}p < 0.001$, according to the post hoc Newman-Keuls test.

Induction of Apoptosis

Hoechst 33342 staining revealed that apoptosis was most pronounced in MCF7 cells treated with the combination of VC and SF. Control cells maintained normal nuclear morphology with low fluorescence intensity, while apoptotic cells showed condensed and fragmented bright blue nuclei. Quantitative analysis confirmed a significantly lower percentage of viable cells in the VC-treated group compared to SF or combination treatments.

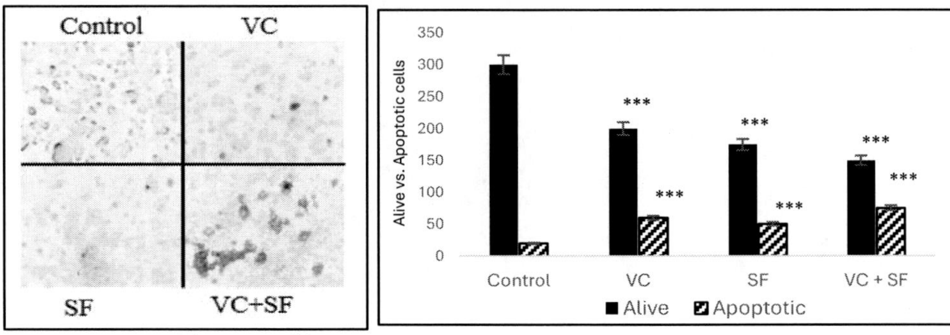

(a) (b)

Figure 4. Apoptosis analysis in MCF7 cells after 24 h. of treatment. (a) Representative fluorescence microscopy images of control, VC, SF, and combination groups stained with Hoechst 33342. Scale bar = 100 μm. (b) Histogram shows the percentage of apoptotic versus viable cells across treatment groups. Data are presented as mean ± SD of three experiments. ***$p < 0.001$ vs control (post hoc Newman–Keuls test).

Intracellular ROS Generation

ROS analysis demonstrated that all treatments induced a marked increase in intracellular ROS generation compared to control cells. This was evident from enhanced fluorescence intensity in VC, SF, and combination-treated groups, indicating elevated oxidative stress in MCF7 cells.

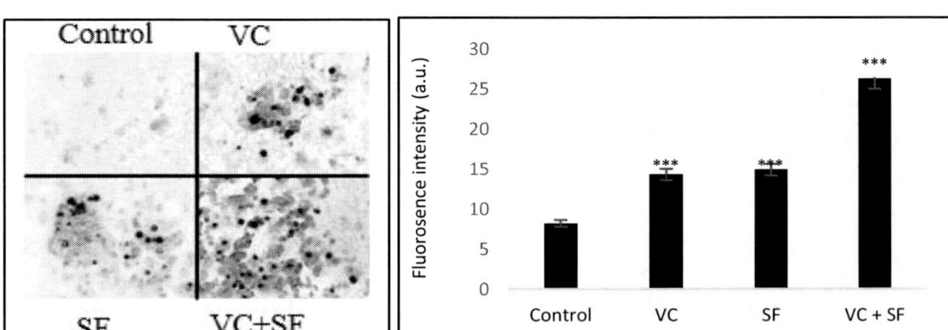

(a) (b)

Figure 5. Intracellular ROS generation in MCF7 cells after 24 h. of treatment. (a) Representative fluorescence microscopy images following H2DCFDA staining. Scale bar = 100 μm. (b) Histogram of fluorescence intensity comparing control, VC, SF, and combination treatments. Data are expressed as mean ± SD of three experiments. ***$p < 0.001$ vs control (post hoc Newman–Keuls test).

Mitochondrial Membrane Potential (Ψ_m)

The generation of ROS in MCF7 cells indicated cell death attributed to the depletion of mitochondrial membrane potential, as detected with Rhodamine 123 staining. Treatments with VC, SF, or the combination of VC and SF induced cell death. Control cells exhibited higher fluorescence intensity, indicating healthy mitochondria, compared to treated cells.

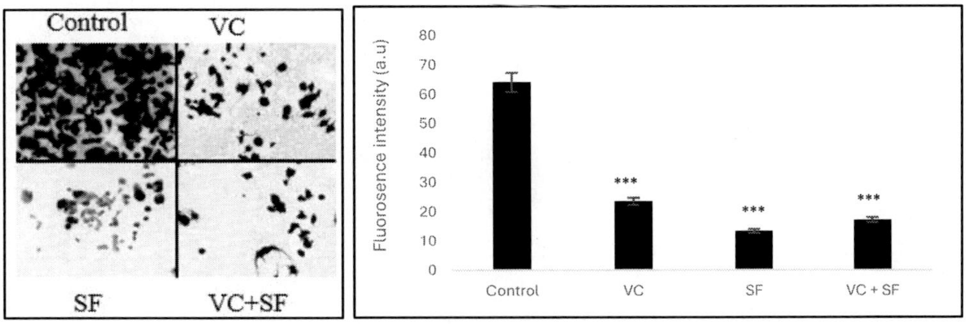

(a) (b)

Figure 6. Mitochondrial membrane potential in MCF7 cells after 24 h. of treatment. (a) Representative fluorescence microscopy images stained with Rhodamine 123, showing reduced fluorescence intensity in VC, SF, and combination groups relative to control. Scale bar = 100 μm. (b) Histogram of fluorescence intensity quantifying mitochondrial depolarization across groups. Data are expressed as mean ± SD of three experiments. ***$p < 0.001$ vs control (post hoc Newman–Keuls test).

Modulation of Bax, Bcl2, AIF, Cytochrome C

ROS generation was associated with modulation of mitochondrial apoptosis regulators. Combination treatment with VC and SF increased Bax expression and decreased BCl2 favoring a pro-apoptotic shift. In parallel, cytochrome c release was enhanced across treatments, consistent with mitochondrial membrane depolarization as well as AIF levels were increased compared to control (see Fig. 7).

Modulation Mitochondrial Signaling Proteins

Mitochondrial apoptosis involves activation of caspases in response to membrane depolarization showed treatment with SF, VC, or the combination led to increase in cas-9, cas-7, cas-3, cas-8, and Apaf-1 compared with the control indicate activation of both intrinsic and extrinsic apoptotic cascades. Combined SF and VC treatment markedly indicate a synergistic induction of mitochonrial apoptosis (see Fig. 8).

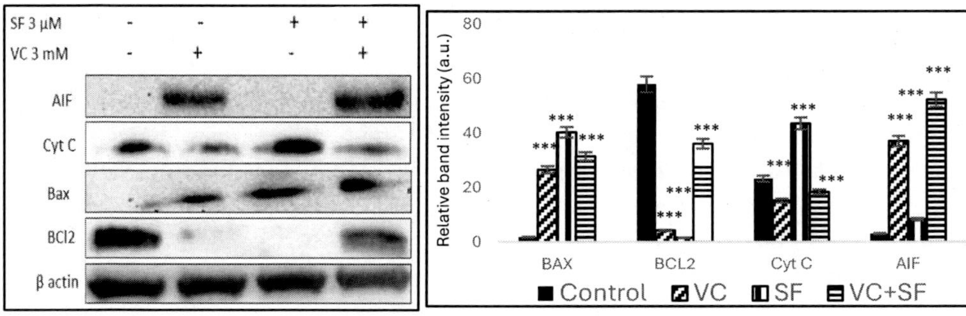

(a) (b)

Figure 7. (a) Western blot analysis showing the expression levels of Bax, Bcl2, cytochrome C, and AIF in MCF7 cells treated with VC, SF, and a combination of both. (b) Densitometric histogram compares relative protein levels normalized to β-actin. Data are presented as mean ± SD (n = 3); Significant changes are indicated by ***p < 0.001, according to the post hoc Newman-Keuls test.

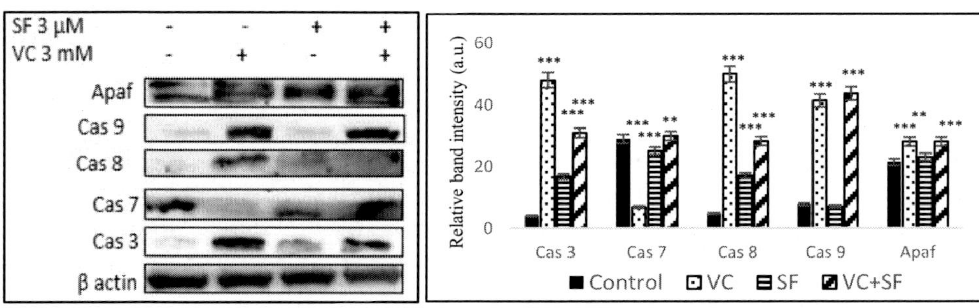

(a) (b)

Figure 8. Western blot analysis of Cas-3, -7, -8, -9, and Apaf in MCF7 cells, following treatment with VC, SF, or their combination. (a) Representative blots showing expression of these proteins. (b) Densitometric histogram compares relative protein levels normalized to β-actin. Data are expressed as mean ± SD (n = 3). Statistical significance was determined using the Newman–Keuls post hoc test (**P < 0.01, ***p < 0.001).

Modulation of MEK Kinase Pathway

To investigate the potential mechanism by which VC, SF, or their combination modulates aberrant cell signaling of mitogen-activated protein kinases (MAPKs), Western blot analysis was performed to assess the active and phosphorylated forms of mitogen-activated protein kinase kinase (MEK). Significant increases in the expressions of MEK-1, MEK-2, MEK-3, and MEK-4 showed unfavorable effect of VC and SF.

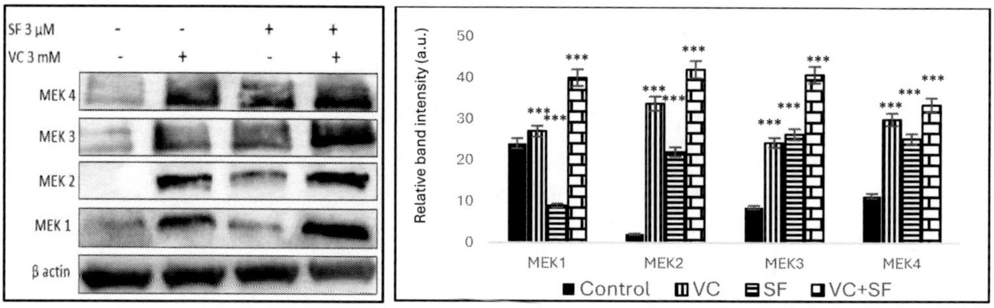

(a) (b)

Figure 9. Western blot analysis of MEK-1, -2, -3, and -4 after treating MCF7 cells with VC, SF, or their combination. (a) Representative blots showing expression of these proteins. (b) Densitometric histogram compares relative protein levels normalized to β-actin. Data are expressed as mean ± SD (n = 3). Significant change indicated by ***p < 0.001, according to the post hoc Newman-Keuls test.

Modulation of Cell Cycle Regulatory Proteins

Inhibition of cell cycle progression is also considered an important strategy in the management of breast cancer. Decreases in proteins involved in cell cycle regulation CDK7, CDK2, cyclin E, B1 and D1 were observed in all treatment of MCF7 with VC, SF or their combination. These proteins play critical roles in driving cell cycle progression through the G1/S and G2/M transitions; thus, their downregulation indicates inhibition of cell proliferation and induction of cell cycle arrest. The observed reductions reflect a favorable effect of VC or SF alone, further enhanced by their combination, suggesting cooperative suppression of cell cycle advancement in MCF7 cells (see Fig.10).

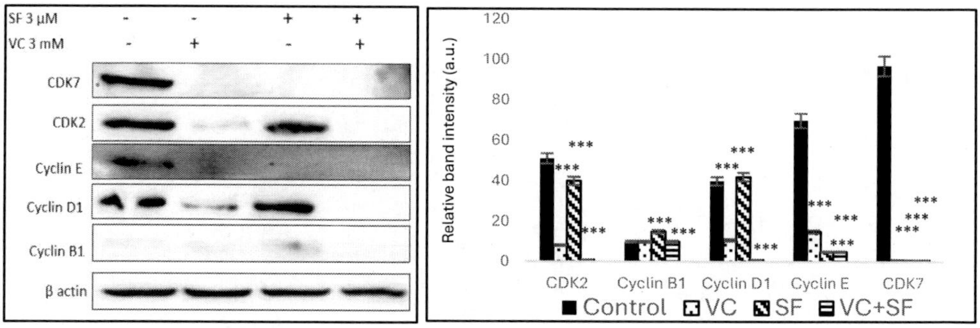

(a) (b)

Figure 10. Western blot analysis of cell cycle regulatory proteins in MCF7 cells after 24 h of treatment. (a) Representative blots of these proteins. (b) Densitometric histogram compares relative protein levels normalized to β-actin. Data are presented as mean ± SD (n = 3); Significant differences are indicated as ***p < 0.001 (post hoc Newman–Keuls test).

Modulation of p21, p53, PTEN, and MDM2

The impact of VC, SF, and their combination on the expression of key regulatory proteins, including p21, p27, PTEN, and MDM2, was assessed. Treatment with VC, SF, or their combination resulted in notable modulation of these proteins. Specifically, there was a significant increase in the expression levels of p21, p27, and PTEN, indicating a positive regulatory effect on cell cycle control and tumor suppression. In addition, the expression of MDM2 decreased, suggesting a potential inhibitory effect on the MDM2 pathway (see Fig. 11).

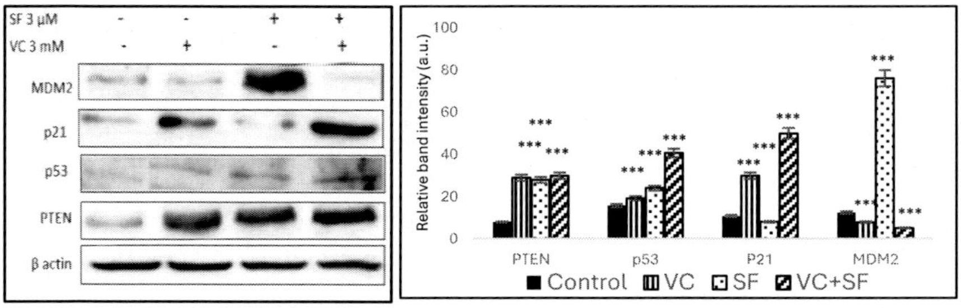

(a) (b)

Figure 11. Western blot analysis of cell cycles regulatory proteins in MCF7 cells after treatment with VC, SF, and their combination. (a) Representative blots showing the expression of these proteins. (b) Densitometric histogram compares relative protein levels normalized to β-actin. Data are expressed as mean ± SD (n = 3). Significant differences are indicated as ***p < 0.001, post hoc Newman–Keuls test.

Modulation of Akt/p85

Decrease in Akt and p85 proteins (also known as p13) after treatment of MCF7 cells with VC, SF or the combination shows favorable results. However, increase in Akt due to SF only showed that treatment of cells with VC overcome this protein that involves cancer progression.

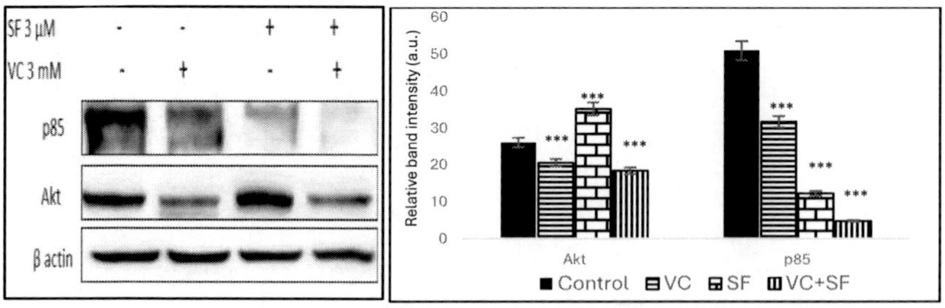

(a) (b)

Figure 12. Western blot analysis of Akt and p85 expressions after treatment of MCF7 cells with VC, SF, or their combination. (a) Representative blots showing expression of these proteins. (b) Densitometric histogram compares relative protein levels normalized to β-actin. Data are expressed as mean ± SD (n = 3). Statistical significance was determined using the Newman–Keuls post hoc test (***p < 0.001).

Modulation of SAPK/JNK and p38

The impact of VC, SF, and their combined treatment on SAPK/JNK and p38 proteins was evaluated. The combination of VC and SF resulted in a decrease in p38 and SAPK/JNK proteins, while individual treatments with SF led to an increase in p38 and SAPK/JNK. VC only treatment cause increased in SAP/JNK. When combined, VC and SF had synergistic effects causing decrease expression of p38 and SAPK/JNK.

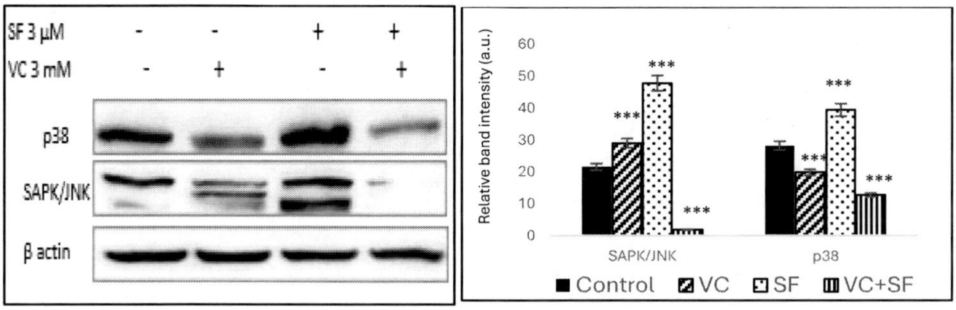

(a) (b)

Figure 13. Western blot analysis data of SAPK/JNK and p38 expressions after treatment of MCF7 cells with VC, SF, or their combination. (a) Representative blots showing expression of these proteins. (b) Densitometric histogram compares relative protein levels normalized to β-actin. Data are expressed as mean ± SD (n = 3). Significant changes are marked as ***p < 0.001, according to the post hoc Newman-Keuls test.

Modulation of ERK 1/2, EGFR, and Histone

Decreased expressions of ERK1/2, EGFR, and histone indicate a favorable effect of VC and SF in MCF7 cells. However, increase in ERK1/2 in SF only treatment was noticed as unfavorable effect of SF.

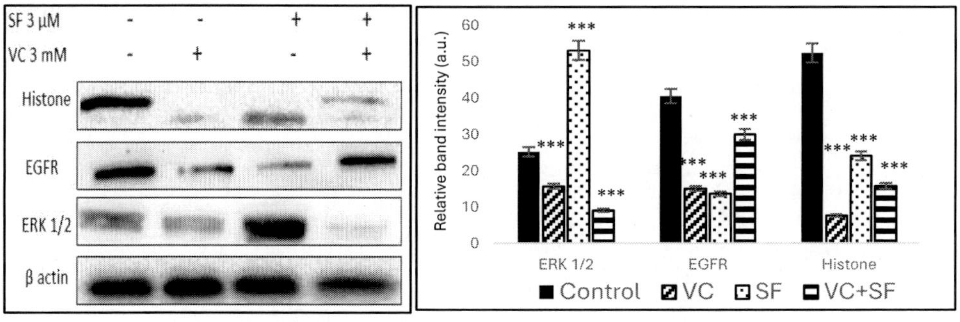

(a) (b)

Figure 14. Western blot analysis expressions of ERK 1/2, histone, and EGFR after the treatment of MCF7 cells with VC, SF, or their combination. (a) Representative blots showing expression of these proteins. (b) Densitometric histogram compares relative protein levels normalized to β-actin. Data are expressed as mean ± SD (n = 3). Significant changes are marked as ***p < 0.001, according to the post hoc Newman-Keuls test.

Modulation of Wnt 1, β-catenin, and ROCK

The effects of VC, AF, and their combination on Wnt, ROCK, and β-catenin proteins were examined in MCF7 cells. Western blot analysis showed that Wnt, ROCK, and β-catenin expression levels were significantly increased across all treatment groups, indicating an unfavorable regulatory effect of VC, SF, or their combination of these signaling proteins. Densitometric quantification confirmed these findings (see Fig. 15).

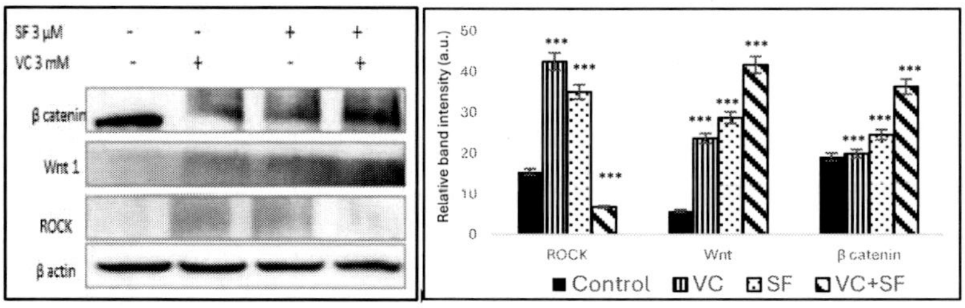

(a) (b)

Figure 15. Western blot analysis data of ROCK, β-catenin, and Wnt expressions after treatment of MCF7 cells with VC, SF, or their combination. (a) Representative blots showing expression of these proteins. (b) Densitometric histogram compares relative protein levels normalized to β-actin. Data are expressed as mean ± SD (n = 3). Significant changes are marked as ***p < 0.001, according to the post hoc Newman-Keuls test.

Modulation of MnSOD, Smac/Diablo, E-Cadherin, and Vimentin

Treatment of MCF-7 breast cancer cells with VC, SF, or their combination led to distinct modulation of apoptosis- and epithelial–mesenchymal transition (EMT)-related proteins. The combination treatment markedly decreased the expression of Smac/DIABLO but increased MnSOD, suggesting activation of mitochondrial oxidative stress responses rather than classical pro-apoptotic signaling. In addition, dual VC and SF exposure caused a pronounced reduction in vimentin and E-cadherin, indicating disruption of both epithelial and mesenchymal integrity. In contrast, SF alone induced an increase in E-cadherin, consistent with partial EMT reversion and limited cytoskeletal recovery (see Fig. 16).

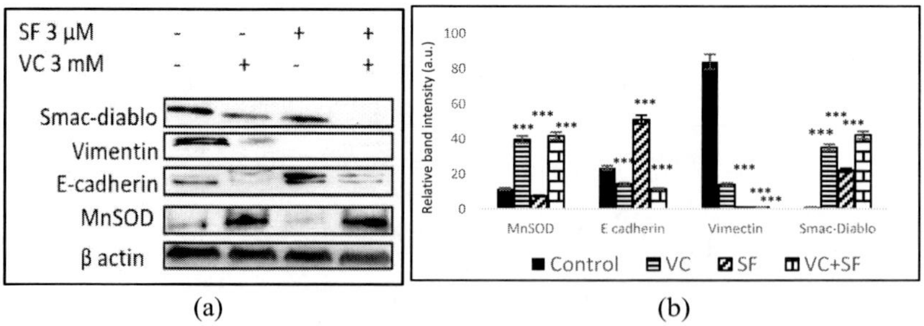

(a) (b)

Figure 16. Western blot analysis of MnSOD, E-cadherin, vimentin, and Smac/DIABLO expression in MCF-7 cells following treatment with VC, SF, or their combination. (a) Representative blots showing differential modulation of apoptotic and EMT-related proteins. (b) Densitometric histogram comparing relative protein levels normalized to β-actin. Data are expressed as mean ± SD (n = 3). Statistical significance was determined using the Newman–Keuls post hoc test (***p < 0.001).

Modulation of HER2, BRCA1, BRCA2, and ERα

Treatment of MCF-7 breast cancer cells with the combination of VC and SF led to a marked downregulation of HER2, BRCA1, BRCA2, and ERα expression compared with individual treatments. In contrast, treatment with VC or SF alone resulted in increased expression of ERα, BRCA1, and BRCA2, indicating potential activation of hormone receptor–associated signaling and DNA repair pathways. The combined VC and SF treatment thus appeared to override these individual effects, promoting a coordinated suppression of proliferative and survival-related markers.

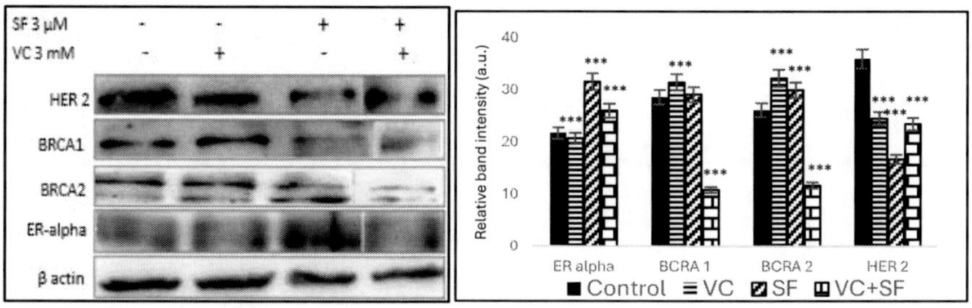

(a) (b)

Figure 17. Western blot analysis data showing the modulation of Erα, HER2, BRCA1 and BRCA2 after treatment of MCF7 cells with VC, SF and the combination. (a) Representative blots showing expression of these proteins. (b) Densitometric histogram compares relative protein levels normalized to β-actin. Data are expressed as mean ± SD (n = 3). Data are expressed as mean ± SD (n = 3). Significant changes are marked as ***p < 0.001, according to the post hoc Newman-Keuls test.

Modulation of MMP2 and MMP9

The effects of VC, SF, and their combination were evaluated in MCF7 cells, revealing a decrease in MMP9 expression with each treatment, while MMP2 slightly changed. MMP9 transcription may respond to oxidative stress and inflammatory signals, whereas MMP2, being less dependent on these pathways, likely maintains stable expression under similar conditions.

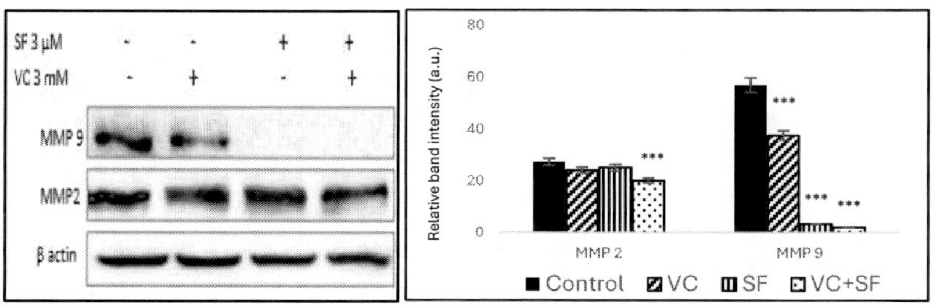

(a) (b)

Figure 18. Western blot analysis expressions of MMP9 and MMP2 in MCF7 after treatment with VC, SF or their combined treatment. (a) Representative blots showing expression of these proteins. (b) Densitometric histogram compares relative protein levels normalized to β-actin. Data are expressed as mean ± SD (n=3). Significant changes are marked as ** p< 0.01, ***p < 0.001, according to the post hoc Newman-Keuls test.

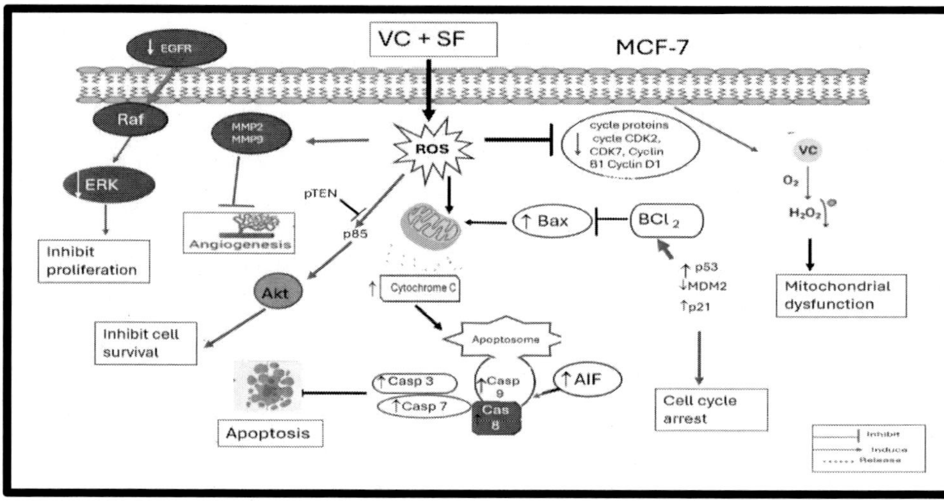

Figure 19. Proposed mechanistic model of VC and SF in breast cancer.

Discussion

As illustrated in Figure 19, the proposed mechanism of VC, SF, and their combination in MCF-7 cells elicits multifaceted effects such as inhibition of proliferation, prevention of angiogenesis, modulation of mitochondrial dysfunction, and apoptosis. Pharmacologic VC and SF individually increased ROS and triggered mitochondrial membrane depolarization, leading to cytochrome c release, Bax up-regulation, Bcl-2 down-regulation, and activation of caspase-9, -8, -7, and -3 together with Apaf-1. When combined, VC and SF produced a synergistic amplification of these mitochondrial apoptotic events, consistent with enhanced oxidative stress and mitochondrial damage. However, the combination caused a reduction in Smac/DIABLO expression, suggesting that despite strong mitochondrial perturbation, the execution of apoptosis may not be fully dependent on the canonical Smac-mediated caspase pathway. Instead, the marked increase in MnSOD implies an adaptive antioxidant response, and the cell death pattern may involve non-canonical oxidative or caspase-independent mechanisms such as necroptosis or paraptosis. These findings still align with previous reports that pharmacologic ascorbate and multi-kinase inhibitors cooperate through redox stress and mitochondrial collapse to promote tumor-cell death, though not always via uniform caspase activation [17–20].

Loss of mitochondrial membrane potential ($\Delta\Psi m$) and accumulation of intracellular ROS confirmed mitochondrial involvement. Increased MnSOD expression likely reflects a compensatory response to high ROS burden, yet the predominance of pro-apoptotic signals (cytochrome c release, Bax induction, and Bcl-2 suppression) indicates that antioxidant defense mechanisms were ultimately overwhelmed. The downregulation of Smac/DIABLO, however, points to a potential feedback restraint on apoptosis signaling - possibly due to mitochondrial exhaustion or altered IAP regulation under severe oxidative conditions. This dual signature of increase in MnSOD and decrease in Smac/DIABLO reinforces that VC and SF elicit a mixed oxidative stress–driven and caspase-modulated death program [18, 21].

Cell-cycle regulation was also affected. The observed decreases in CDK7, CDK2, and cyclins E, B1, and D1 after all treatments indicate suppression of proliferative capacity. Similar reductions in CDKs and cyclins following VC or SF exposure have been documented in other cancer models, supporting cell-cycle arrest as a secondary anticancer mechanism complementary to mitochondrial stress [22–23].

Signaling analysis revealed complex MAPK and PI3K/Akt responses. Individual VC or SF treatments elevated MEK isoforms and, in the case of SF, transiently increased ERK1/2, p38, and SAPK/JNK - patterns consistent with compensatory stress or survival signaling frequently reported after RAF- or RTK-targeted therapy [8]. VC alone enhanced SAPK/JNK activation, likely via ROS-mediated stress, whereas the combined VC and SF treatment reversed these increases, yielding decreased p38 and SAPK/JNK levels. Similarly, both agents reduced total Akt and p85 (PI3K) expression, but SF alone occasionally produced a rebound Akt increase that was abrogated by VC co-treatment. Together, these data suggest that VC suppresses adaptive pro-survival signaling provoked by SF, thereby strengthening the oxidative-stress-induced cell-death response. Such interplay between MAPK and PI3K/Akt pathways under redox stress has been widely documented [24–26].

Vitamin C and SF also modulated markers associated with EMT and invasion. Combination treatment reduced both vimentin and E-cadherin expression, whereas SF alone increased E-cadherin, indicating partial EMT reversal. The dual loss of vimentin and E-cadherin likely reflects cytoskeletal collapse during oxidative-mediated cell death, rather than a clean EMT switch [27]. Wound-healing assays showed enhanced migration in some conditions, though proliferation effects cannot be excluded. Previous work demonstrates that low oxidative doses of VC can promote, while high doses inhibit migration; thus dose- and time-dependent responses should be considered [28]. Moreover, the decrease in MMP9 with relatively stable MMP2 levels suggests that both VC and SF selectively suppress inducible matrix-degrading enzymes responsive to oxidative and inflammatory cues [29–30].

At the genomic and receptor-signaling level, VC or SF alone increased ERα, BRCA1, and BRCA2 expression, while the combination down-regulated these proteins together with HER2. Single-agent up-regulation likely represents a transient stress-response or hormone-receptor feedback; conversely, the combination's suppression of HER2 and ERα indicates effective inhibition of proliferative signaling. This dual regulation aligns with earlier findings that pharmacologic VC can create a "BRCAness" phenotype by attenuating homologous-recombination repair genes [31], whereas SF has been shown to promote BRCA1 degradation via TRIM21 [32]. Therefore, combined treatment may synergistically compromise DNA-repair capacity and hormonal growth signaling, enhancing cytotoxic efficacy.

Despite predominantly favorable apoptotic and anti-proliferative outcomes, several "unfavorable" responses were detected. MEK1–4 up-regulation and increased Wnt/β-catenin and ROCK expression across treatments could represent adaptive survival pathways. Wnt/β-catenin activation is a recognized resistance mechanism to kinase inhibitors, and persistent MEK elevation can mediate ERK reactivation ("RAF-paradox" signaling). The fact that VC and SF reduced ERK, p38, and SAPK/JNK but not Wnt components suggests partial escape through alternative pathways. Targeting these compensatory networks - such as combining with MEK or Wnt inhibitors - may further enhance therapeutic efficacy [33–35].

Collectively, these findings outline a coherent mechanism: VC and SF generate oxidative stress leading to mitochondrial depolarization, cytochrome c release, and caspase activation. However, the reduction of Smac/DIABLO and concurrent MnSOD elevation indicates that the combination invokes an oxidative-stress-dominant, partially caspase-independent pathway rather than pure intrinsic apoptosis. The combination treatment amplifies mitochondrial dysfunction while concurrently suppressing Akt, ERK, HER2, and ERα signaling and reducing cell-cycle regulators. The outcome is profound growth inhibition accompanied by redox imbalance and cytoskeletal collapse. Yet residual pro-survival signaling via MEK and Wnt/β-catenin underscores dynamic adaptation to combined oxidative and kinase stress. Further studies should explore antioxidant modulation, timing of Smac depletion, and the contribution of non-canonical death modes such as necroptosis or ferroptosis.

Conclusion

Pharmacologic VC potentiates SF-induced cytotoxicity in MCF-7 cells through oxidative stress–mediated mitochondrial damage, suppression of proliferative and survival signaling, and modulation of hormone- and DNA-repair pathways. The downregulation of Smac/DIABLO reframes this synergy as redox-driven rather than classical apoptosis-dominant, emphasizing the diverse cell-death modalities initiated by this promising combination therapy.

Key Findings

Combined treatment of VC and SF in MCF-7 breast cancer cells produced a distinct pattern of oxidative stress–driven cytotoxicity characterized by mitochondrial dysfunction, cell-cycle arrest, and modulation of multiple signaling pathways. Although both agents independently activated intrinsic apoptotic markers such as Bax, cytochrome c, and caspases, their combination resulted in reduced Smac/DIABLO expression and elevated MnSOD, suggesting a shift from canonical caspase-dependent apoptosis toward oxidative, caspase-independent cell death. The dual treatment also suppressed proliferative regulators (CDK2, CDK7, cyclins B1, D1, E) and growth-promoting signals (HER2, ERα, BRCA1/2, Akt, and ERK), while decreasing EMT markers (vimentin, E-cadherin) and matrix-degrading enzymes (MMP9). Collectively, these results indicate that VC potentiates SF cytotoxicity through amplified oxidative stress, mitochondrial destabilization, and suppression of survival and repair pathways, providing a mechanistic rationale for the therapeutic synergy of VC and SF in hormone-responsive breast cancer.

Acknowledgments

The author thanks Union University for the source and support of research funding as well as colleagues and editing tools for assistance with improving the clarity of the manuscript.

References

[1] Orrantia-Borunda E., Nuñez P.A., Acuña-Aguilar L.E., Gómez-Valles F.O., Ramírez-Valdespino C.A. Breast Cancer. In: Mayrovitz HN, editor. *Subtypes of Breast Cancer*. Brisbane, Exon Publications 2022.

[2] American Cancer Society. "Breast Cancer Facts & Figures 2022-2023." Atlanta: *American Cancer Society*, 2022. Available at: (https://www.cancer.org).

[3] Perou C.M., Eisen M.B., Jeffrey S.S., Rees C.A., Pollack J.R. Molecular portraits of human breast tumours. *Nature* 2000; 406: 747-752.

[4] Ductal Carcinoma in Situ and Invasive Ductal Carcinoma." Breastcancer.org, 2022. Available at: *https://www.breastcancer.org/symptoms/types/idc.*

[5] Goldhirsch A., Winer E.P., Coates A.S., Gelber R.D., Thurlimann B., Senn H.J. Personalizing the treatment of women with early breast cancer: highlights of the St Gallen International Expert Consensus on the Primary Therapy of Early Breast Cancer. *Annals of Oncology* 2013; 24: 2206-2223.

[6] Slamon D., Wiermann W., Robert N., Martin M., Press M., Mackey J. Adjuvant trastuzumab in HER2-positive breast cancer. *N Engl J Med* 2011; 365: 1273-1283.

[7] Harbeck N., Penault-Llorca F., Cortes J., Gnant M., Poortmans P., Ruddy K. Breast cancer. *Nature Reviews Disease Primers* 2019; 5: 66.

[8] Llovet J.M., Ricci S., Mazzaferro V., Hilgard P., Gane E. Sorafenib in advanced hepatocellular carcinoma. *N Engl J Med* 2008; 359: 378-390.

[9] Escudier B., Eisen T., Stadler W.M., Audard S., Negrier S. Sorafenib in advanced clear-cell renal-cell carcinoma. *N Engl J Med* 2007; 356: 125-134.

[10] Brose M.S., Nutting C.M., Elisei R., Siena S., Bastholt L. Sorafenib in radioactive iodine-refractory, locally advanced or metastatic differentiated thyroid cancer : a randomized, double-blind, phase 3 trial. *The Lancet* 2014 ; 384 : 319-328.

[11] Wilhelm S.M., Adnane L., Newell P., Villanueva A., Llovet J.M., Lynch M. Preclinical overview of sorafenib, a multikinase inhibitor that targets both RAF/MEK/ERK pathway and receptor tyrosine kinases involved in tumor progression and angiogenesis. *Cancer Research* 2004 ; 64: 7099-7109.

[12] Chen Q., Espey M.G., Krishna M.C., Mitchell J.B., Corpe C.P., Buettner G.R., et al., Pharmacological ascorbic acid concentrations selectively kill cancer cells : action as a pro-drug to deliver hydrogen peroxide to tissues. *PNAS* 2005 ; 102 : 13604-13609.

[13] Chen Q., Espey M.G., Sun A.Y., Lee J.H., Buettner G.R., Levine M. Ascorbate in pharmacologic concentration selectively generate ascorbate radical and hydrogen peroxide in extracellular fluid *in vivo*. *PNAS* 2007 ; 104 : 8749-8754.

[14] Olney K.E., Du J., Van Erve T.J., Witmer J.R., Wagner B.A., Buettner G.R., et al., Inhibitors of hydroperoxide metabolism enhance ascorbate-induce cytotoxicity. *Free Radic Res* 2013 ; 47 :154-163.

[15] Soule H.D., Vazquez J., Long A., Albert S., Brennan M. A human cell line from a pleural effusion derived from a breast carcinoma. *J of the Nat Cancer Inst* 1973 ; 51 (5) : 1409–1416.

[16] Horwitz K.B., Costlow M.E., McGuire W.L. MCF-7 : A human breast cancer cell line with estrogen, androgen, progesterone, and glucocorticoid receptors. *Steroids* 1975 ;26(6) :785-795.

[17] Rouleau L., Antony A.N., Bisetto S., Newberg A., Doria C., Levine M., et al., Synergistic effects of ascorbate and sorafenib in hepatocellular carcinoma: New insights into ascorbate cytotoxicity. *Free Rad Biol & Med* 2016 ; 95 : 308-322.

[18] Böttger F., Valles-Marti A., Cahn L., Jimenez C.R. High-dose intravenous vitamin C, a promising multi-targeting agent in the treatment of cancer. *J Exper & Clin Cancer Res* 2021 ; 40 : 343.

[19] Redza-Dutordoir M., Averill-Bates D. Activation of apoptosis signaling pathways by reactive oxygen species. *BBA* 2016 ; 1863 : 2977-2992.

[20] Mustafa M., Ahmad R., Tantry I.Q., Ahmad W., Siddiqui S., Alam M., et al., Apoptosis: A Comprehensive Overview of Signaling pathways, morphological changes, and physiological significance and therapeutic implications. *Cells* 2024 ; 13(22) : 1838.

[21] Rafat S., Hakami M.A., Hazazi A., Alsairi A.A., Rashid S., Hasan M.R., et al., Inhibition of autophagy and the cytoprotective role of Smac mimetic against ROS induced cancer: A potential therapeutic strategy in relapse and chemoresistance cases in breast cancer. *Curr Issues Mol Biol* 2023 ; 45(7) : 5752-5762.

[22] El Banna N., Hatem E., Masurel A.H., Leger T., Baille D., Vernis L., et al., Redox modifications of cysteine-containing proteins, cell cycle arrest and translation inhibition: involvement in vitamin C-induced breast cancer cell death. *Redox Biology* 2019 ; 26 : 101290.

[23] Bennett L.L., Mondal A. Curcumin and afatinib synergistically inhibit growth of human osteosarcoma cells by inhibition of matrix metallo proteinases, mitogen activated kinases 1-4, and reactive oxygen species. *J of Pharm and Drug Dev* 2021 ; 3, 1.

[24] Lohmeyer J., Nerreter T., Dotterweich J., Einsele H., Bernhardt R.S. Sorafenib paradoxically activates the RAS/RAF/ERK pathway in polyclonal human NK cells during expansion and thereby enhances effector functions in a dose- and time-dependent manner. *Clin Exp Immunol* 2018 ; 193 : 64-72.

[25] Zheng H., Xu Y., Liehn E.A., Rusu M. Vitamin C as scavenger of reactive oxygen species during healing after myocardial infarction. *Int J Mol Sci* 2024 ; 25(6), 3114.

[26] Panka D.J., Cho D.C., Atkins M.B., Mier J.W. GSK-3β inhibition enhances sorafenib-induced apoptosis in melanoma cell lines. *J Biol Chem* 2008 ; 2, 283.

[27] Zeng L.H., Wang Q.M., Feng L.Y., Ke Y.D., Xu Q.Z., Wei A.Y., et al., High dose vitamin C suppresses the invasion and metastasis of breast cancer cells via inhibiting epithelial-mesenchymal transition. *Oncol Target & Ther* 2019 ; 10 : 7405-7413.

[28] Kashif M., Yao H., Schmidt S., Chen X., Truong M., Tuksammel E., et al., ROS-lowering doses of vitamin C - Accelerate malignant melanoma metastasis. *Redox Biol* 2023 ; 60, 102619.

[29] Wei J., Meng F.D., Qu K., Wang Z., Wu Q., Zhang L., et al., Sorafenib inhibits proliferation and invasion of human hepatocellular carcinoma cells via up-regulation of p53 and suppress FoxM1. *Acta Pharmacologica Sinica* 2015 ; 36 : 241-251.

[30] Bennett L.L. Effects of pharmacological dose of vitamin C on MDA-MB-231 cells. *Biomedicines* 2025 ; 13(3) : 640.

[31] Ma Y., Chen P., Driskon J.A., Khabele D., Godwin A.K., Chen Q. Pharmacological ascorbate induces 'BRCAness' and enhances the effects of Poly (ADP-ribose) polymerase inhibitors against BRCA1/2 wild-type ovarian cancer. *Oncol Lett* 2020 ; 19(4) : 2629-2638.

[32] Huang N., Li P., Sun X., Tong L., Dong X., Zhang X., et al., TRIM21 mediates the synergistic effect of olaparib and sorafenib by degrading BRCA1 through ubiquitination in TNBC. *NPJ Breast Cancer* 2023 ; 9, 85.

[33] Hong R.Y., Min S., Huang J., Zou M., Zhou D.Y., Liang Y. High-dose vitamin C promotes mitochondrial biogenesis in HCT116 colorectal cancer cells by regulating the AMPK/PGC-1α. *J Cancer Res Oncol* 2025 ; 151, 167.

[34] Kim J.H., Hwang S., Lee J.H., Im S.S., Son J. Vitamin C suppresses pancreatic carcinogenesis through the inhibition of both glucose metabolism and Wnt signaling. *Int J Mol Sci* 2022 ; 23 (20), 12249.

[35] Merikhian P., Eisavand M.R., Farahmand L. Triple-negative breast cancer: understanding Wnt signaling in drug resistant. *Cancer Cell Inter* 2021 ; 21, 419.

Chapter 12

Expert Commentary: Vitamin C in Triple-Negative Breast Cancer (MDA-MB-231)

Lunawati L. Bennett*, PhD, PharmD
Union University, College of Pharmacy, Jackson, Tennessee, USA

Introduction

Triple-negative breast cancer (TNBC) remains among the most treatment-resistant and aggressive forms of breast malignancy. It is characterized by the absence of estrogen receptor (ER-), progesterone receptor (PR-), and human epidermal growth factor receptor 2 (HER2-) expression; therefore, it is lacking molecular targets using existing therapies. Because of this, TNBC continues to pose major clinical challenges and carries a poorer prognosis than other subtypes of breast cancers.

In chapter 11, I discussed the interaction of pharmacological vitamin C (VC) with standard antineoplastic agents in hormone-receptor-positive MCF7 cells. To extend these findings into a more resistant model, I investigated the direct effect of high-dose VC on MDA-MB-231, a representative of TNBC line. This study, later published in *Biomedicines,* offered an opportunity to examine how VC alone might influence cell survival, redox balance, and metastatic potential in an inherently aggressive phenotype [1].

Insights from the Published Study

The investigation revealed several striking features of pharmacological VC in TNBC cells. When MDA-MB-231 cells were exposed to concentrations between 4 mM and 16 mM, a clear dose-dependent decline in cells viability was observed, reaching roughly 50% reduction at the highest dose. Morphological changes typical of apoptosis appeared within 24 h of exposure.

Molecular analyses confirmed activation of both intrinsic and extrinsic apoptotic pathways, marked by increased expression of caspases 7, 8, 9 and Apaf-1. VC also enhanced p53 and p21 expression, consistent with DNA-damage signaling and cell-cycle arrest. Interestingly, metastatic regulators MMP-2 and MMP-9 were markedly reduced, implying that VC may suppress matrix degradation and limit invasive behavior.

---

* Corresponding Author's Email: llbennett@uu.edu

Equally important, parallel exposure of non-cancerous HEK 293 cells showed minimal toxicity at comparable concentrations, suggesting a measure of tumor selectivity. Together, these findings indicate that pharmacological VC alone can trigger apoptosis and dampening metastatic signaling in TNBC cells without broadly harming normal counterparts.

Comparison with MCF7 Observations

When viewed alongside the MCF7 results (Chapter 12), several patterns emerge. While MCF7 cells responded to lower VC concentrations, MDA-MB-231 cells required higher doses to achieve comparable cytotoxicity - reflecting their notorious resistance and altered redox metabolism. Yet both cell types converged on similar terminal pathways: activation of caspases, induction of p53/p21, and reduction in pro-metastatic proteins.

This suggests that the fundamental antineoplastic mechanism of vitamin C - oxidative stress induction leading to apoptotic signaling - operates across distinct molecular backgrounds, though the sensitivity threshold varies with tumor subtype.

Reflections and Future Directions

The MDA-MB-231 study was intentionally designed to isolate the intrinsic molecular actions of VC without additional pharmacologic interference. Combination trials with antineoplastic drugs were not pursued at that stage due to laboratory contamination and scheduling constraints. Rather than a limitation, this separation provided a valuable opportunity to observe VC's independent effects within a highly aggressive model.

Future work will integrate VC with standard chemotherapeutics to determine whether synergistic activity extends to receptor-negative contexts. Such studies are particularly relevant given the urgent need for new therapeutic strategies in TNBC, where conventional treatments often fail to produce durable responses.

Expert Perspective

Reflecting on these findings, I am convinced that VC's anticancer potential lies in its ability to modulate redox-dependent survival signaling and restore apoptotic competence even in resistant cells. While MCF7 and MDA-MB-231 differ in receptor status and molecular phenotype, both demonstrate that pharmacological VC can disrupt key hallmarks of malignancy - proliferation, invasion, and evasion of cell death.

The body of evidence from these studies emphasizes a unifying theme: VC is not merely a nutritional compound but a powerful biochemical modulator with context-dependent anticancer properties. Continued research exploring its combination with targeted or cytotoxic agents may open new possibilities for managing aggressive and treatment-refractory tumors such as TNBC.

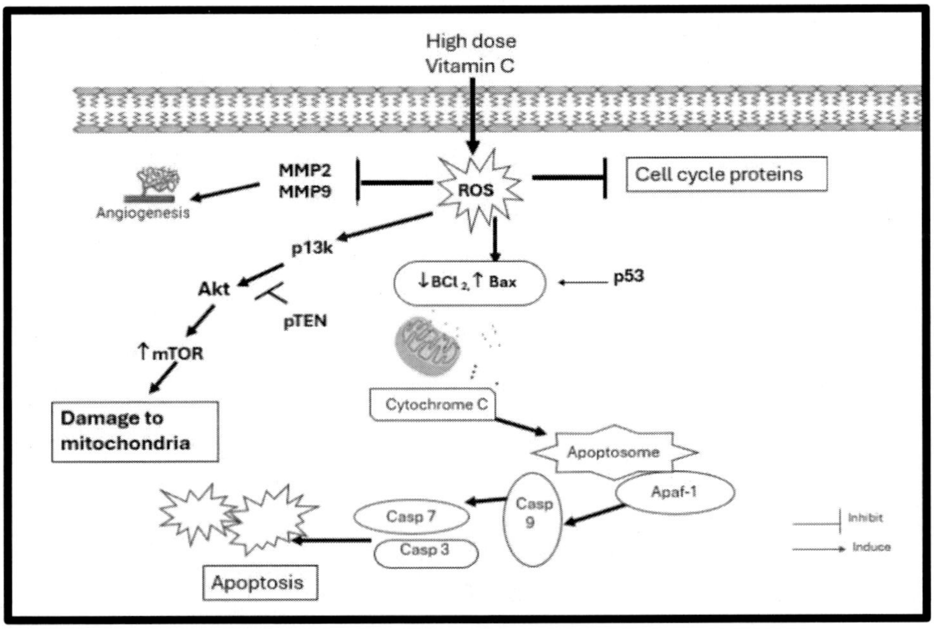

Figure 1. The inhibit is ROS inhibit MMP2, MMP9. ROS inhibit cell cycle progression. PTEN inhibit conversion p13k to Akt.

Reference

[1] Bennett L.L. Pharmacological Vitamin C Induces Apoptosis and Suppresses Metastatic Pathways in MDA-MB-231 Cells. *Biomedicines* 2025 ; 13(3) : 640.

Chapter 13

Redox Modulation and Kinase Signaling Crosstalk by Vitamin C and Sorafenib in Metastatic Prostate Cancer Cells

Lunawati L. Bennett*, PhD, PharmD
Union University, College of Pharmacy, Jackson, Tennessee, USA

Abstract

Prostate cancer remains a leading cause of cancer-related mortality among men, with metastatic disease presenting significant therapeutic challenges due to resistance and limited treatment responsiveness. This study investigated whether pharmacologic concentrations of vitamin C enhance the anticancer efficacy of low dose sorafenib in LNCaP clone FGC prostate cancer cells. Cell viability (SRB), mitochondrial membrane potential (Rhodamine 123), nuclear morphology (Hoechst 33342), and Western blot analyses were used to evaluate treatment effects.

Vitamin C alone and sorafenib alone each reduced cell viability and induced apoptotic signaling. When combined, vitamin C enhanced sorafenib-induced pro-apoptotic responses, including increased Bax, p21, PTEN, and p53 expression, along with decreased Bcl-2, Akt, p85, MDM2, and MEK1–4 levels, indicating mitochondrial-dependent apoptosis and partial suppression of survival signaling. However, the combination also activated compensatory pathways, including elements of the MAPK/PI3K-Akt and Wnt/β-catenin networks, which attenuated the extent of final apoptotic commitment despite effect-level synergy.

These findings suggest that vitamin C can potentiate sorafenib-induced apoptotic signaling, but that adaptive survival feedback limits full synergistic cytotoxicity. Therefore, optimal therapeutic benefit in prostate cancer may require co-targeting of compensatory pathways alongside vitamin C and sorafenib.

Keywords: prostate cancer, vitamin C, sorafenib, metastatic prostate cancer, crosstalk

Abbreviations

MAPKs	Mitogen-activated protein kinases;
MEKs	Mitogen-activated protein kinase kinases;
MDM2	Mouse double minute 2 homolog;

* Corresponding Author's Email: llbennett@uu.edu

MnSOD	Manganese superoxide dismutase;
p85	Phosphatidylinositol-3-kinase;
PTEN	Phosphatase and tensin homolog;
ROCK	Rho-associated kinase;
ROS	Reactive oxygen species.

Introduction

Prostate cancer (PC) is a significant malignancy affecting men over the age of 70 and is a major contributor to global mortality rates [1-2]. This cancer caused 358,989 deaths worldwide with about 1.3 million new diagnoses [3]. Currently, about 10 million men globally live with PC, with roughly 700,000 having metastatic forms, the more deadly form, of the disease [4-5].

Prostate cancer is divided into central, transitional, and peripheral regions. More than 95% of PC cases are adenocarcinomas, primarily of acinar origin, with a few being of ductal origin [6]. If diagnosed at an early stage, the survival rate for men with localized PC can be as high as 99% [7]. Late-stage PC with distant metastases have a poor five-year survival rate. The mortality rate is expected to double by 2040 [4].

Docetaxel (Taxotere ®) is the chemotherapy used for PC [8]. This agent inhibits microtubule depolymerization, suppressing mitotic cell division thus causing apoptosis [9] However, resistance and relapses due to multidrug resistance (MDR1) highlight the need for using more efficacious drug or combination therapy with other antineoplastics [10].

High dose intravenous vitamin C combined with docetaxel in metastatic castration-resistant PC had been tried in phase II trial. The study was suspended early due to VC did not improving prostate specific antigen (PSA) response [11]. VC had also been used with pantoprazole in metastatic resistant PC with better therapeutic outcomes than treatment with VC or pantoprazole alone [12].

To evaluate the cytotoxic potential of high-dose VC, various antineoplastic agents - including paclitaxel, doxorubicin, etoposide, temsirolimus, bortezomib, afatinib, and sorafenib - were tested on human pancreatic cancer using the model LNCaP clone FGC cell line. For combination studies, the lowest concentrations of each antineoplastic and high-dose VC that yielded a synergistic reduction in cell viability were selected. General experimental procedures followed the protocols outlined in Chapter 3 (Materials and Methods), while methodological details specific to this study are described below.

Cell Culture

The LNCaP clone FGC (ATCC CRL-1740) was cultured in RPMI-1640 medium supplemented with 10% fetal bovine serum (FBS) and 1% penicillin-streptomycin. Cells were maintained in T75 flasks at 37°C in a humidified atmosphere containing 5% CO_2. It is a well-established human prostate adenocarcinoma cell line derived from a lymph node metastasis of a 50-year-old patient. It is androgen-sensitive and widely used as a model for metastatic prostate cancer, particularly for studies of androgen receptor signaling, apoptosis, and therapeutic responses. LNCaP FGC cells exhibit epithelial morphology.

Results

Cell Viability and Selection of Doses

Treatment of LNCaP clone FGC cells with increasing concentrations of VC (0.3–20 mM) for 24 h revealed a dose-dependent reduction in cell viability. Cell survival remained approximately 50% across concentrations ranging from 0.3 to 10 mM but dropped sharply to about 40% at 20 mM VC. Based on this pattern, 10 mM was selected as the optimal working concentration for subsequent assays to assess molecular and cellular responses. Similarly, treatment with SF alone caused a concentration-dependent decline in viability, with approximately 50% cell death observed at 0.6 μM. This dose was therefore chosen for the combination studies. When VC (10 mM) was combined with SF (0.6 μM), cell viability was further reduced compared to either treatment alone, indicating a potential synergistic interaction that enhanced cytotoxicity in prostate cancer cells. The Chou–Talalay analysis indicates effect-level synergy in drug interaction, but downstream compensatory survival signaling limited the net apoptotic response.

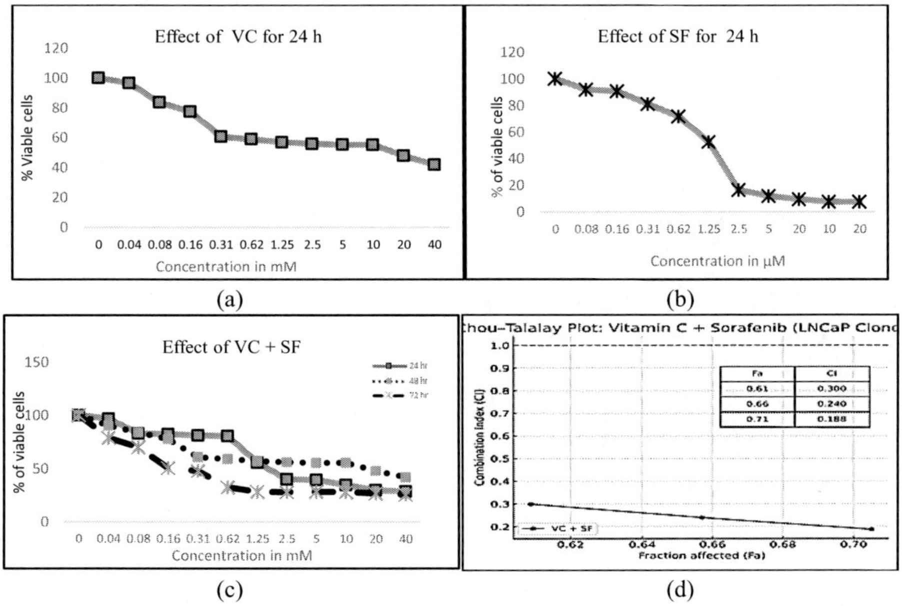

Figure 1. Effect of VC and SF on cell viability of LNCaP clone FGC cells. (a) Cells were treated with increasing concentrations of VC (0.04–40 mM). (b) Dose–response curve of SF (0.1– 20 μM). (c) Combined treatment with VC (10 mM) and SF (0.6 μM) further reduced viability compared to either VC or SF alone. Data is expressed as mean ± SD of triplicate experiments. (d) Chou-Talalay plot showed VC and SF interactions were limited due to feedback survival signaling.

Changes in Cell Morphology

VC and SF resulted in alteration morphologies of LNCaP clone FGC cells. While control cells remained healthy, showing increased numbers and adherence after 24 h, cells treated with VC or ET alone exhibited reduced viability and morphological changes. The combination treatment led to even greater cell death, with many cells appearing floating in the culture dish.

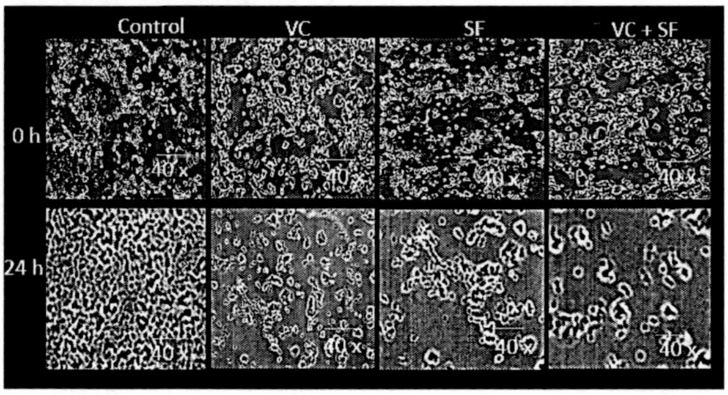

Figure 2. Inverted microscopic images of cells (40X) after 24 h treatment with VC, SF, or the combination.

Wound-Healing

After 24 h treatment of LNCaP clone FGC cells, the combination of VC and SF led to significantly reduced migration of cells, resulting in a wider wound gap compared to treatments with VC or SF alone. In contrast, control cells migrated closer together, indicating early signs of invasion and potential cancer metastasis. The histogram comparing the wound widths across control, VC, SF, and combination treatments.

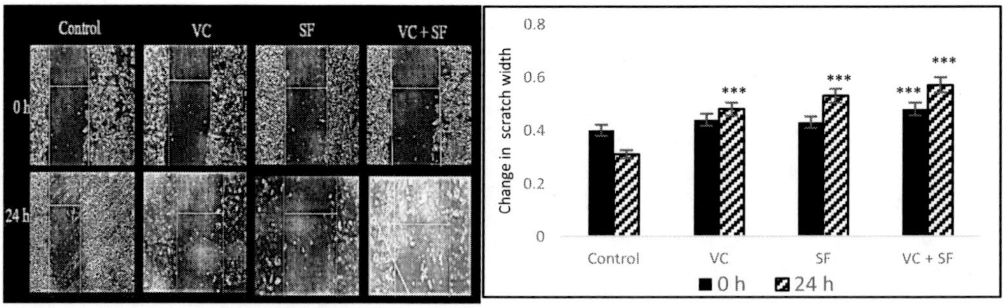

(a) (b)

Figure 3. (a) Presents the results of the wound healing assay for LNCaP clone FGC cells comparing 0 and 24 h. (b) Shows a histogram comparing wound widths across different treatment groups. Data is expressed as mean ± SD of triplicate experiments. Significant difference indicated by ***$p < 0.001$, according to the post hoc Newman-Keuls test.

Induction of Apoptosis

The combination of VC and SF resulted in a higher rate of apoptosis in LNCaP clone FGC cells compared to treatment with VC or SF alone. This finding, confirmed by Hoechst 33342 staining and observed in fluorescence microscopy images shown that control had less apoptotic cells than the treatments.

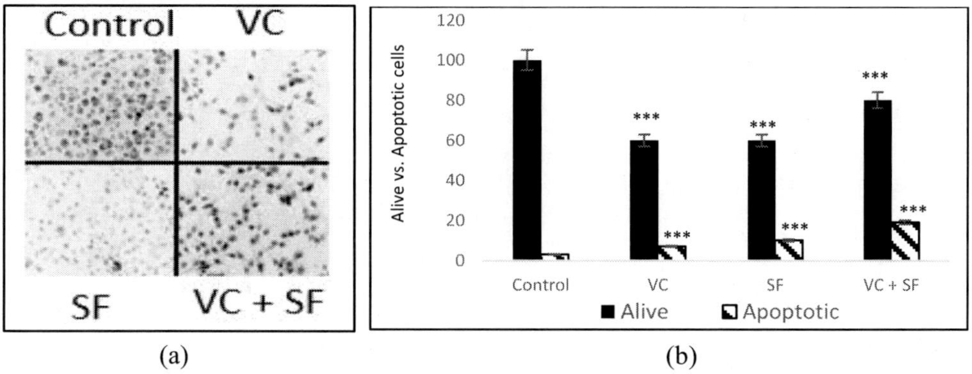

Figure 4. (a) Shows fluorescence microscopic images of LNCaP clone FGC cells treated for 24 h with VC, SF, or their combination. (b) Presents a histogram of the percentage of apoptotic cells relative to alive cells. Data is expressed as mean ± SD of triplicate experiments. A significant increase in apoptotic cells was observed, with ** $p < 0.01$, ***$p < 0.001$, as determined by the post hoc Newman-Keuls test.

Intracellular ROS Generation

The generation of intracellular ROS in LNCaP clone FGC cells following treatment with VC, SF, or their combination, using H2DCFDA staining. Higher ROS generation indicated by increased fluorescence intensity, with darker colors indicating lower ROS generation. Histogram of fluorescence intensity corresponding to the VC, SF, and combined treatments (see Fig 5).

Mitochondrial Membrane Potential (Ψ_m)

The generation of ROS in LNCaP clone FGC indicated cell death attributed to the depletion of mitochondrial membrane potential, as detected with Rhodamine 123 staining. Treatments with VC, SF, or the combination induced cell death, as shown in the fluorescence microscopic images. Control cells exhibited higher fluorescence intensity, indicating healthy mitochondria (see Fig. 6).

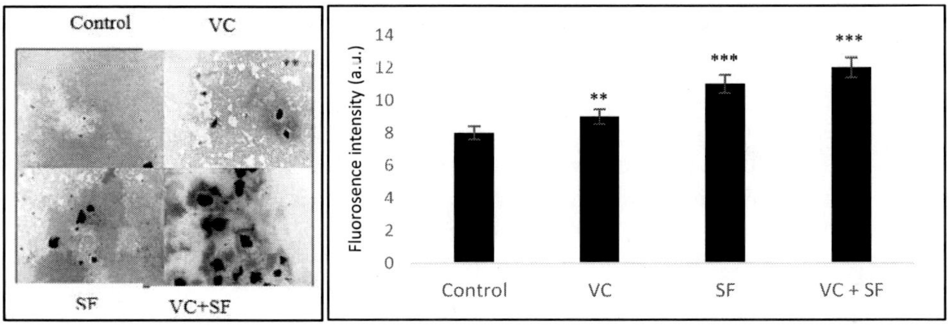

(a) (b)

Figure 5. (a) Shows the results of intracellular ROS generation assessed with H2DCF staining, with a scale bar indicating 100 μm. Figure 5(b) Presents a histogram illustrating the band intensity corresponding to treatments with VC, SF or their combination versus the control of LNCaP clone FGC. Data is expressed as mean ± SD of triplicate experiments. A significant change in ROS levels was observed, indicated by ** $p < 0.01$, ***$p < 0.001$, according to the post hoc Newman-Keuls test.

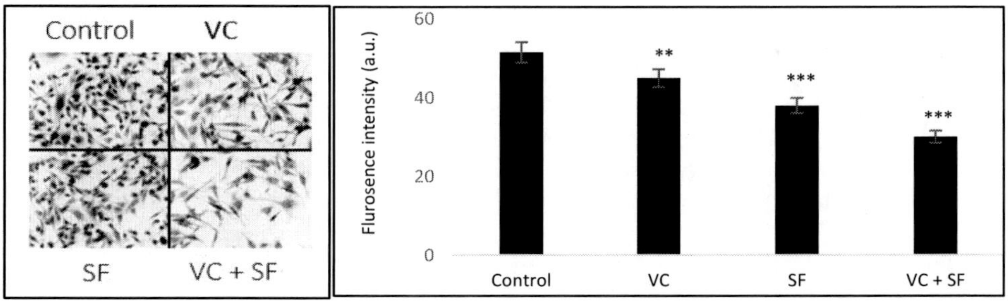

(a) (b)

Figure 6. (a) Shows the results of fluorescence microscopic examination depicting changes in mitochondrial membrane depolarization in treated cells compared to LNCaP clone FGC control cells. The scale bar represents 100 μm. (b) Presents a histogram illustrating the fluorescence intensity corresponding to the control, VC, SF, or combination treatments, with a significant decrease indicated by ***$p < 0.001$, according to the post hoc Newman-Keuls test. Data is expressed as mean ± SD of triplicate experiments.

Modulation of Bax, Bcl2, AIF, and Cytochrome C

In apoptotic cells, the intracellular generation of ROS is linked to alterations in the expressions of Bax and Bcl2 proteins. The Western blot analysis shows an increase in Bax, a decrease in Bcl2, and an increased release of cytochrome C into the cytosol, which further induced apoptosis in LNCaP clone FGC cells. An increase in the expression of apoptosis-inducing factor (AIF) was observed in all treated cells.

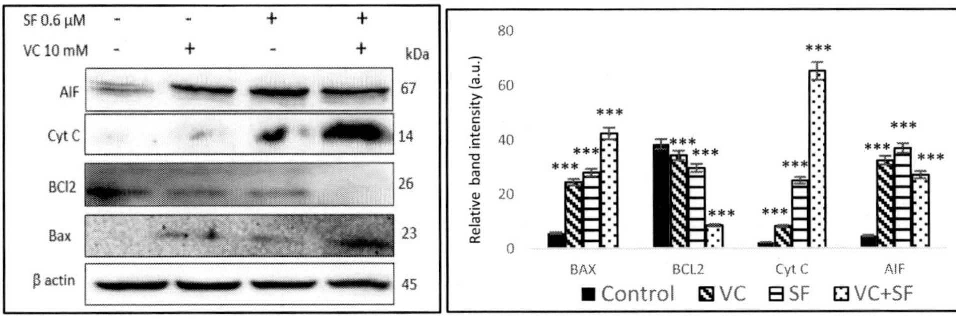

(a) (b)

Figure 7. Western blot analysis of Bax, Bcl2, AIF, and cyt C expressions in LNCaP clone FGC cells following treatment with VC, SF, or their combination (a) Representative blots showing expression of these proteins. (b) Densitometric histogram compares relative protein levels normalized to β-actin. Data is expressed as mean ± SD of triplicate experiments. Significant changes are indicated by ***$p < 0.001$, according to the post hoc Newman-Keuls test.

Modulation Mitochondrial Signaling Proteins

Mitochondrial apoptosis resulting from a decline in membrane potential is linked to various crucial proteins, including caspases (Cas-9, -3, -7, and -8). Treatment with VC, SF caused increase in caspases expression, indicate activation of both intrinsic and extrinsic apoptotic cascades, with the combination caused further increasement. The decrease in XIAP (X-linked inhibitor of apoptosis) confirmed the effect of VC and SF on LNCaP clone FGC cells.

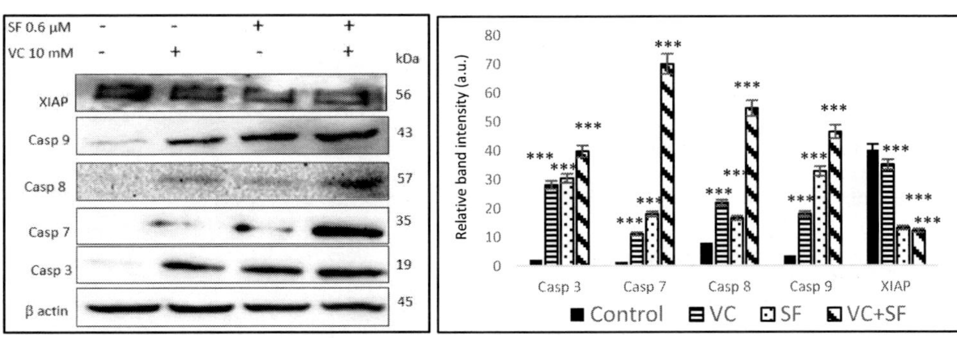

(a) (b)

Figure 8. Western blot analysis results of Cas-3, -7, -8, -9, and XIAP after treatment of cells with VC, SF, and the combination. (a) Representative blots showing expression of these proteins. (b) Densitometric histogram compares relative protein levels normalized to β-actin. Data is expressed as mean ± SD of triplicate experiments. Significant changes ***$p < 0.001$, according to the post hoc Newman-Keuls test.

Modulation of MEK Kinase Pathway

To investigate the potential mechanism of VC, SF, or the combination in modulating aberrant cell signaling of mitogen-activated protein kinases (MAPKs), Western blot analysis was conducted to assess the active and phosphorylated forms of mitogen-activated protein kinase kinase (MEK). Significant decreases in MEK-1, -2, -3, and -4 expressions were observed in LNCaP clone FGC cells.

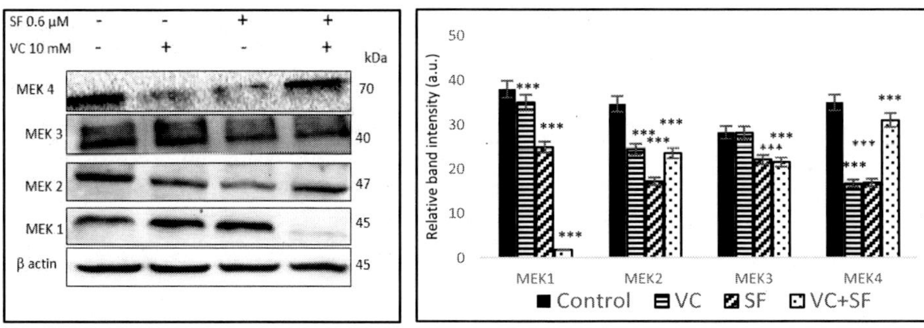

(a) (b)

Figure 9. Western blot analysis of MEK-1, -2, -3, and -4 after treating LNCaP clone FGC cells with VC, SF, or their combination. (a) Representative blots showing expression of these proteins. (b) Densitometric histogram compares relative protein levels normalized to β-actin. Data are expressed as mean ± SD (n = 3), with a significant change indicated by ***p < 0.001, according to the post hoc Newman-Keuls test.

Modulation of Cell Cycle Regulatory Proteins

Inhibition of cell cycle progression is also considered an important strategy in the management of PC. Increases in proteins involved in cell cycle regulation CDk7, CDk2, cyclin B1 and cyclin D1 were observed in all treatment of LNCaP clone FGC cells with VC, SF or their combination showing unfavorable effect.

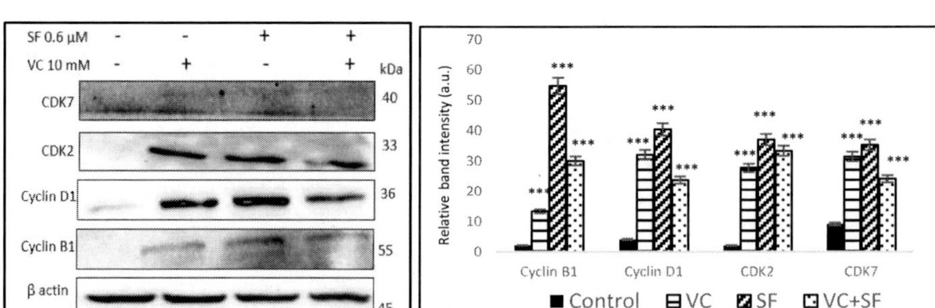

(a) (b)

Figure 10. Western blot analysis of cyclin B1, cyclin D1, CDK2, and CDK7 expressions after treating LNCaP clone FGC cells with VC, SF, or the combination. (a) Representative blots showing expression of these proteins. (b) Densitometric histogram compares relative protein levels normalized to β-actin. Data are expressed as mean ± SD (n = 3). Significant increases are indicated as ***p < 0.001, according to the post hoc Newman-Keuls test.

Modulation of p21, p27, PTEN, and MDM2

The impact of VC, SF, and their combination was tested on LNCaP clone FGC cells for key regulatory proteins of p21, p27, PTEN, and MDM. Treatment with VC, SF, or their combination resulted in notable modulation of these proteins. There was a significant increase in the expression levels of p21, p27 and PTEN indicative of a positive regulatory effect on cell cycle control and tumor suppression. Conversely, the expression of MDM2 decreased, suggesting a potential inhibitory effect on the MDM2 pathway.

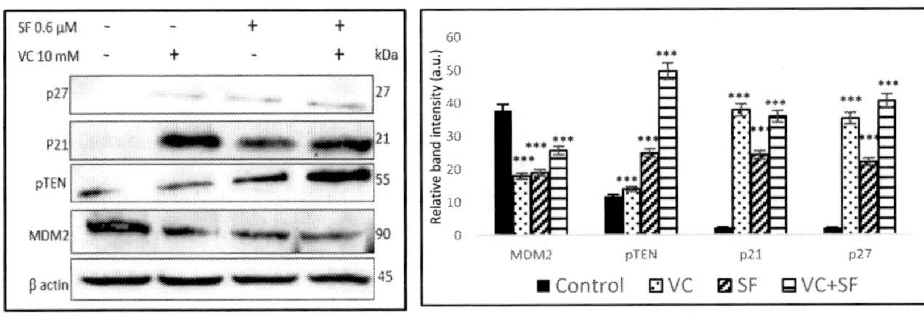

(a) (b)

Figure 11. Western blot analysis of p21, p27, PTEN, and MDM expressions in LNCaP clone FGC cells after treatment with VC, SF, and their combination. (a) Representative blots showing expression of these proteins. (b) Densitometric histogram compares relative protein levels normalized to β-actin. Data is expressed as mean ± SD of triplicate experiments. Significant changes are marked as ***$p < 0.001$, according to the post hoc Newman-Keuls test.

Modulation of Akt/p85

The effect of VC, SF, and their combination on Akt and p85 proteins was assessed. An increase in p85 (also known as p13) and Akt expressions showed unfavored effect of VC, SF on the combination on LNCaP clone FGC cells. These findings suggest that prostate cancer subtypes may activate compensatory survival signaling in response to treatment, highlighting the importance of dose optimization and pathway-specific therapeutic targeting.

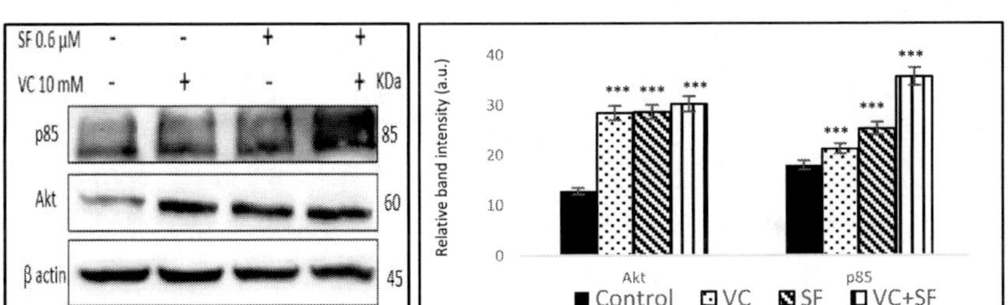

(a) (b)

Figure 12. Western blot analysis of Akt and p 85 expressions after treatment of LNCaP clone FGC cells with VC, SF, or their combination. (a) Representative blots showing expression of these proteins. (b) Densitometric histogram compares relative protein levels normalized to β-actin. Data is expressed as mean ± SD of triplicate experiments. Significant changes are indicated as ***$p < 0.001$, according to the post hoc Newman-Keuls test.

Modulation of SAPK/JNK and p38

The impact of VC, SF, and their combined treatment on SAPK/JNK and p38 proteins was evaluated in LNCaP clone FGC cells. SF alone and the combination treatment caused a decrease in p38 and SAPK/JNK expressions, while VC only treatment caused increase the expression. This contrasting response suggests that VC alone may trigger cellular stress signaling, while SF and the combination suppress these pathways, reflecting a complex and model-specific regulatory interaction.

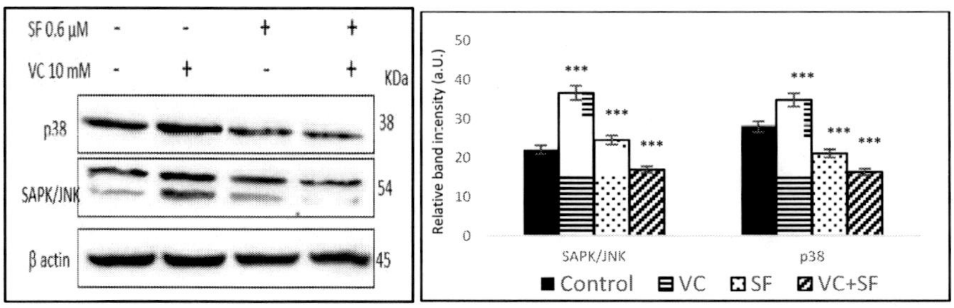

(a) (b)

Figure 13. Western blot analysis of SAPK/JNK and p38 expressions after treatment of cells with VC, SF, or their combination. (a) Representative blots showing expression of these proteins. (b) Densitometric histogram compares relative protein levels normalized to β-actin. Data is expressed as mean ± SD (n = 3). Significant changes are marked as ***p < 0.001, according to the post hoc Newman-Keuls test.

Modulation of ERK, Raf, and EGFR

The impact of VC, SF, and their combined treatment on ERK, Raf, and EGFR showed increase their expressions in all treatments indicate an unfavorable effect in LNCaP clone FGC cells. Activation of the ERK and EGFR signaling axis is commonly associated with enhanced cell survival and proliferation; however, its concurrent activation with elevated ROS and apoptotic markers suggests a compensatory stress response rather than a true pro-survival mechanism.

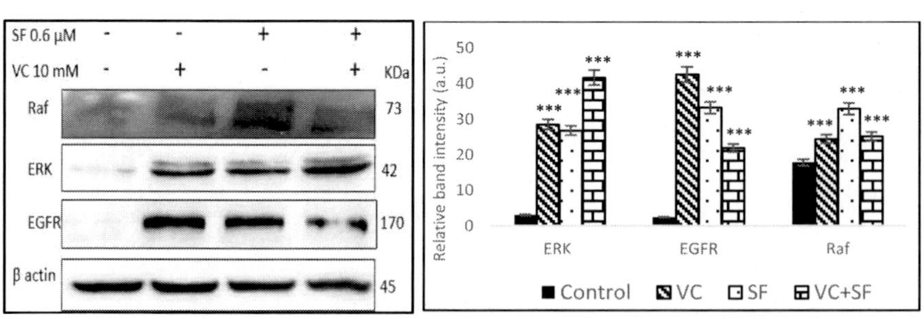

(a) (b)

Figure 14. Western blot analysis expressions of ERK, Raf, and EGFR after the treatment of cells with VC, SF, or their combination. (a) Representative blots showing expression of these proteins. (b) Densitometric histogram compares relative protein levels normalized to β-actin. Data is expressed as mean ± SD (n=3). Significant changes are marked as ***p < 0.001, according to the post hoc Newman-Keuls test.

Modulation of Wnt, β-catenin, and ROCK

The impact of VC, SF, and their combined treatment on β-catenin, Wnt, and ROCK proteins was assessed in LNCaP clone FGC cells. An increase in Wnt, β-catenin and ROCK expressions was observed in all treatments. This increase in these oncogenic proteins signifies a non- favorable effect of using VC and SF, either alone or in combination with the prostate cancer.

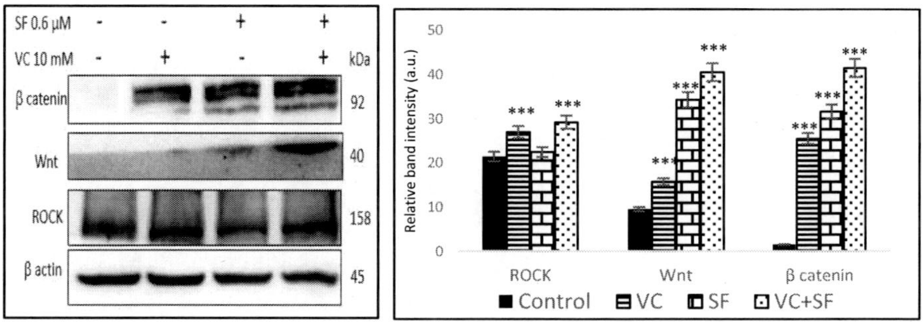

(a) (b)

Figure 15. Western blot analysis expressions of ROCK, β-catenin, and Wnt after treatment of cells with VC, SF, or their combination. (a) Representative blots showing expression of these proteins. (b) Densitometric histogram compares relative protein levels normalized to β-actin. Data is expressed as mean ± SD of triplicate experiments. Significant changes are marked as ***$p < 0.001$, according to the post hoc Newman-Keuls test.

Modulation of MnSOD, Smac/Diablo, E-Cadherin, and Histone

The impact of VC, SF, and their combined treatment on MnSOD, Smac/Diablo, E-cadherin and histone were assessed in LNCaP clone FGC cells. Increase in Smac/Diablo, MnSOD and E-cadherin expressions were identified, while decrease in histone expression was observed in all treatments.

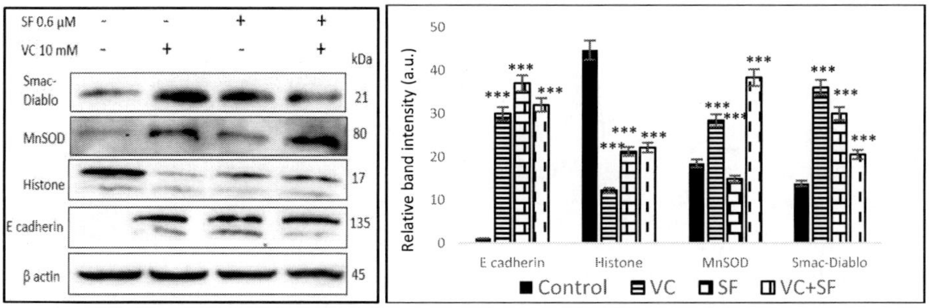

(a) (b)

Figure 16. Western blot analysis of MnSOD, Smac/Diablo, E-cadherin, and histone expressions after treatment of cells with VC, SF, or their combination. (a) Representative blots showing expression of these proteins. (b) Densitometric histogram compares relative protein levels normalized to β-actin. Data is expressed as mean ± SD ($n = 3$). Significant changes are marked as ***$p < 0.001$, according to the post hoc Newman-Keuls test.

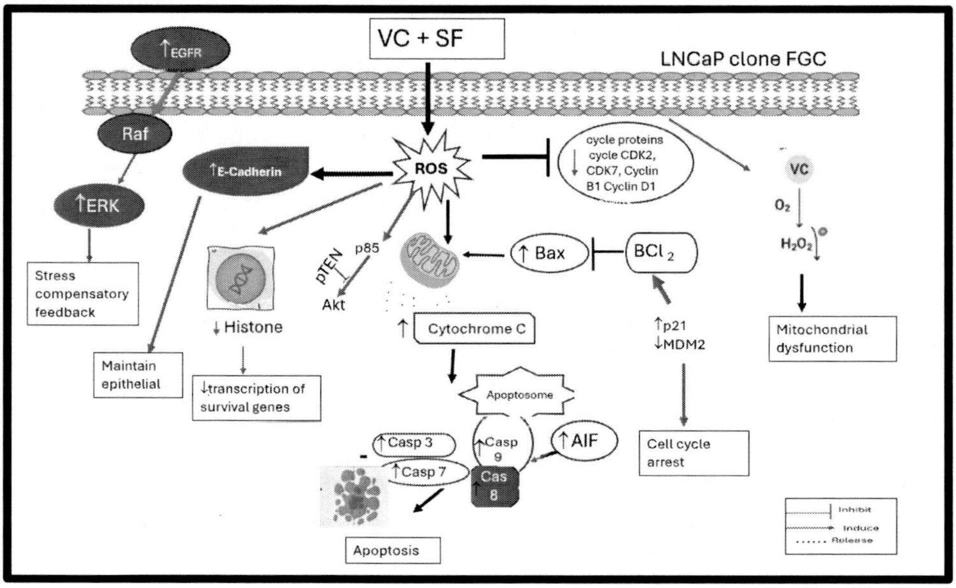

Figure 17. Proposed mechanistic model of VC and SF in prostate cancer.

Discussion

As illustrated in Figure 17, treatment of LNCaP clone FGC prostate cancer cells with pharmacologic vitamin C, sorafenib, or their combination resulted in a dual molecular response characterized by activation of mitochondrial apoptosis together with concurrent induction of compensatory survival signaling. Pro-apoptotic markers were consistently elevated: Bax increased while Bcl-2 decreased, cytochrome-c translocated into the cytosol, and both AIF and Smac/DIABLO levels rose. Caspase-3, -7, -8, and -9 were also upregulated, accompanied by reduced XIAP, supporting apoptosome assembly and caspase-dependent apoptotic execution. In parallel, increased p21 and p27 and decreased MDM2 suggested checkpoint activation and cell-cycle restraint.

However, this apoptotic program occurred alongside activation of major survival and proliferative signaling nodes, including PI3K/Akt, MEK/ERK, EGFR, Raf, and Wnt/β-catenin pathways, as well as elevated cyclins and CDKs. Increased MnSOD further suggests a mitochondrial antioxidant response aimed at buffering treatment-induced oxidative stress [11-12]. Together, these findings indicate that while VC and SF initiate mitochondrial injury and apoptotic signaling, LNCaP cells simultaneously activate feedback pathways to restore homeostasis and promote survival.

This mechanistic coexistence can be explained by adaptive signal rewiring in response to oxidative and kinase perturbation. Pharmacologic VC increases mitochondrial ROS, promoting MOMP and release of cytochrome-c and Smac to trigger caspase activation. Yet ROS and kinase inhibition can also induce compensatory RTK/MAPK/PI3K pathway upregulation as part of a cellular damage-survival balancing response. Additionally, the mixed pattern of cyclin/CDK accumulation with elevated p21/p27 may reflect cell-cycle arrest with stalled or inactivated kinase complexes, or heterogeneity in which only a subset of cells attempts to re-enter the cell cycle under stress, generating a population-averaged signal in Western blot analysis.

The elevation of Wnt/β-catenin and ROCK suggests activation of pathways associated with structural integrity and survival, while changes in E-cadherin expression reflect context-dependent epithelial stress responses rather than simple EMT reversal. Together, these adaptive features help explain why the combination treatment produces enhanced apoptotic signaling but does not yield a fully synergistic cytotoxic outcome [13-14].

Although VC and SF reduced viability more than either agent alone, the simultaneous activation of survival pathways likely attenuated the extent of final apoptotic commitment, consistent with the dose-response and protein expression data [15]. Because these findings are based on a single treatment duration and fixed concentration, cell-to-cell heterogeneity cannot be fully resolved. Future work should evaluate time-dependent changes and co-inhibition of compensatory pathways to determine whether sustained synergy can be achieved.

Conclusion

Pharmacologic VC enhances sorafenib-induced mitochondrial apoptosis in LNCaP FGC cells, but adaptive activation of MAPK, PI3K/Akt, and Wnt/β-catenin signaling limits overall cytotoxic synergy. These data suggest that co-targeting survival feedback pathways may be necessary to fully realize the therapeutic potential of VC in prostate cancer.

Key Findings

While VC enhances SF-induced apoptotic signaling in LNCaP prostate cancer cells, compensatory activation of MAPK, PI3K/Akt, and Wnt/β-catenin survival pathways limits the extent of final cytotoxic response. Thus, VC functions as a biologically active redox modulator in this model, but co-inhibition of adaptive survival feedback may be necessary to achieve meaningful therapeutic synergy in prostate cancer.

Acknowledgments

The author thanks Union University for the source and support of research funding as well as colleagues and editing tools for assistance with improving the clarity of the manuscript.

References

[1] Wasim S., Lee S.Y., Kim J. Complexities of prostate cancer. *Int J Mol Sci* 2022 ; 23, 14257.

[2] American Cancer Society. Global Cancer Statistics, *https://pressroom.concer.org* 4/4/2024.

[3] Rawla P. Epidemiology of Prostate Cancer. *World J Oncol* 2019, 10 : 63–89.

[4] Sandhu S., Moore C.M., Chiong E., Beltran H., Bristow R.G., Williams S.G. Prostate cancer. *Lancet* 2021; 398: 1075–1090.

[5] Siegel R.L., Miller K.D., Jemal A. Cancer Statistics. *CA Cancer J Clin* 2018; 68: 7–30.

[6] Virgo K.S., Basch E., Loblaw D.A., Oliver T.K., Rumble R.B., Carducci M.A, et al., Second-Line Hormonal Therapy for Men with Chemotherapy-Naive, Castration-Resistant Prostate Cancer: American Society of Clinical Oncology Provisional Clinical Opinion. *J Clin Oncol* 2017 ; 35 : 1952–1964.

[7] Crew B.A. Closer look at a revered robot. *Nature* 2020 ; 580 : S5–S7.

[8] Jain K.K. Personalized medicine for cancer: From drug development into clinical practice. *Expert Opin Pharmacother* 2005 ; 6 : 1463–1476.

[9] Zhu Y., Liu C., Nadiminty N., Lou W., Tummala R., Evans C.P., et al., Inhibition of ABCB1 Expression Overcomes Acquired Docetaxel Resistance in Prostate Cancer. *Mol Cancer Ther* 2013 ; 12 : 1829–1836.

[10] Abidi A. Cabazitaxel: A novel taxane for metastatic castration-resistant prostate cancer-current implications and prospects. *J Pharmacol Pharmacother* 2013 ; 4 : 230–237.

[11] Paller C.J., Zahurak M.L., Mandl A., Metri N.A., Lalji A., Heath E., et al., High-dose intravenous vitamin C combined with docetaxel in men with metastatic castration-resistant prostate cancer : A randomized placebo-controlled phase II trial. *Cancer Res Commun* 2024 ; 1 : 2174-2182.

[12] Li Z., He P., Long Y., Yuan G., Shen W., Chen Z., et al., Drug repurposing of pantoprazole and vitamin C targeting tumor microenvironment conditions improves anticancer effect in metastatic castration resistant prostate cancer. *Front Oncol* 2021 ; 11 :660320.

[13] Bottger F., Valles-Marti A., Cahn L., Jimenez C.R. High-dose intravenous vitamin C, a promising multi-targeting agent in the treatment of cancer. *J Exp & Clin Cancer Res* 2021 ; 40 : 343.

[14] Ullen A., Farnebo M., Thyrell L., Mahmoudi S., Kharaziha P., Lennartsson L., et al., Sorafenib induces apoptosis and autophagy in prostate cancer cells in vitro. *Int J of Oncol* 2010 ; 37 : 15-20.

[15] Guz J., Xarakowska E., Mijewski P., Wasilow A., Lesniewski F., Foksinski M., et al., Epigenetic DNA modifications and vitamin C in prostate cancer and benign prostatic hyperplasia : exploring similarities, disparities, and pathogenic implications. *Neoplasia* 2024 ; 58 : 101079.

Chapter 14

The Synergistic Antileukemic Effects of Vitamin C and Sorafenib in Chronic Myelogenous Leukemia

Lunawati L. Bennett*, PhD, PharmD
Union University, College of Pharmacy, Jackson, Tennessee, USA

Abstract

Chronic myelogenous leukemia is cancer that primarily affects adults between 45 to 65 years old. CML rarely occurs in younger individuals or in children. This cancer represents about 15-20% of adult leukemias in Western countries, with an estimated incidence of 1-2 cases per 100,000 people annually in the US. CML affect males more than females with ratio approximately 1.5 to 1. Historically, the median survival for CML patients was approximately 3-5 years following diagnosis.
The aim of this study was to evaluate whether the addition of vitamin C to the current standard chemotherapy regimen provides additional therapeutic benefits. Specifically, the study investigates whether vitamin C alone or in combination with a low dose of the chemotherapeutic agent sorafenib is more effective in treating this leukemia using K562 as the model. Results from SRB assays, Rhodamine 123, Hoechst 33342 staining, and Western blot analysis showed that the addition of vitamin C to sorafenib produced a synergistic reduction in cell viability, accompanied by increased mitochondrial dysfunction and enhanced apoptotic signaling in leukemia cells. Collectively, these findings suggest that vitamin C amplifies sorafenib-induced cytotoxicity by promoting intrinsic apoptotic pathways and disrupting survival signaling, supporting the therapeutic potential of this combination as a more effective strategy for managing chronic myelogenous leukemia.

Keywords: chronic myelogenous leukemia, vitamin C, sorafenib, synergistic, blood cancer

Abbreviations

APAF	Apoptotic peptidase activating factor;
Bax	Bcl2 Associated X-protein;
Bcl2	B cell lymphoma 2;

* Corresponding Author's Email: llbennett@uu.edu

Cas	Caspase;
CDK7	Cyclin dependent kinase 7;
Cyt C	Cytochrome C;
EGFR	Epidermal growth factor receptor;
ERK	Extracellular signal-regulated kinase
MAPKs	Mitogen-activated protein kinases;
MEKs	Mitogen-activated protein kinase kinases;
MDM2	Mouse double minute 2 homolog.

Introduction

Chronic myelogenous leukemia (CML) is cancer that primarily affects adults between 45 to 65 years old affect male than female [1-2]. CML progresses through three distinct phases known as chronic phase, accelerated phase and blast crisis. Each of the phases signifies poor prognosis and typically signals resistance to standard treatment [3-5]. Treatment Options include tyrosine kinase inhibitors (TKIs), hematopoietic stem cell transplantation (HSCT), Interferon-alpha (IF-α), and chemotherapy. TKIs are now the mainstay of CML treatment. Imatinib, the first TKI approved for CML, revolutionized CML therapy by targeting the BCR-ABL tyrosine kinase. Subsequent TKIs, such as dasatinib, nilotinib, bosutinib, and ponatinib, provide options for patients with imatinib resistance or intolerance [6]. TKIs have transformed CML from a fatal disease to a manageable chronic condition for most patients [7].

Sorafenib Has been used for the treatment of hepatocellular carcinoma, renal -cell carcinoma and thyroid cancer [8-10]. It works by inhibiting several key kinases involved in cancer growth and angiogenesis. It targets serine/threonine kinases in the RAF/MEK/ERK pathway, particularly RAF-1 and BRAF, that regulate cell proliferation and inhibit cancer growth [11].

Pharmacological vitamin C (VC) concentration has been observed to enhance the activity of the ten-eleven translocation (TET) family of enzymes, which are involved in DNA demethylation. This process plays a role in the regulation of cancer stem cells, particularly in leukemias. In CML, the activity of TET enzymes is often reduced, leading to aberrant DNA methylation that can promote cancer cell proliferation. Vitamin C's role in enhancing TET activity can, therefore, potentially help restore normal gene expression patterns and reduce the leukemia stem cell population [12]. In addition, VC may enhance the efficacy of TKIs by promoting oxidative stress in CML cells while also acting on pathways that support leukemia cell death [13]. VC may also promote differentiation in leukemia stem cells, potentially making them more susceptible to standard therapies and reducing the risk of relapse [14].

High-dose intravenous vitamin C (VC) to attain plasma levels of $\geq$ 20 mM, has recently emerged as a potential non-toxic adjuvant to standard care radio-chemotherapy-based cancer therapies across various disease sites [15-16]. The proposed anti-cancer mechanism of pharmacological VC involves redox-active metal-mediated or auto-oxidation of ascorbate, resulting in the formation of O_2 and H_2O_2 [16-17].

This study was designed to evaluate the chemo-enhancing potential of VC in combination with low-dose SF for treating CML, utilizing K562 cells as the model. The findings of this investigation reveal that the use of VC with SF demonstrated greater efficacy in the treatment of CML. This marks a novel discovery in the field.

To evaluate the cytotoxic potential of high-dose VC, various antineoplastic agents - including paclitaxel, doxorubicin, etoposide, temsirolimus, bortezomib, afatinib, and sorafenib - were tested on human CML using the model K562 cell line. For combination studies, the lowest concentrations of each antineoplastic and high-dose VC that yielded a synergistic reduction in cell viability were selected. General experimental procedures followed the protocols outlined in Chapter 3 (Materials and Methods), while methodological details specific to this study are described below.

Cell Culture

Chronic myelogenous leukemia K562 (ATCC CRL-3344) was established in 1970 from the pleural effusion of a 53-year-old female patient with CML in blast crisis that carries the Philadelphia chromosome (BCR–ABL fusion gene). It was cultures as suspension non-adherent cells that exhibit characteristics of undifferentiated hematopoietic progenitors of the erythroid–myeloid lineage in RPMI-1640 medium supplemented with 10% fetal bovine serum (FBS), 1% streptomycin/penicillin and maintained at 37°C in a humidified atmosphere with 5% CO_2

Results

Cell Viability and Selection of Doses

Cells treated with VC alone showed approximately 50% viability at a concentration of 10 mM, while treatment with SF alone induced 50% cell death at 6 μM. Based on these findings, 5 μM SF was selected for combination studies with VC to evaluate potential synergistic effects on K562 cell viability. The combined treatment of VC and SF produced a greater reduction in cell viability than either agent alone in a time-dependent manner at 24, 48, and 72 h, indicating a synergistic interaction. According to the SRB assay results, 5 μM SF, 9 mM VC, and their combination were chosen for subsequent molecular analyses. The cells are more sensitive when treated with both VC and SF - likely because VC increases oxidative pressure and weakens cellular defenses, allowing sorafenib to act more effectively on survival pathways.

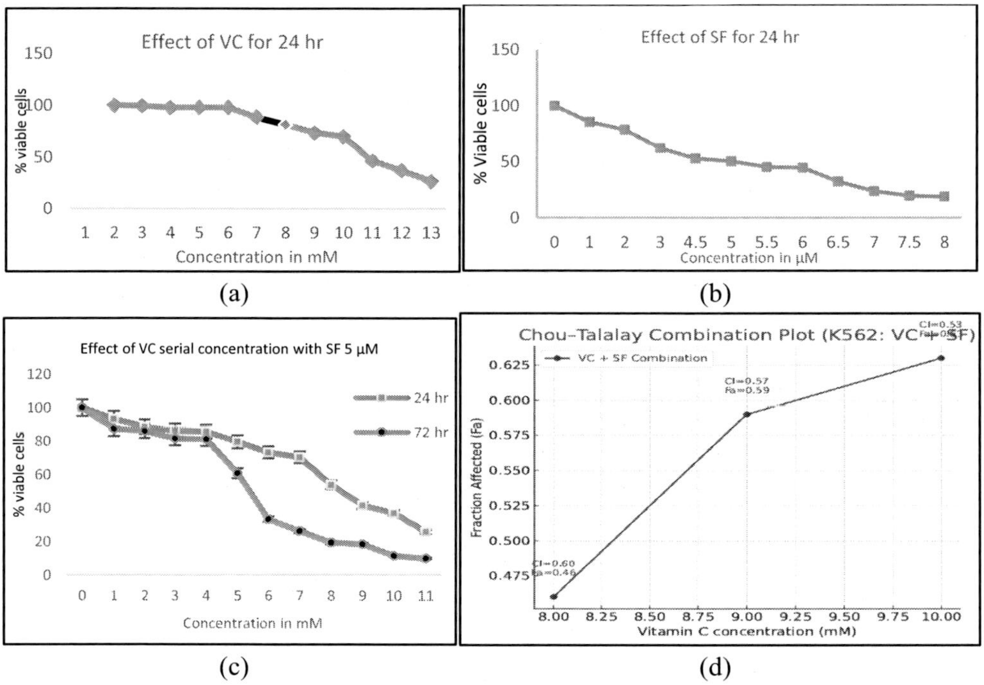

Figure 1. Effect of VC, SF, and their combination on the viability of K562 cells. (a-b) Cells were treated with increasing concentrations of VC (0–13 mM) or SF (0–10 μM).VC alone caused ~50% reduction in viability at 10 mM, while SF alone induced 50% cell death at 6 μM. (c)The combination of 9 mM VC and 5 μM SF produced a synergistic decrease in cell viability across all time points. Data are presented as mean ± SD of three independent experiments. (d) Based on Chou-Talalay plot, the combination showed synergistic effect with Fa=0.59, CI=0.71.

Changes in Cell Morphology

VC and SF resulted in alteration of K562 morphologies in the number of cells. Control cells remained healthy, showing increased in numbers after 24 h, while cells treated with VC or SF alone exhibited reduced viability and morphological changes. The combination of VC and SF led to even greater cell death.

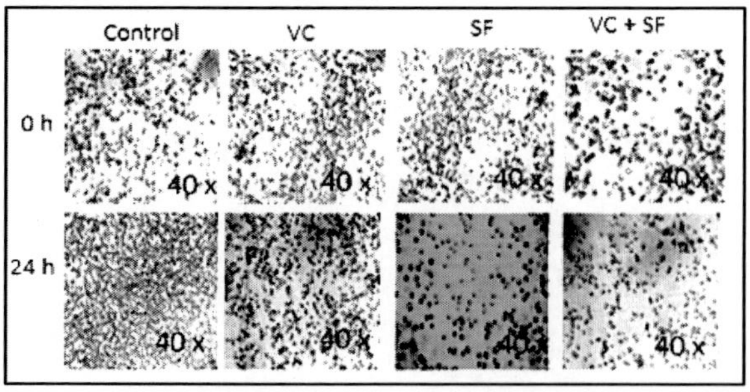

Figure 2. Inverted microscopic images of K562 cells (40X) after 24 h treatment with VC, SF or their combination.

Death and Alive Cell

The number of cell death in K562 cells treated with individual SF, VC, or their combination were evaluated with nuclear-ID red/green cell viability. Red fluorescent indicated cells were death impermeable to nucleic acid dye while green fluorescent indicated cells were alive permeable to nucleic acid dye. When the image from red dye and green dye were merged, cells that were death had red or dark orange color, while alive cells showed yellow/greenish color.

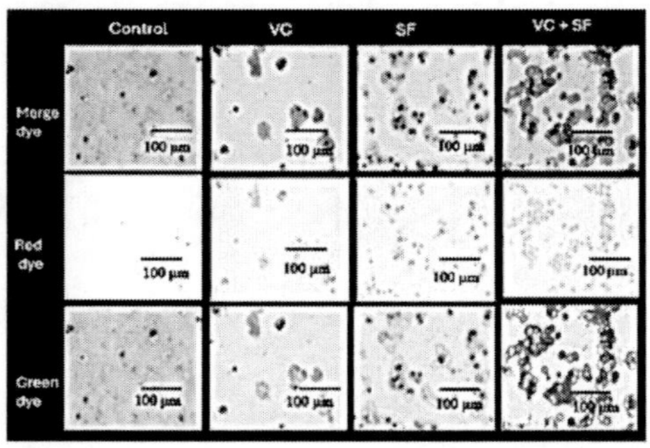

Figure 3. Fluorescence microscope of K562 cells treated with VC, SF, or their combination. The scale bar represents 100 μm. Data are expressed as mean ± SD (n = 3).

Induction of Apoptosis

The combination of VC and SF resulted in a higher rate of apoptosis in K562 cells compared to treatment with VC or SF alone, as confirmed by Hoechst 33342 staining and observed in fluorescence microscopy images. The nuclei of control cells exhibited lower fluorescence intensity, indicating normal and healthy. In contrast, cells undergoing apoptosis displayed a bright blue color due to nuclear condensation and fragmentation, with histogram comparing normal and apoptotic cells.

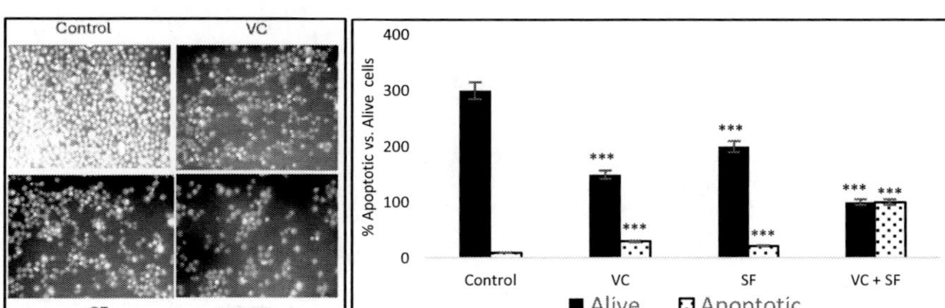

(a) (b)

Figure 4. Intracellular induction of apoptosis in K562 cells treated for 24 h with VC, SF, or their combination. (a) Fluorescence microscopic images following Hoechst 33342 staining. The scale bar represents 100 μm. (b) Histogram of fluorescence intensity comparing control, VC, AF, and combination treatments. Data are expressed as mean ± SD (n = 3); with ***$p < 0.001$, as determined by the post hoc Newman-Keuls test.

Intracellular ROS Generation

The generation of intracellular ROS was assessed in K562 cells following treatment with VC, SF, or their combination, using H2DCFDA staining. Variations in fluorescence intensity through microscopic images showed higher ROS generation indicated by increased fluorescence intensity in VC, SF and the combination. The control showed darker colors indicating lower ROS generation.

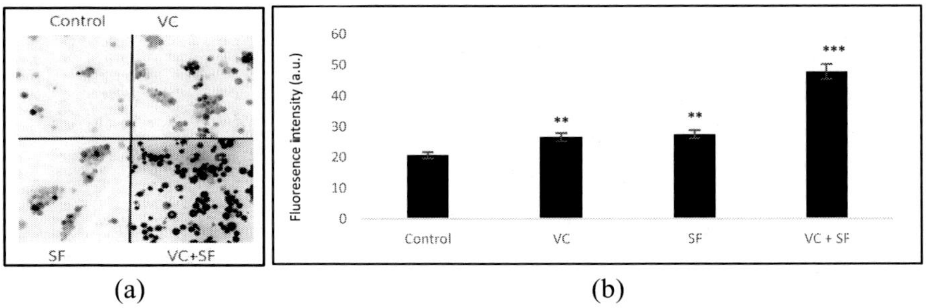

Figure 5. Intracellular ROS generation in K562 cells after 24 h. of treatment. (a) Representative fluorescence microscopy images following H2DCFDA staining. Increased fluorescence intensity corresponds to higher ROS levels. Scale bar = 100 μm. (b) Histogram of fluorescence intensity comparing control, VC, SF, and combination treatments. Data are expressed as mean ± SD (n = 3); ** p<0.01, ***p < 0.001 post hoc Newman–Keuls test.

Mitochondrial Membrane Potential (Ψ_m)

The generation of ROS in K562 cells indicated cell death attributed to the depletion of mitochondrial membrane potential, as detected with Rhodamine 123 staining. Treatments with VC, SF, or the combination induced cell death, as shown in darker the fluorescence microscopic images. Control cells exhibited higher fluorescence intensity, indicating healthy mitochondria, compared to treated cells.

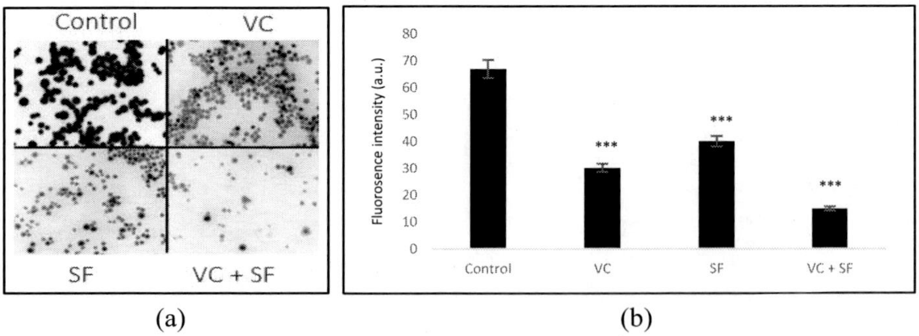

Figure 6. Intracellular mitochondrial membrane potentially change in K562 after 24 h. of treatment. (a) Representative fluorescence microscopy images following Rhodamine 123 staining. Scale bar = 100 μm. (b) Histogram of fluorescence intensity comparing control, VC, SF, and combination treatments. Data are expressed as mean ± SD (n = 3); ***p < 0.001 according to post hoc Newman–Keuls test.

Modulation of Bax, Bcl2, AIF, and Cytochrome C

In apoptotic cells, the intracellular generation of ROS is linked to alterations in the expressions of Bax and Bcl2 proteins. Increase in Bax only observed in combination treatment. Decrease in Bcl2 expressions VC and the combination. Treatment with VC alone had a favorable effect on Bcl-2 and Bax. ROS generation also led to a reduction in mitochondrial membrane potential, resulting in an increased release of cytochrome C into the cytosol, which further induced apoptosis. Slight increase in the expression of apoptosis-inducing factors (AIF) was observed in cells treated with SF only, while slight decrease in VC or the combination treatment.

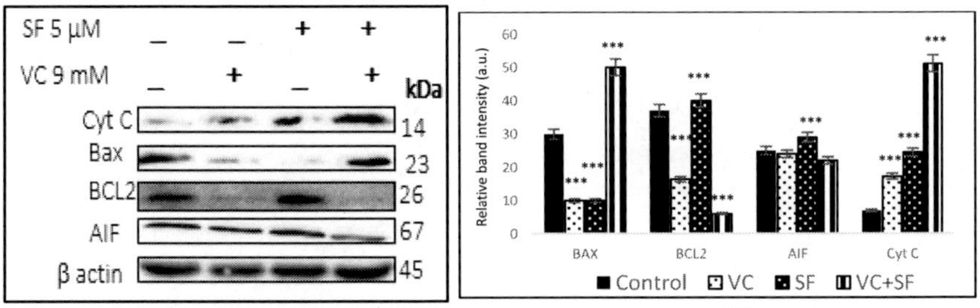

(a) (b)

Figure 7. Western blot analysis of Bax, Bcl2, AIF, and cyt C expressions in K562 cells following treatment with VC, SF, or their combination. (a) Representative blots showing expression of these proteins. (b) Densitometric histogram compares relative protein levels normalized to β-actin. Data are expressed as mean ± SD (n=3). Statistical significance was determined using the Newman–Keuls post hoc test (***$p < 0.001$).

Modulation Mitochondrial Signaling Proteins

Mitochondrial apoptosis resulting from a decline in membrane potential is linked to various crucial proteins, including caspases (Cas-9, -3, -7, and -8) and apoptotic peptidase activating factor (Apaf). Significant increase in Cas-3, -7, -8, -9, and Apaf following VC-only or the combination in all treatment, while SF only caused decrease expression of Cas -9 and -7.

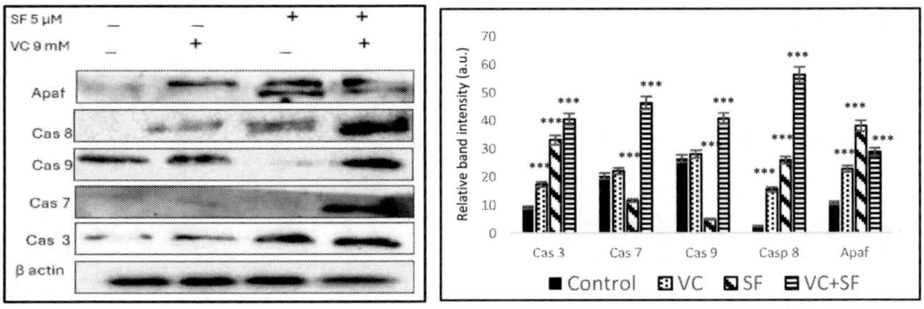

(a) (b)

Figure 8. Western blot analysis results of Apaf, Cas-3, -7, -8, and -9 expressions in K562 cells. (a) Representative blots showing expression of these proteins. (b) Densitometric histogram compares relative protein levels normalized to β-actin. Data are expressed as mean ± SD (n = 3). Statistical significance was determined using the Newman–Keuls post hoc test (***$p < 0.001$).

Modulation of MEK Kinase Pathway

To investigate the potential mechanism of VC, SF, or their combination in modulating aberrant cell signaling of mitogen-activated protein kinases (MAPKs), Western blot analysis was conducted to assess the active and phosphorylated forms of mitogen-activated protein kinase kinase (MEK). Significant decreases in MEK-1, -2, -3, and -4 expressions were observed in cells treated with VC, SF, or their combination.

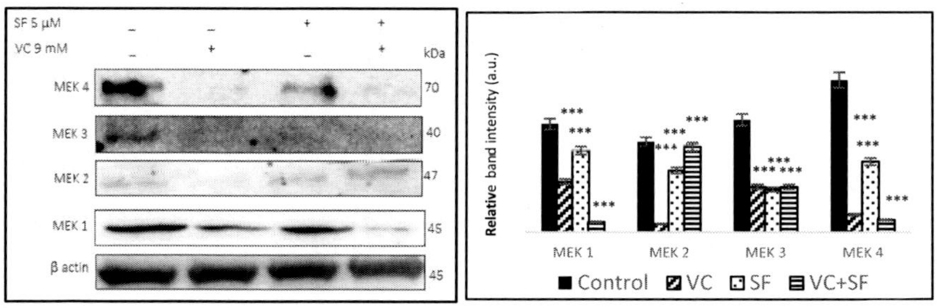

(a) (b)

Figure 9. Western blot analysis results of MEK-1, -2, -3, and -4 after treating K562 cells with VC, SF, or their combination. (a) Representative blots showing expression of these proteins. (b) Densitometric histogram compares relative protein levels normalized to β-actin. Data are expressed as mean ± SD (n = 3). Statistical significance was determined using the Newman–Keuls post hoc test (***$p < 0.001$).

Modulation of Cell Cycle Regulatory Proteins

Inhibition of cell cycle progression is also considered an important strategy in the management of CML. Decreases in proteins involved in cell cycle regulation CDk7, CDk2, cyclin B1 and cyclin D1 were observed in all treatment of K562 with VC, SF or their combination These proteins play critical roles in driving cell cycle progression through the G1/S and G2/M transitions; thus, their downregulation indicates inhibition of cell proliferation and induction of cell cycle arrest.

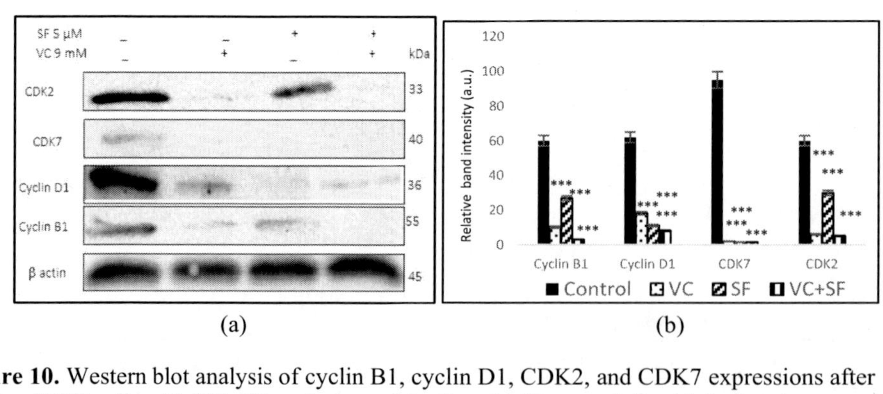

(a) (b)

Figure 10. Western blot analysis of cyclin B1, cyclin D1, CDK2, and CDK7 expressions after treating K562 cells with VC, SF, or their combination. (a) Representative blots showing expression of these proteins. (b) Densitometric histogram compares relative protein levels normalized to β-actin. Data are expressed as mean ± SD (n = 3). Significant increases are indicated as ***$p < 0.001$, according to the post hoc Newman-Keuls test.

Modulation of p21, p53, PTEN, and MDM2

The impact of VC, SF, and their combination on the expression of key regulatory proteins, including p21, p53, PTEN, and MDM2, was assessed in K562 cells. Treatment with VC, SF, or their combination resulted in notable increase of p21, p53, and PTEN, with decrease in MDM2 in all treatment. Decrease of PTEN was observed in SF only treatment.

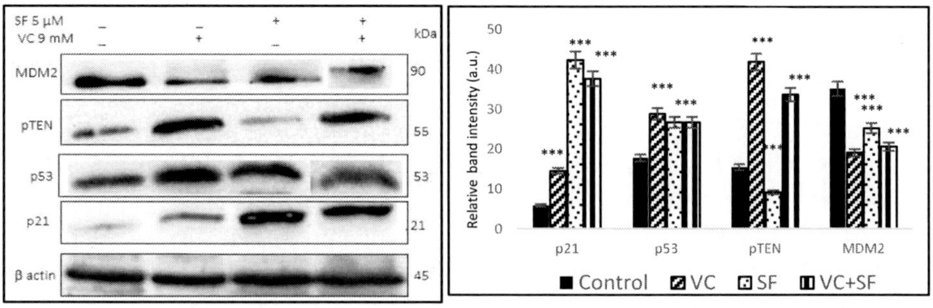

(a) (b)

Figure 11. Western blot analysis of p21, p53, PTEN, and MDM2 expression in K562 cells following treatment with VC, SF, or their combination. (a) Representative blots showing expression of these proteins. (b) Densitometric histogram compares relative protein levels normalized to β-actin. Data are expressed as mean ± SD (n = 3). Statistical significance was determined using the Newman–Keuls post hoc test (***p < 0.001).

Modulation of Akt/p85

The effect of VC, SF, and their combination on Akt and p85 proteins was assessed. A decrease in Akt expressions was observed in VC only, while increase in p85 and Akt were observed in all other treatments compared to the control, indicating unfavorable effect of the treatment compared to the control.

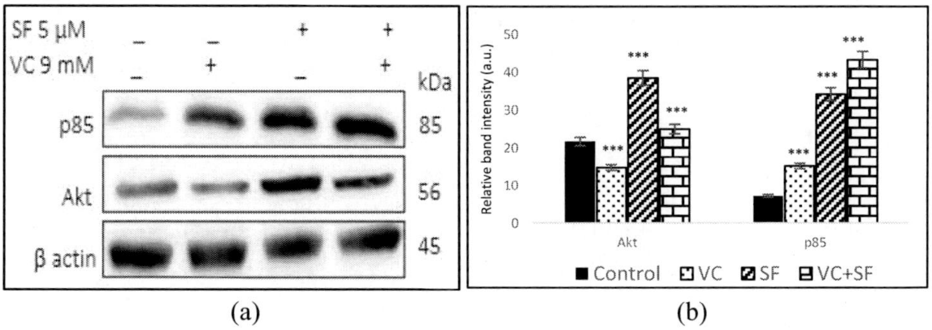

(a) (b)

Figure 12. Western blot analysis data showing the modulation of Akt and p85 expression after treatment of K562 cells with VC, SF, or their combination. (a) Representative blots showing expression of these proteins. (b) Densitometric histogram compares relative protein levels normalized to β-actin. Data are expressed as mean ± SD (n = 3). Statistical significance was determined using the Newman–Keuls post hoc test (***p < 0.001).

Modulation of SAPK/JNK and p38

The impact of VC, SF, and their combined treatment on SAPK/JNK and p38 proteins was evaluated in K562 cells. Decrease in p38 and SAP/JNK expression were observed in all treatment suggests the combination treatment effectively suppresses stress-induced signaling pathways, potentially contributing to enhanced apoptotic sensitivity (see Fig. 13).

Modulation of MnSOD, Smac/Diablo, and Vimentin

The impact of VC, SF, and their combined treatment on MnSOD, Smac/Diablo, and Vimentin protein expression was evaluated in K562 cells. Treatment with VC, SF, or the combination resulted in a marked increase in Smac/Diablo levels, corresponding to enhanced pro-apoptotic signaling through mitochondrial pathway activation. A reduction in MnSOD expression suggested diminished antioxidant defense, thereby promoting intracellular oxidative stress and sensitizing cells to apoptosis. Decreased Vimentin expression reflected a suppression of cytoskeletal remodeling and mesenchymal characteristics, which may correspond to reduced migratory or invasive potential. VC, SF, and particularly their combination, exert favorable anticancer effects by promoting apoptosis while simultaneously reducing oxidative resistance and invasive phenotypes in K562 cells (see Fig. 14).

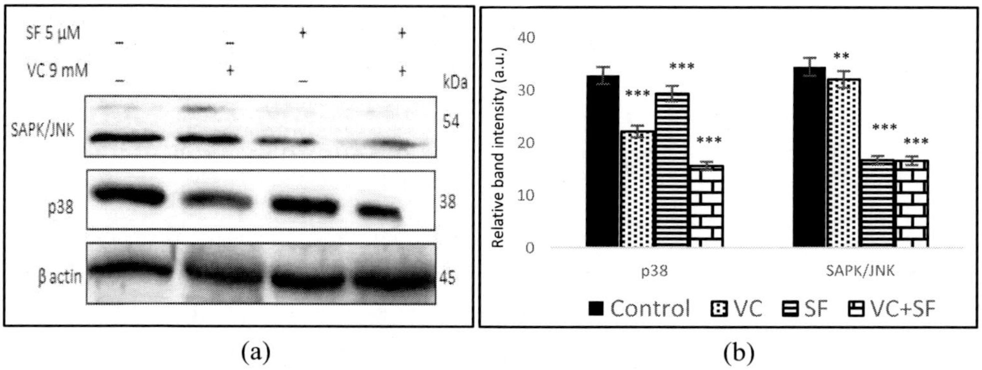

Figure 13. Western blot analysis data showing the modulation of SAPK/JNK and p38 expressions after treatment of K562 cells with VC, SF, or their combination. (a) Representative blots showing expression of these proteins. (b) Densitometric histogram compares relative protein levels normalized to β-actin. Data are expressed as mean ± SD (n = 3). Significant changes are marked as ** $p < 0.01$, ***$p < 0.001$, according to the post hoc Newman-Keuls test.

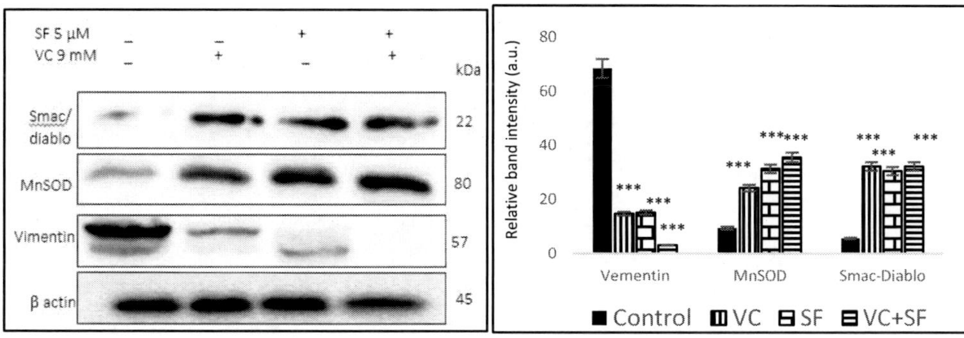

(a) (b)

Figure 14. Western blot analysis data showing the modulation of MnSOD, Smac/Diablo, and Vimentin proteins after treatment of K562 cells with VC, SF, or their combination. (a) Representative blots showing expression of these proteins. (b) Densitometric histogram compares relative protein levels normalized to β-actin. Data are expressed as mean ± SD (n = 3). Significant changes are marked as ***p < 0.001, according to the post hoc Newman-Keuls test.

Modulation of MDR-ABC and Histone

The impact of VC, ET, and their combined treatment on MDR-ABC (multi-drug resistance) and histone proteins were assessed in k562 cells revealing differential modulation of drug efflux and chromatin-associated regulatory pathways that may contribute to the observed therapeutic response.

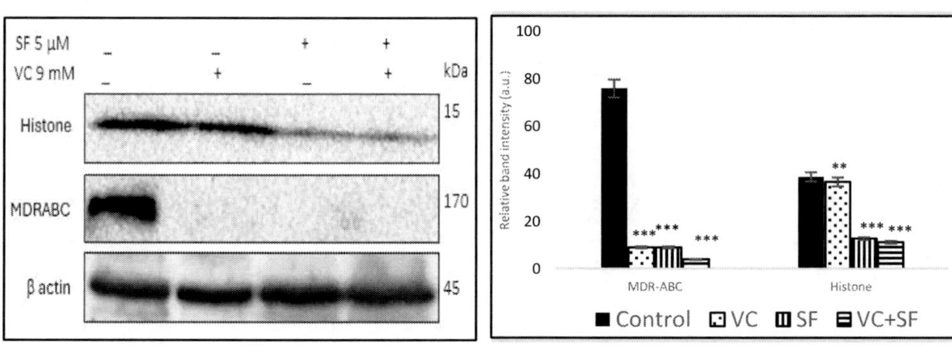

(a) (b)

Figure 15. Western blot analysis of MDR-ABC and histone expressions after treatment of cells with VC, SF, or their combination. (a) Representative blots showing expression of these proteins. (b) Densitometric histogram compares relative protein levels normalized to β-actin. Data are expressed as mean ± SD (n = 3). Significant changes are marked as ** p< 0.01, ***p < 0.001, according to the post hoc Newman-Keuls test.

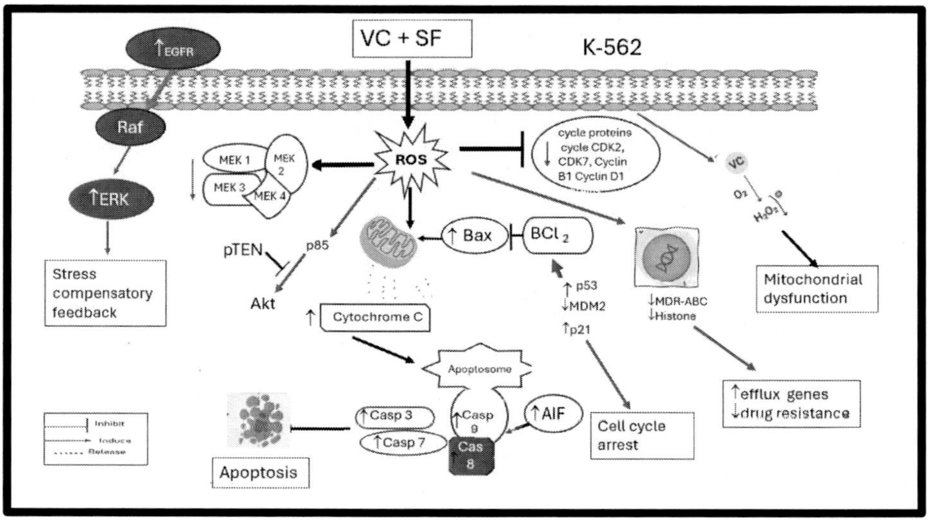

Figure 16. Proposed mechanistic model of VC and SF in CML.

Discussion

As illustrated in Figure 16, the proposed mechanism of VC, SF, and their combination in CML elicits complex multifaceted pathways such as mitochondrial dysfunction, decreased drug resistance, cell cycle arrest, and induction of apoptosis. Despite significant therapeutic advances, the emergence of drug resistance and incomplete eradication of leukemic stem cells remain major challenges in CML therapy due to constitutively active BCR-ABL oncoprotein which sustains aberrant cell proliferation and survival through activation of MAPK and PI3K/AKT signaling cascades. Redox-active compounds such as high dose of VC have gained renewed attention for their ability to selectively induce oxidative stress and sensitize malignant cells to targeted therapies.

Morphological and viability assays revealed that VC or SF alone reduced K562 cell viability, while their combination caused extensive cell death. Fluorescence imaging using nuclear-ID and Hoechst 33342 staining confirmed a higher apoptotic index in the combination group compared to monotherapy. These morphological changes were accompanied by a pronounced increase in intracellular ROS generation establishing oxidative stress as an early event in treatment response. The increase in ROS coincided with a marked reduction of mitochondrial membrane potential ($\Delta\Psi m$), indicating mitochondrial depolarization and loss of function. Such mitochondrial perturbations are consistent with oxidative injury that initiate intrinsic apoptosis.

At the molecular level, combined VC and SF treatment increased the expression of pro-apoptotic Bax while decreasing anti-apoptotic BCl2, thereby tilting the mitochondrial rheostat toward apoptosis. This was associated with cytosolic release of cytochrome c and increased expression of Smac/Diablo, both of which activate the caspase cascade. In parallel, the combination prominently upregulated caspase-3, -7, -8, -9, and Apaf-1, confirming execution of the intrinsic apoptotic pathway. SF alone modestly reduced cas-9 and -7 levels, suggesting a dose- or time-dependent modulation of caspase turnover, whereas VC alone or in combination robustly enhanced caspase activation. Together, these data establish that the VC and SF combination engages mitochondria-dependent apoptosis driven by ROS accumulation and caspase activation.

Disruption of redox homeostasis was further supported by a decrease in MnSOD, an essential antioxidant enzyme, which would amplify intracellular ROS burden. Concurrently, the observed downregulation of vimentin implies a suppression of mesenchymal-like, migratory phenotypes, aligning with a less aggressive cellular behavior under combination treatment. These effects resonate with prior findings that pharmacologic VC selectively induces oxidative stress in malignant but not normal cells, generating hydrogen peroxide through metal-catalyzed oxidation processes that overwhelm leukemic antioxidant defenses [18-19].

Beyond oxidative injury, the treatments significantly altered oncogenic signaling networks. Western blot analysis revealed marked reductions in MEK-1 through -4, suggesting suppression of the RAF-MEK-ERK axis - a critical pathway downstream of BCR-ABL that supports CML proliferation and survival. SF, a known RAF and multi-kinase inhibitor, likely contributed directly to this effect, while VC-induced oxidative stress may have further inactivated kinases through redox modification. Downregulation of cell-cycle regulators CDK2, CDK7, cyclin B1, and cyclin D1 corroborates a cell-cycle arrest phenotype, which was reinforced by increased expression of the tumor suppressors p53, p21, and PTEN, alongside reduced MDM2. Activation of the p53–p21 axis likely mediates G1 or G2/M arrest, facilitating apoptotic commitment rather than survival. Interestingly, PTEN reduction observed in SF-only treatment suggests potential compensatory signaling, whereas VC preserved or enhanced PTEN expression, indicating a stabilizing effect on tumor-suppressive pathways [11, 20].

The stress-activated kinases SAPK/JNK and p38 were decreased in all treatments, reflecting either late-phase downregulation following transient early activation or proteolytic degradation during apoptosis. This aligns with previous reports showing that the effect of SF on JNK/p38 is context-dependent, with transient activation followed by decline once apoptosis is established. Additional studies using phospho-specific antibodies and time-course analyses would clarify these dynamics [21].

Importantly, the combination treatment also downregulated multidrug resistance (MDR) transporters and histone proteins, implying both improved chemosensitivity and chromatin destabilization under oxidative stress. Inhibition of MDR expression could have therapeutic implications by resensitizing CML cells to tyrosine kinase inhibitors or other chemotherapeutic agents [22].

The integrated results suggest that pharmacologic VC potentiates the antileukemic action of SF through dual mechanisms: (1) induction of oxidative mitochondrial apoptosis via ROS overproduction, Bax/Bcl-2 modulation, $\Delta\Psi m$ loss, cytochrome c release, and caspase cascade activation, and (2) suppression of proliferative and survival pathways, including RAF/MEK/ERK and CDK/cyclin signaling, accompanied by stabilization of tumor suppressors such as p53, p21, and PTEN. This mechanistic synergy converges on irreversible mitochondrial damage and apoptosis in K562 cells [22-23].

These findings are in strong agreement with studies showing that high-dose ascorbate acts as a pro-oxidant and enhances cytotoxicity of kinase inhibitors and chemotherapeutics [23-24]. However, they contrast with reports that low-dose antioxidant forms of VC may protect tumor cells or antagonize certain drugs emphasizing the critical importance of concentration and route of administration [25]. Moreover, the dependence of VC cytotoxicity on redox-active metals and extracellular catalase activity indicates that the cellular microenvironment can significantly modulate efficacy. These nuances should be addressed in future studies by assessing metal availability, antioxidant enzyme levels, and pharmacologic dosing achievable through intravenous administration [26-27].

Conclusion

The data underscore the promise of VC and SF combination therapy as a potential strategy to overcome resistance and improve apoptosis induction in CML. Further, in vivo studies using appropriate animal models are warranted to validate the translational potential of this combination and to define optimal dosing, timing, and safety parameters.

Key Findings

The combination of pharmacologic VC and SF exhibited a synergistic antileukemic effect in myelogenous cells by promoting oxidative stress–mediated mitochondrial dysfunction and apoptosis. This effect was characterized by elevated ROS generation, loss of mitochondrial membrane potential, cytochrome c and Smac release, activation of multiple caspases, and modulation of Bax/Bcl-2 balance. Concurrent suppression of MEK/MAPK and CDK/cyclin signaling, along with increased p53, p21, and PTEN expression, reinforced apoptotic commitment and cell-cycle arrest. The dual action of redox stress induction and oncogenic pathway inhibition highlights the therapeutic potential of combining vitamin C with kinase inhibitors to enhance efficacy and overcome drug resistance in CML.

Acknowledgments

The author thanks Union University for the source and support of research funding as well as colleagues and editing tools for assistance with improving the clarity of the manuscript.

References

[1] Kantarjian H., O'Brien S., Shan J., Huang X. Cytogenetic and molecular responses and outcomes in chronic myelogenous leukemia: need for new response definitions? *Cancer* 2008.

[2] Sampaio M.M., Santos M.L.C., Marques H.S., de Sa Santos L.K., Santos M.N., et al., Chronic myeloid leukemia-from the Philadelphia chromosome to specific target drugs" A literature review. *World J of Clin Oncol* 2021 ; 12 : 69-94.

[3] Flis S., Chojnacki T. Chronic myelogenous leukemia, a still unsolved problem: pitfalls and new therapeutic possibilities. *Drug Des Dev Ther* 2019; 13: 825–843.

[4] Apperley J.F. Part II: Management of chronic myeloid leukemia. *The Lancet Oncol* 2007 ; 8(12): 1116–1128.

[5] Senapati J., Jabbour E., Kantarjian H., Short N.J. Pathogenesis and management of accelerated and blast phases of chronic myeloid leukemia. *Leukemia* 2023 ; 37 : 5-17.

[6] Hochhaus A., Breccia M., Saglio G., García-Gutiérrez V. Expert opinion management of chronic myeloid leukemia after resistance to second-generation tyrosine kinase inhibitors. *Leukemia* 2020; 34: 1495-1502.

[7] Bhatia R. Novel approaches to therapy in CML. *Am Soc Hematol Educ Program* 2017; (1): 115–120.

[8] Llovet J.M., Ricci S., Mazzaferro V., Hilgard P., Gane E. Sorafenib in advanced hepatocellular carcinoma. *N Engl J Med* 2008; 359: 378-390.

[9] Escudier B., Eisen T., Stadler W.M., Audard S., Negrier S. Sorafenib in advanced clear-cell renal-cell carcinoma. *N Engl J Med* 2007; 356: 125-134.

[10] Brose M.S., Nutting C.M., Elisei R., Siena S., Bastholt L. Sorafenib in radioactive iodine-refractory, locally advanced or metastatic differentiated thyroid cancer : a randomized, double-blind, phase 3 trial. *The Lancet* 2014 ; 384 : 319-328.

[11] Wilhelm S.M., Adnane L., Newell P., Villanueva A., Llovet J.M., Lynch M. Preclinical overview of sorafenib, a multikinase inhibitor that targets both RAF/MEK/ERK pathway and receptor tyrosine kinases involved in tumor progression and angiogenesis. *Cancer Res* 2004 ; 64 : 7099-7109.

[12] Agathocleous M. Vitamin C promotes stem cell function and reduces blast crisis in CML. *Nature* 2017; 549(7673): 476-479.

[13] Pires D.A., Brandão-Rangel M.A.R., Silva-Reis A., Olímpio F.R.S., Oliveira C.R., Silva J.R., et al., Vitamin C inhibits lipopolysaccharide-induced hyperinflammatory state of chronic myeloid leukemia cells through purinergic signaling and autophagy. *Nutrients* 2024 ; 16, 383.

[14] Isola S., Gammeri L., Furci F., Gangemi S., Pioggia G., Allegra A. Vitamin C Supplementation in the Treatment of Autoimmune and Onco-Hematological Diseases: From Prophylaxis to Adjuvant Therapy. *Int J Mol Sci* 2024, 25, 7284.

[15] Chen Q., Espey M.G., Krishna M.C., Mitchell J.B., Corpe C.P., Buettner G.R., et al., Pharmacological ascorbic acid concentrations selectively kill cancer cells : action as a pro-drug to deliver hydrogen peroxide to tissues. *PNAS* 2005 ; 102 : 13604-13609.

[16] Chen Q., Espey M.G., Sun A.Y., Lee J.H., Buettner G.R., Levine M. Ascorbate in pharmacologic concentration selectively generate ascorbate radical and hydrogen peroxide in extracellular fluid *in vivo*. *PNAS* 2007 ; 104 : 8749-8754.

[17] Olney K.E., Du J., Van Erve T.J., Witmer J.R., Wagner B.A., Buettner G.R., et al., Inhibitors of hydroperoxide metabolism enhance ascorbate-induce cytotoxicity. *Free Radic Res* 2013 ; 47 :154-163.

[18] Giansanti M., Karimi T., Faraoni I., Graziani G. High-dose vitamin C : Preclinical evidence for tailoring treatment in cancers patients. *Cancer* 2021 ; 13 (6), 1428.

[19] Nigam M., Punia B., Dimri D.B., Mishra A.P., Radu A.F., Bungau G. Reactive oxygen species: A double-edged sword in the modulation of cancer signaling pathway dynamics. *Cells* 2025 ; 14(15), 1207.

[20] Kurosu T., Ohki M., Wu N., Kagechika H., Miura O. Sorafenib induces apoptosis specifically in cells expressing BCR/ABL by inhibiting it kinase activity to activate the intrinsic mitochondrial pathway. *Cancer Res* 2009 ; 69 (9) : 3927-2936.

[21] Yan H., HeL., Lv D., Yang J., Yuan Z. The role of the dysregulated JNK signaling pathway in the pathogenesis of human diseases and its potential therapeutic strategies: A comprehensive review. *Biomol* 2024 ; 14 (2), 243.

[22] Ge M., Chen X.Y., Huang P., Fleishman J.S., Yng D.H., Wu Z.H., et al., Understanding and overcoming multidrug resistance in cancer. *Nature Rev Clin Oncol* 2025 ; 22 : 760-780.

[23] Bottger F., Marti A.V., Jimenez C.R. High-dose intravenous vitamin C, a promising multi-targeting agent in the treatment of cancer. *J Exp Clin Cancer Res* 2021 ; 49, 343.

[24] Danboyi T., Jimoh A., Danboyi E.H., Teru G.A.D. Vitamin C dosage in health and disease. In: Kukurt A, Gelen V editors. *Ascorbic Acid-Biochemistry and Functions* 2024.

[25] Calder P.C., Kreider R.B., McKay D.L. Enhanced vitamin C delivery: A systemic literature review assessing the efficacy and safety of alternative supplement forms in healthy adults. *Nutrients* 2026 ; 17 (2), 279.

[26] Li W.N., Zhang S.J., Feng J.Q., Jin W.L. Repurposing vitamin C for cancer treatment: Focus on targeting the tumor microenvironment. *Cancer* 2022 ; 14 (11), 2608.

[27] Cao X., Yi Y., Ji M., Liu Y., Wang D., Zhao H. The dual role of vitamin C in cancer: from antioxidant prevention to prooxidant. *Front in Med* 2025 ; 12 :1633447.

Chapter 15

The Synergistic Cytotoxicity of Vitamin C and Sorafenib via Mitochondrial Apoptosis and Signaling Modulation in Chronic Lymphocytic Leukemia

Lunawati L. Bennett*, PhD, PharmD
Union University, College of Pharmacy, Jackson, Tennessee, USA

Abstract

Chronic lymphocytic leukemia is cancer that primarily affects older adults, characterized by the accumulation of impaired but mature B-lymphocytes in the blood, bone marrow, and lymphoid tissues. CLL is most common form of leukemia in adults in Western countries, it accounts for approximately 25-30% of all leukemia cases. CLL is due to the clonal expansion of $CD5^+$ B cells that are arrested at an intermediate stage of differentiation. The leukemic cells evade apoptosis process due to genetic mutations and alterations in the B-cell receptor signaling pathway which plays a critical role in the survival and proliferation of CLL cells. Overactivity of this pathway promotes cancer growth and progression. Additionally, CLL cells create an immunosuppressive microenvironment that can impair T-cell function, allowing the leukemia cells to evade immune surveillance. The aim of this study was to evaluate whether the addition of vitamin C to the current standard chemotherapy regimen provides additional therapeutic benefits. Specifically, the study investigates whether VC alone or in combination with a low dose of the chemotherapeutic agent sorafenib is more effective in treating CLL using Z138 as the model. Results from SRB assays, Rhodamine 123, Hoechst 33342 staining, and Western blot analysis showed that the addition of vitamin C to sorafenib amplified oxidative stress and apoptotic signaling, while suppressing oncogenic proteins such as MEK -1, -2, -3, -4, ERK, Akt, and EGFR. These findings suggest that vitamin C enhances sorafenib's anticancer efficacy by simultaneously promoting mitochondrial-mediated apoptosis and inhibiting key survival pathways, supporting its potential as a complementary therapeutic strategy in chronic myelogenous leukemia.

Keywords: chronic lymphocytic leukemia, vitamin C, tyrosine kinase inhibitor, adult cancer

---

* Corresponding Author's Email: llbennett@uu.edu

Abbreviations

MAPKs	Mitogen-activated protein kinases;
MEKs	Mitogen-activated protein kinase kinases;
MDM2	Mouse double minute 2 homolog;
MnSOD	Manganese superoxide dismutase;
p85	Phosphatidylinositol-3-kinase;
PTEN	Phosphatase and tensin homolog;
ROCK	Rho-associated kinase;
ROS	Reactive oxygen species;
SAPK/JNK	Stress-activated protein kinase/c-Jun N-terminal kinase;
Smac/DIABLO	Second mitochondria-derived activator of caspases/ Direct IAP-Binding protein with Low pI.

Introduction

Chronic lymphocytic leukemia (CLL) is the most common adult leukemia in Western countries, representing about 25–30% of all leukemia cases, with an annual incidence of approximately 4–5 per 100,000 persons. The disease primarily affects elderly individuals (median age ~70 years) and is characterized by the clonal accumulation of $CD5^+$ B cells arrested at an intermediate stage of differentiation. These malignant cells evade apoptosis through genetic

and signaling alterations, particularly hyperactivation of the B-cell receptor (BCR) pathway - and by fostering an immunosuppressive microenvironment that impairs T-cell surveillance [1–3].

Despite major advances with targeted therapies such as ibrutinib (BTK inhibitor) and venetoclax (BCL-2 inhibitor), treatment resistance and relapse remain frequent, underscoring the need for novel adjuvant approaches that enhance therapeutic response and overcome apoptotic resistance [4]. Sorafenib, a multi-kinase inhibitor targeting RAF, VEGFR, and PDGFR signaling, exhibits antileukemic activity through MAPK inhibition and mitochondrial stress induction [5]. However, its clinical application in hematologic malignancies is limited by dose-dependent toxicity and compensatory redox adaptation. Vitamin C (VC), at pharmacologic concentrations, functions as a pro-oxidant in cancer cells by generating reactive oxygen species (ROS), disrupting mitochondrial integrity, and promoting apoptotic signaling while sparing normal cells [6-8].

Given these complementary mechanisms, combining VC with SF may potentiate oxidative stress, amplify apoptosis, and attenuate pro-survival signaling in CLL cells. This study therefore investigates the molecular effects of VC and SF - alone and in combination - on CLL-derived Z-138 cells, focusing on ROS generation, mitochondrial dysfunction, caspase activation, and modulation of survival pathways. The goal is to determine whether redox modulation via VC enhances the antineoplastic efficacy of SF in a leukemia context, offering insights into potential translational synergy.

To evaluate the cytotoxic potential of high-dose VC, various antineoplastic agents - including paclitaxel, doxorubicin, etoposide, temsirolimus, bortezomib, afatinib, and sorafenib - were tested on chronic lymphocytic leukemia model using Z-138 cells. For combination studies, the lowest concentrations of each antineoplastic and high-dose VC that yielded a synergistic reduction in cell viability were selected. General experimental procedures followed the protocols outlined in Chapter 3 (Materials and Methods), while methodological details specific to this study are described below.

Cell Culture

Human mantle-cell lymphoma Z-138 (ATCC® CRL-3001™) was derived from a male patient with CLL that progressed to lymphoma blastoid variant. The line carries cytogenetic abnormalities characteristic of mantle-cell lymphoma. Cells were maintained in Iscove's Modified Dulbecco's Medium (IMDM) supplemented with 10% fetal bovine serum and 1% penicillin/streptomycin at 37°C in a humidified atmosphere containing 5% CO_2.

Results

Cell Viability and Selection of Doses

Cells treated with VC alone showed approximately 50% viability at a concentration of 12.5 mM, while treatment with SF alone induced 50% cell death at 5 μM. Based on these findings, 5 μM SF was selected for combination studies with VC to evaluate potential synergistic effects on Z138 cell viability. The combined treatment of VC and SF produced a greater reduction in cell viability than either agent alone, indicating a synergistic interaction. Chou-Talalay analysis indicates a strong synergistic cytotoxic effect of VC and SF in CLL Z138 cells, which is far greater than expected from either agent alone.

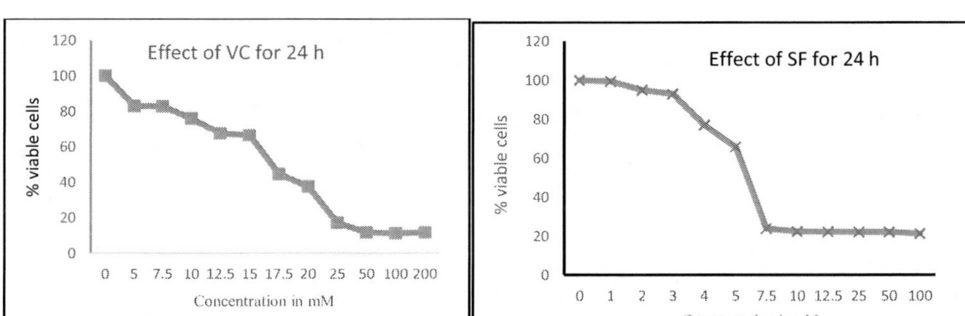

(a) (b)

Figure 1. (Continued).

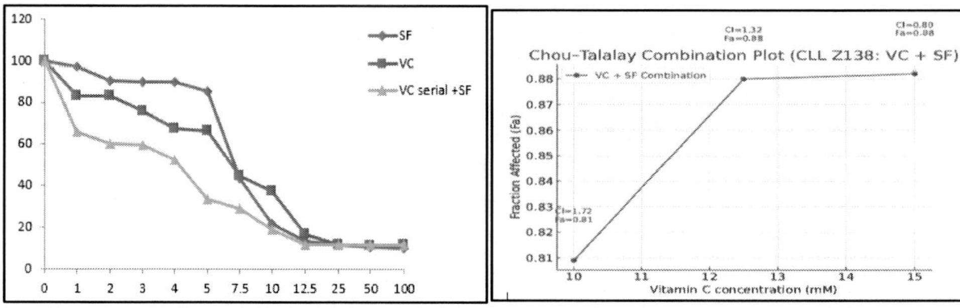

(c) (d)

Figure 1. (a) shows that Z-138 cell viability decreased with increasing VC concentrations (0 to 200 mM) after 24 h (b) indicates a reduction in cell viability with SF achieved IC 50 at 5μM. 1(c) highlights the combined effect of VC at 12.5 mM and SF at 5 μM. Data represents SD from three independent experiments. (d). Strong synergistic effects with CI 0.61 and Fa = 0.81.

Changes in Cells Morphology

VC and SF resulted in alteration of morphologies Z-138 cell. While control cells remained healthy, showing increased numbers and more rounded appearance after 24 h of incubation, cells treated with VC or SF alone exhibited reduced viabilities with shrink and morphological changes. VC and SF treatment caused significant changes in the cell number and appearance.

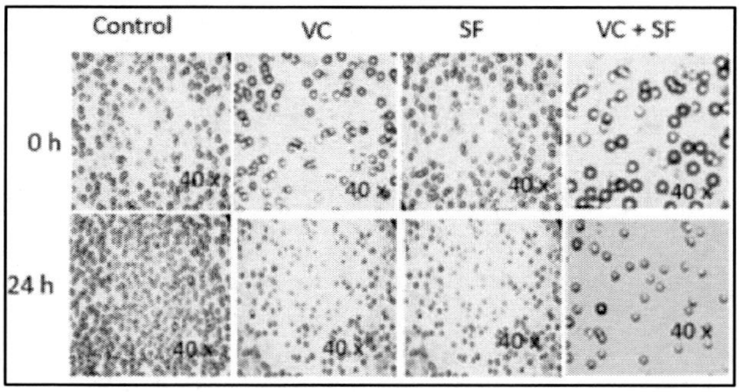

Figure 2. Inverted microscopic images of Z-138 cells (40X) after 24 h treatment with VC, SF, or a combination revealed alterations in cell morphologies versus control cell increase in numbers with healthy appearances.

Dead and Alive Cells

Cell viability after treatment of VC and SF was further examined using Nuclear-ID Red/Green staining to distinguish live and dead cells. Control Z-138 cells exhibited predominantly green fluorescence, consistent with high viability. Treatment with SF and VC induced relatively greater reddish/yellowish fluorescence signal, indicating cell death (see Fig.3).

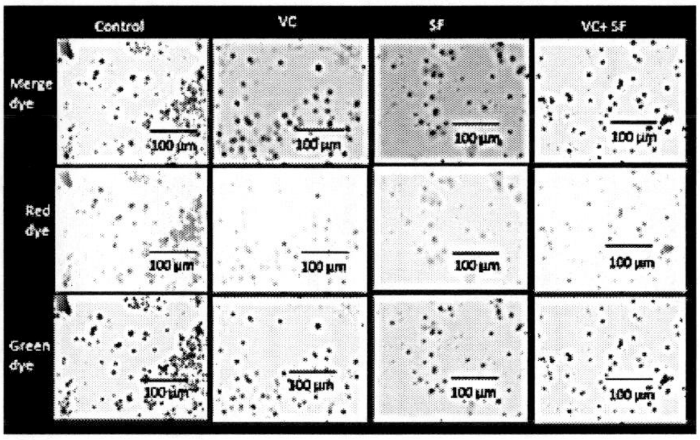

Figure 3. Presents the results of the fluorescence image of Z-138 cells stained with nuclear Red/green.

Induction of Apoptosis

The combination of VC and SF resulted in a higher rate of apoptosis in Z-138 cells compared to treatment with VC or SF alone. This finding confirmed by Hoechst 33342 staining and observed in fluorescence microscopy images which reveals control cells had more alive cells, while apoptotic cells exhibited bright blue fluorescence due to nuclear condensation and fragmentation (see Fig.4).

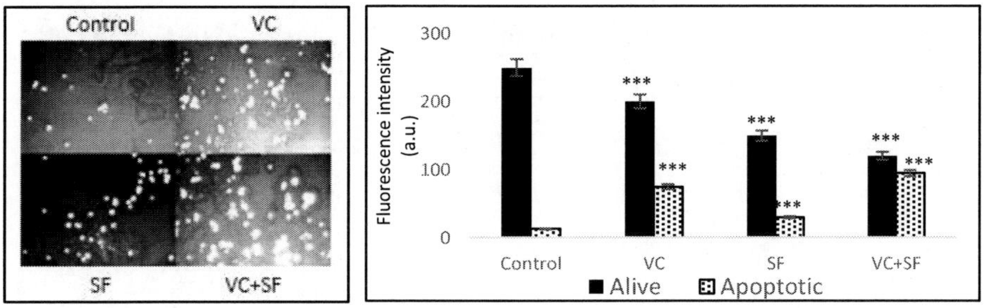

(a) (b)

Figure 4. (a) Fluorescence microscopic images of Z-138 cells treated for 24 h with VC, SF, or their combination. The images reveal a significantly higher number of apoptotic cells, indicated by bright nuclei, in the treatments versus control (b). The scale bar represents 100 µm. Data represents SD from three independent experiments. A significant increase in apoptotic cells was observed, with $**p < 0.01$, $***p < 0.001$, as determined by the post hoc Newman-Keuls test.

Intracellular ROS Generation

The generation of intracellular ROS was assessed in Z-138 cells following treatment with VC, SF, or their combination, using H2DCFDA staining. Variations in fluorescence intensity through microscopic images were observed with higher ROS generation as indicated by increase in fluorescence intensity. Control with darker colors indicates lower ROS generation.

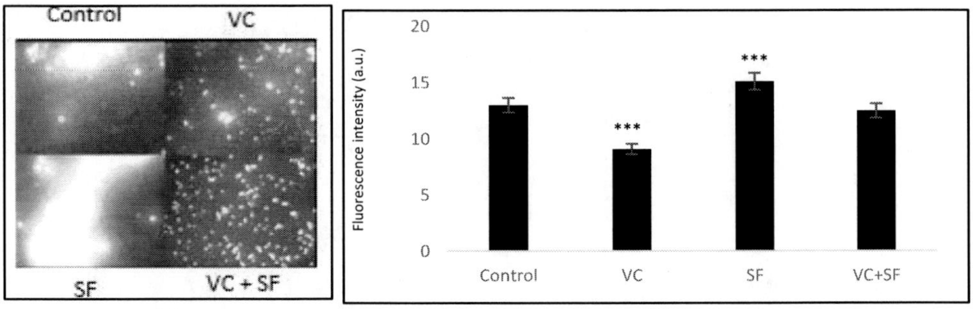

(a) (b)

Figure 5. Intracellular ROS generation in Z-138 cells after 24 h. of treatment. (a) Representative fluorescence microscopy images following H2DCFDA staining. Increased fluorescence intensity corresponds to higher ROS levels. Scale bar = 100 µm. (b) Histogram of fluorescence intensity comparing control, VC, SF, and combination treatments. Data are expressed as mean ± SD (n = 3); ***p < 0.001 vs control (post hoc Newman–Keuls test).

Mitochondrial Membrane Potential (Ψ_m)

The generation of ROS in Z-138 cells indicated cell death attributed to the depletion of mitochondrial membrane potential, as detected with Rhodamine 123 staining. Treatments with VC, SF, or the combination induced cell death, as shown in the fluorescence microscopic with darker images. Control cells exhibited higher fluorescence intensity, indicating healthy mitochondria, compared to treated cells.

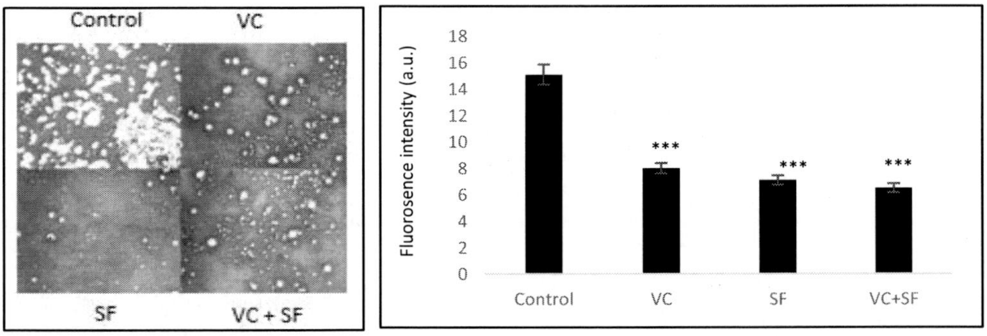

(a) (b)

Figure 6. The mitochondrial membrane potential of Z-138 cells after 24 h. of treatment with VC, SF, or the combination. (a) Representative fluorescence microscopy images following H2DCFDA staining. Increased fluorescence intensity corresponds to higher ROS levels. Scale bar = 100 µm. (b) Histogram of fluorescence intensity comparing control, VC, SF, and combination treatments. Data are expressed as mean ± SD (n = 3); ***p < 0.001 vs control (post hoc Newman–Keuls test).

Modulation of Bax, Bcl2, AIF, and Cytochrome C

In apoptotic cells, the intracellular generation of ROS is linked to alterations in the expressions of Bax and Bcl2 proteins. Increase in Bax and a decrease in Bcl2 expressions in Z-138 cells treated with a combination of VC and SF also resulting in an increased release of cytochrome C (cyt) into the cytosol, which further induced apoptosis. A slight increase in the expression of apoptosis-inducing factor (AIF) was observed in cells treated with VC alone.

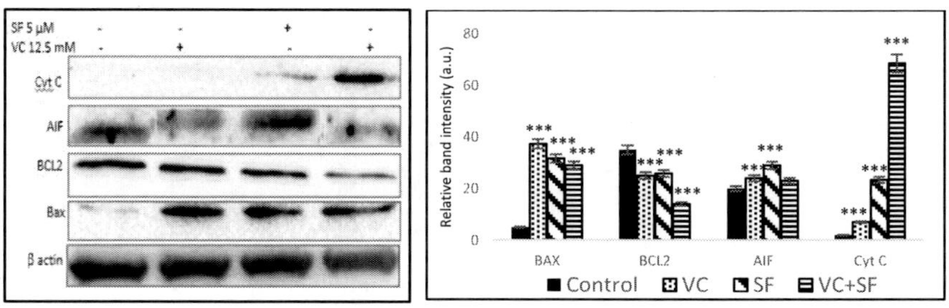

(a) (b)

Figure 7. Western blot analysis of Bax, Bcl2, AIF, and cyt C expressions in Z-138 cells following treatment with VC, SF, or their combination. (a) Representative blots showing expression of these proteins. (b) Densitometric histogram compares relative protein levels normalized to β-actin. Data are expressed as mean ± SD (n = 3). Statistical significance was determined using the Newman–Keuls post hoc test (***$p < 0.001$).

Modulation Mitochondrial Signaling Proteins

Mitochondrial apoptosis resulting from a decline in membrane potential is linked to various crucial proteins, including caspases (Cas-9, -3, -7, and -8) and apoptotic peptidase activating factors (Apaf-1). Marked increases in caspase-9, -7, -3, -8, and Apaf-1 compared with the control indicate activation of both intrinsic and extrinsic apoptotic cascades. The combined SF and VC treatment produced the most pronounced response, demonstrating a synergistic induction of mitochondrial apoptosis.

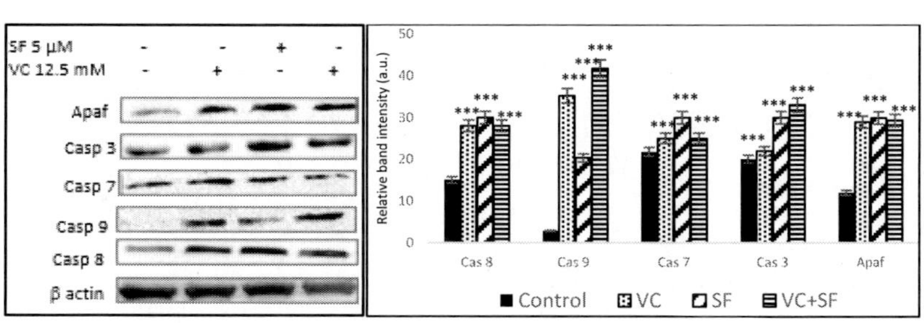

(a) (b)

Figure 8. Western blot analysis results of various mitochondrial signaling proteins in Z-138 cells after treatment with VC, SF or the combination. (a) Representative blots showing expression of these proteins. (b) Densitometric histogram compares relative protein levels normalized to β-actin. Data are expressed as mean ± SD (n = 3). Significant changes are indicated by ***$p < 0.001$, according to the post hoc Newman-Keuls test.

Modulation of MEK Kinase Pathway

To investigate the potential mechanism of VC, SF, or their combination in modulating aberrant cell signaling of mitogen-activated protein kinases (MAPKs), Western blot analysis was conducted to assess the active and phosphorylated forms of mitogen-activated protein kinase kinase (MEK). Significant decreases in MEK-1, -2, -3, and -4 expressions were observed in Z-138 cells. The corresponding band intensity is depicted in the histogram compared to control.

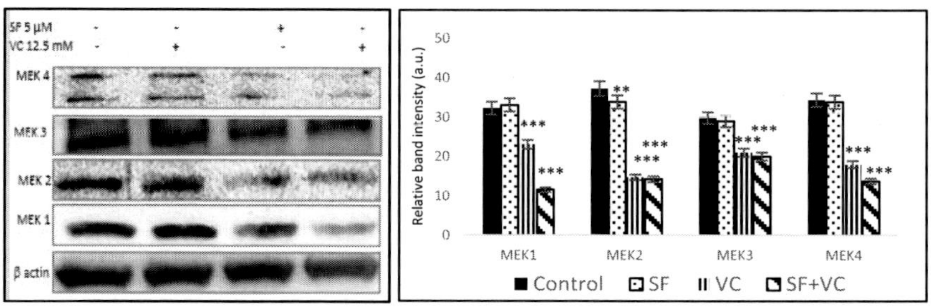

(a) (b)

Figure 9. Western blot analysis results of MEK-1, -2, -3, and -4 after treating Z-138 cells with VC, SF, or their combination. (a) Representative blots showing expression of these proteins. (b) Densitometric histogram compares relative protein levels normalized to β-actin. Data are expressed as mean ± SD (n = 3). Significant change indicated by ***$p < 0.001$, according to the post hoc Newman-Keuls test.

Modulation of Cell Cycle Regulatory Proteins

Modulation of cell cycle progression is also considered an important strategy in the management of CLL. Decreases in proteins involved in cell cycle regulation CDK2, cyclin B1 and cyclin D1 were observed in VC only treated cells of Z-138, while SF caused increase expression of cyclin B1 and CDK2 showing unfavorable effect of SF only treatment. Combination of VC and SF cause decrease in all these proteins showing synergistic effect.

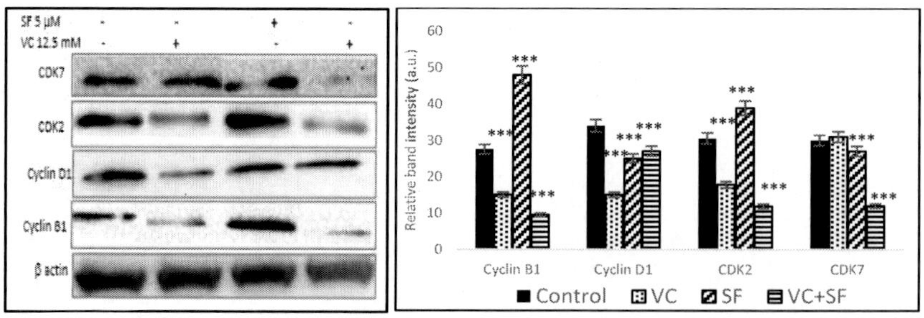

(a) (b)

Figure 10. Western blot analysis of cyclin B1, cyclin D1, CDK2, and CDK7 expressions after treating Z-138 cells with VC, SF, or their combination. (a) Representative blots showing expression of these proteins. (b) Densitometric histogram compares relative protein levels normalized to β-actin. Data are expressed as mean ± SD (n = 3). Significant increases are indicated as ***$p < 0.001$, according to the post hoc Newman-Keuls test.

Modulation of p21, p53, PTEN, and MDM2

The impact of VC, SF, and their combination on the expression of key regulatory proteins, including p21, p53, PTEN, and MDM2 were assessed in Z-138 cells. Treatment with VC, SF, or their combination resulted in notable modulation of these proteins. Specifically, there was a significant increase in the expression levels of p21, indicative of a positive regulatory effect on cell cycle control and tumor suppression. Conversely, the expression of MDM2 decreased, suggesting a potential inhibitory effect on the MDM2 pathway. Slight increase in p53 and PTEN levels was identified in cells treated with VC and SF combination, with significant increase in PTEN expression in cells treated with SF only.

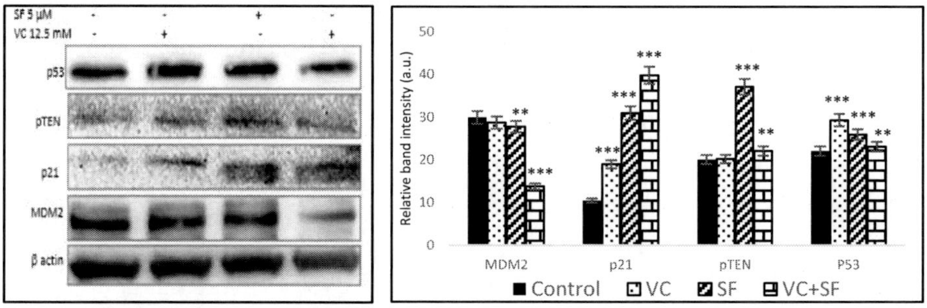

(a) (b)

Figure 11. Western blot analysis of MDM2, p21, PTEN, p53 expressions in Z-138 cells treated with VC, SF, and their combination. (a) Representative blots showing expression of these proteins. (b) Densitometric histogram compares relative protein levels normalized to β-actin. Data are expressed as mean ± SD (n = 3). Significant changes are marked as **p < 0.01 and ***p < 0.001, according to the post hoc Newman-Keuls test.

Modulation of Akt/p85/mTOR

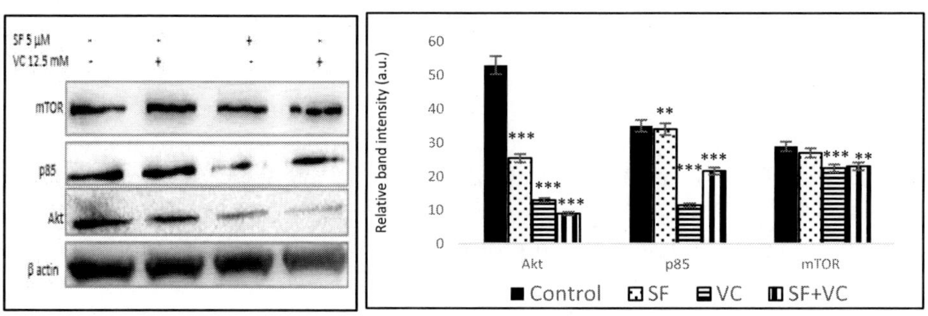

(a) (b)

Figure 12. Western blot analysis of Akt, p85, and mTOR expressions after treatment of Z-138 cells with VC, SF, or their combination. (a) Representative blots showing expression of these proteins. (b) Densitometric histogram compares relative protein levels normalized to β-actin. Data are expressed as mean ± SD (n = 3). Significant changes are indicated as **p < 0.01 and ***p < 0.001, according to the post hoc Newman-Keuls test.

The effect of VC, SF, and their combination on Akt, p85 and mTOR expression was assessed with Western blot. A decrease in Akt expression was observed in all treatments compared to the control, indicating a favorable effect of VC, SF, or their combination. In addition, slight decrease in p85 and mTOR showed favorable effect of combining VC to SF treatment in Z-138 cells.

Modulation of SAPK/JNK and p38

The impact of VC, SF, and their combined treatment on SAPK/JNK and p38 proteins was evaluated in Z-138 cells. The combination treatment caused more pronounce decrease in p38 and SAP/JNK proteins, while SF only causes increase in SAPK/JNK expression. The combination treatment showed favorable effect on CLL. The reduction in stress-activated kinases suggests that VC, either alone or in combination with SF, effectively suppresses stress-induced signaling pathways, thereby attenuating cellular responses associated with oxidative or mitogenic stress.

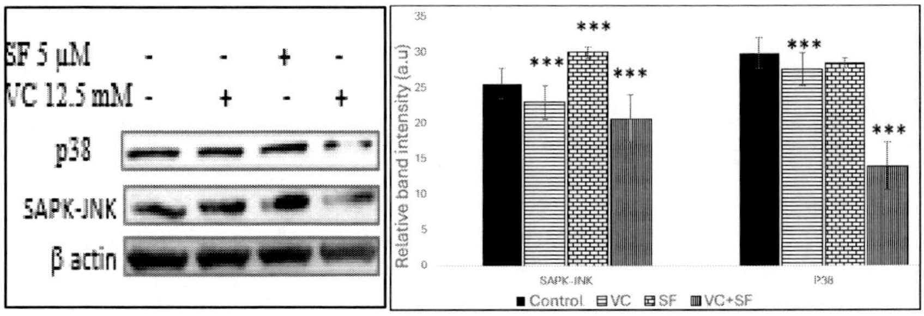

(a) (b)

Figure 13. Western blot analysis of SAPK/JNK and p38 expressions after treatment of Z-138 cells with VC, SF, or their combination. (a) Representative blots showing expression of these proteins. (b) Densitometric histogram compares relative protein levels normalized to β-actin. Data are expressed as mean ± SD (n = 3). Significant changes are marked as***p < 0.001, according to the post hoc Newman-Keuls test.

Modulation of ERK and EGFR

The impact of VC, SF, and their combined treatment on ERK1/2 and EGFR was assessed in Z-138 cells. Decreased expressions of ERK1/2 and EGFR in all treatments indicate inhibition of cell survival and proliferation of cancerous cells by VC and ET in CLL (see Fig. 14).

Modulation of Histone and ABCG2

The impact of VC, SF, and their combined treatment on histone and ABCG2 proteins was assessed in Z-138 cells. A decrease in both proteins indicates that the combination may suppress drug resistance of leukemic cells by ABCG2, a key ATP-binding cassette transporter, which is often upregulated in malignant cells and alter chromatin regulation. VC contributes to enhanced cytotoxic effects of SF in CLL (see Fig.15).

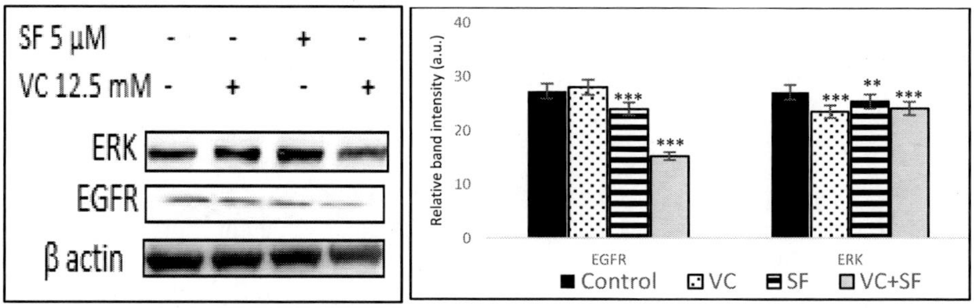

(a) (b)

Figure 14. Western blot analysis of ERK and EGFR expressions after treatment of Z-138 cells with VC, SF, or their combination. (a) Representative blots showing expression of these proteins. (b) Densitometric histogram compares relative protein levels normalized to β-actin. Data are expressed as mean ± SD (n = 3). Significant changes are marked as $^{**}p < 0.01$, $^{***}p < 0.001$, according to the post hoc Newman-Keuls test.

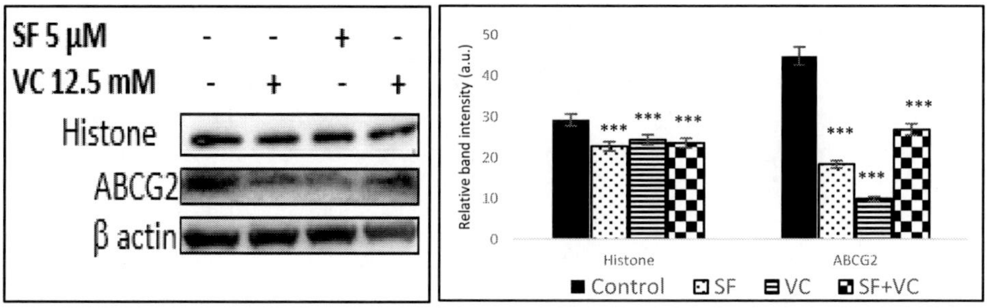

(a) (b)

Figure 15. Western blot analysis of histone and ABCG2 expressions after treatment of Z-138 cells with VC, SF, or their combination. (a) Representative blots showing expression of these proteins. (b) Densitometric histogram compares relative protein levels normalized to β-actin. Data are expressed as mean ± SD (n = 3). Significant changes are marked as $^{***}p < 0.001$, according to the post hoc Newman-Keuls test.

Modulation of MnSOD, Smac/Diablo, and Vimentin

Both VC and SF alone increased the expression of Smac/Diablo and MnSOD, suggesting enhanced pro-apoptotic signaling and elevated antioxidant defense. The combination treatment further amplified these effects, indicating potential synergistic activation of mitochondrial apoptotic pathways. In contrast, Vimentin expression, a marker of cytoskeletal integrity and epithelial–mesenchymal transition (EMT), was significantly reduced across all treatment groups, with the combination showing the most pronounced decrease. This reduction in Vimentin suggests that VC and SF, especially together, may suppress metastatic potential in Z-138 cells.

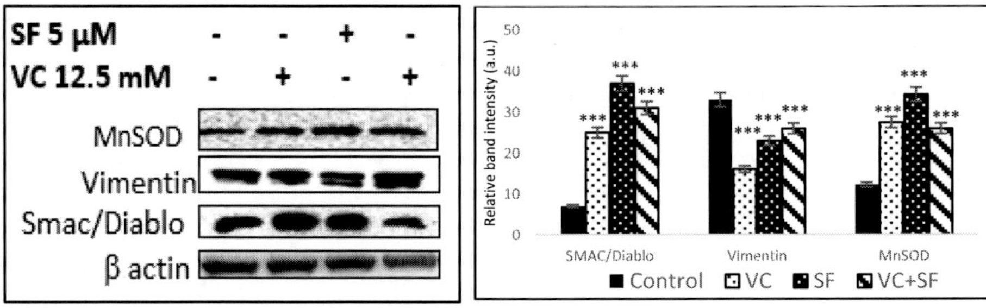

(a) (b)

Figure 16. Western blot analysis of MnSOD, Smac/Diablo, and Vimentin expressions after treatment of Z-138 cells with VC, SF, or their combination. (a) Representative blots showing expression of these proteins. (b) Densitometric histogram compares relative protein levels normalized to β-actin. Data are expressed as mean ± SD (n = 3). Data represents SD from three independent experiments. Significant changes are marked as ***p < 0.001, according to the post hoc Newman-Keuls test.

Modulation of MMP9 and MMP2

The impact of VC and SF combined treatment on MMP2 and MMP 9 Showed favorable effect in Z-138 cells, while VC or SF treatment alone cause increased in the expression of MMP9. The combination markedly reduced both MMP2 and MMP9 levels, suggesting a synergistic suppression of extracellular matrix degradation and metastatic potential, which may contribute to the overall antitumor efficacy in CLL (see Fig. 17).

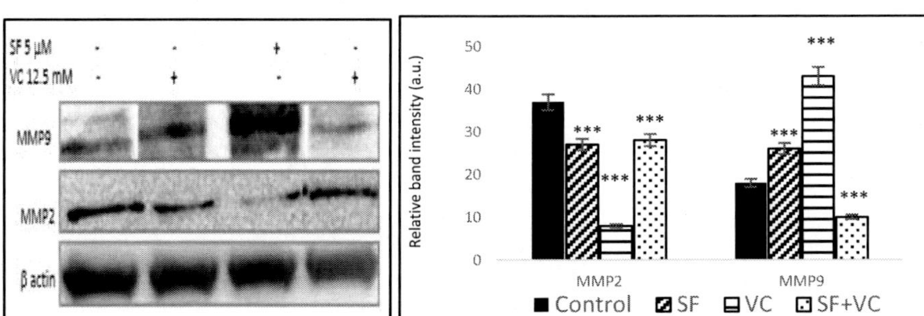

(a) (b)

Figure 17. Western blot analysis of MMP2 and MMP9 expressions after treatment of Z-138 cells with VC, SF, or their combination. (a) Representative blots showing expression of these proteins. (b) Densitometric histogram compares relative protein levels normalized to β-actin. Data are expressed as mean ± SD (n = 3). Significant changes are marked as ***p < 0.001, according to the post hoc Newman-Keuls test.

Modulation of PDL1 and PDK1

The effect of VC and SF on PD-L1 and PDK1 expressions was evaluated in Z-138 cells. While VC alone led to an increase in PD-L1 and PDK1 levels, the combined VC and

SF treatment resulted in a marked reduction of both proteins, indicating a more favorable therapeutic effect through suppression of immune evasion and metabolic survival signaling (see Fig. 18).

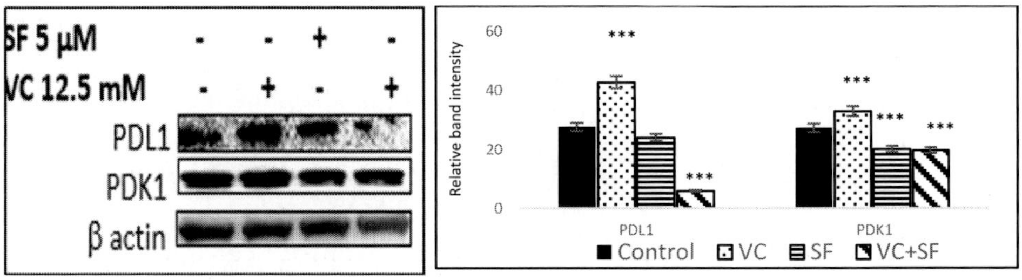

(a) (b)

Figure 18. Western blot analysis of PDL1 and PDK1 expressions after treatment of Z-138 cells with VC, SF, or their combination. (a) Representative blots showing expression of these proteins. (b) Densitometric histogram compares relative protein levels normalized to β-actin. Data are expressed as mean ± SD (n = 3). Significant changes are marked as ***p < 0.001, according to the post hoc Newman-Keuls test.

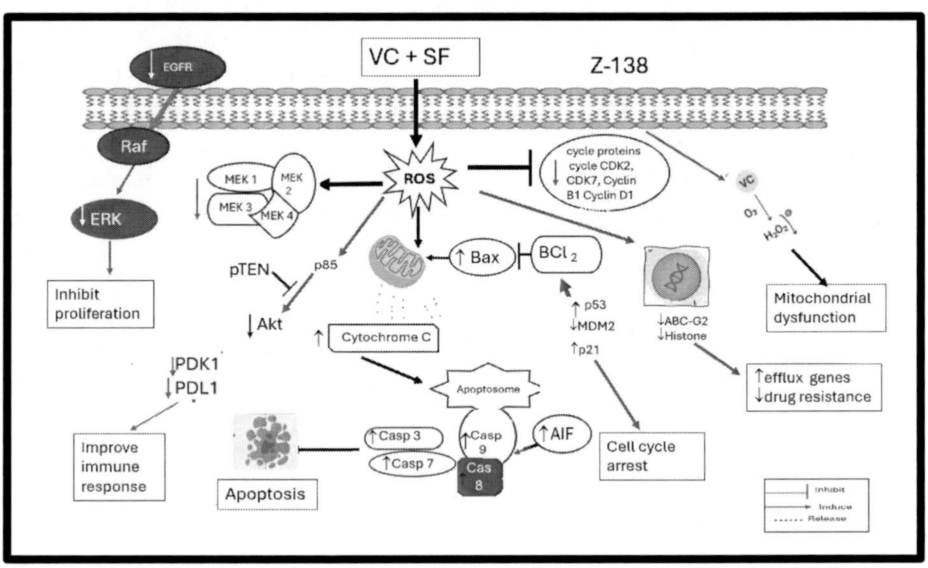

Figure 19. Proposed mechanistic model of VC and SF in CLL.

Discussion

As illustrated in Figure 19, VC, SF, and their combined treatment exert cytotoxic effects on Z-138 CLL cells, by synergistic induce apoptosis, inhibit cells proliferation, arrest cell cycle proteins, and cause mitochondria dysfunction. Nuclear-ID and Hoechst 33342 staining clearly showed that the combination of VC and SF increased apoptotic morphology compared with either treatment alone. The higher proportion of red fluorescence in the live/dead assay, coupled with the condensed and fragmented nuclei in Hoechst staining, confirmed apoptosis as the dominant mode of cell death. This cytotoxic effect coincided with a marked rise in intracellular ROS detected by H_2DCFDA and a decline in mitochondrial membrane potential ($\Delta\Psi m$) observed with Rhodamine 123 staining. ROS overproduction is a known mechanism through which high-dose VC induces selective cancer cell death by generating H_2O_2 and depleting antioxidant defenses [10]. Similar mechanisms have been reported in hematologic malignancies, where pharmacologic VC selectively kills leukemic cells by impairing mitochondrial respiration. In their study, Darwiche et al used VC with approved drug for CLL such as ibrutinib, venetoclax. This combination showed synergism in CLL cells [11].

Western blot analysis supported these findings, showing upregulation of Bax and downregulation of Bcl-2, accompanied by cytosolic release of cytochrome C and increased expression of AIF. These molecular events signify activation of intrinsic apoptosis and mitochondrial outer membrane permeabilization. Parallel elevation of caspases -9, -3, -7, and -8, together with enhanced Apaf-1, reinforces that the VC and SF combination triggers both intrinsic and extrinsic apoptotic cascades. A reduction in XIAP (X-linked inhibitor of apoptosis) further confirms the loss of survival checkpoints. Comparable activation of caspase cascades has been observed when SF was combined with oxidative stressors in leukemia models [12-13].

Aberrant MAPK activity contributes to leukemogenesis and chemoresistance. The observed decreases in MEK-1, -2, -3, and -4 expression after VC and SF treatment indicate effective suppression of the MAPK cascade, which likely contributes to the reduced ERK1/2 phosphorylation seen in parallel assays. Inhibition of this pathway can diminish cell proliferation and promote apoptosis in CLL [14]. Decreases in p38 and SAPK/JNK proteins, especially under combination treatment, suggest that VC augments the kinase-inhibitory effect of SF, possibly by modulating ROS-dependent phosphorylation feedback loops. While SF typically inhibits Raf/MEK/ERK signaling [15], the data show that VC further amplifies this suppression, consistent with reports that VC can inactivate MAPK and PI3K/Akt pathways in hematologic cancers [16].

Interestingly, the combined treatment also reduced Akt, p85, and mTOR levels, pointing to downregulation of the PI3K/Akt/mTOR axis. In CLL, constitutive activation of this pathway drives survival and therapy resistance [17]. The observed decreases indicate that VC may sensitize leukemic cells to SF by concurrently attenuating both MAPK and PI3K pathways, a dual blockade that may underline the synergistic apoptotic effect.

Cell-cycle dysregulation is central to CLL pathogenesis. In Z-138 cells, VC alone decreased cyclin B1, cyclin D1, and CDK2, suggesting partial arrest, whereas SF alone increased some of these proteins, consistent with stress-induced compensatory proliferation. The combination, however, suppressed all tested cyclins and CDKs, implying a cooperative inhibition of G_1/S and G_2/M transitions. These changes align with the upregulation of p21 and p53, both key mediators of checkpoint arrest and apoptosis. Enhanced PTEN expression, particularly in SF-treated cells, further supports restoration of negative regulation on PI3K/Akt signaling [18-19] The decrease in MDM2, an E3 ligase that normally suppresses p53, indicates stabilization of tumor-suppressor signaling. Together, these findings suggest that the VC and SF combination restores cell-cycle control and promotes apoptosis through the p53–p21–PTEN axis, a mechanism consistent with prior reports showing VC-induced demethylation and reactivation of tumor-suppressor genes [20-21].

The elevation of MnSOD and Smac/Diablo proteins suggests that, while oxidative stress is initiated, the mitochondrial antioxidant response and apoptosome formation are simultaneously enhanced. Smac release neutralizes IAPs, reinforcing caspase activation [22-23]. Increased E-cadherin and reduced Vimentin further indicate reversal of epithelial–mesenchymal transition (EMT), implying that VC and SF may reduce invasiveness. These effects are comparable to observations in other cancers where SF suppressed EMT markers and VC restored epithelial integrity [24].

Decreases in histone and ABCG2 expression also imply reduced chromatin condensation and lower drug-efflux activity, potentially enhancing intracellular retention of SF. Reduced PDK1 and PD-L1 levels observed under combined treatment point toward inhibition of metabolic adaptation and immune-evasion mechanisms, which may further potentiate antileukemic effects [25].

The Wnt/β-catenin and ROCK pathways, often aberrantly activated in leukemias, regulate cell migration and survival. The data demonstrated that combination treatment maintained low expression of these proteins, consistent with impaired cytoskeletal dynamics and diminished motility. Downregulation of MMP-2 and MMP-9 in the combined group supports reduced extracellular-matrix degradation and metastatic potential. These results mirror prior findings that SF downregulates MMPs and Wnt signaling in melanoma and hepatoma cells, while VC antagonizes β-catenin activation by modulating redox status [26-27].

Future work should evaluate in vivo efficacy of VC and SF in CLL xenograft models while assessing pharmacodynamics and oxidative stress biomarkers; synergistic selectivity to understand if normal lymphocytes are spared from ROS-mediated cytotoxicity, exploring dose ratios that maximize apoptosis while minimizing off-target kinase inhibition, and clinical feasibility using high-dose VC infusion with SF in CLL patients.

Conclusion

Combination of VC and SF exerts a synergistic antileukemic effect in Z-138 cells through activation of intrinsic and extrinsic apoptotic pathways, suppression of MEK/ERK and PI3K/Akt/mTOR signaling, and modulation of cell-cycle and redox-regulatory proteins. VC enhances SF efficacy by promoting ROS-dependent apoptosis and reducing prosurvival kinases, EMT markers, and efflux transporters. These findings provide a mechanistic rationale for integrating VC as an adjuvant to kinase inhibitors in the treatment of CLL. Together, these findings reveal that oxidative stress–mediated mitochondrial apoptosis, coupled with inhibition of survival and proliferative kinases, underlies the favorable effects of this combination in leukemic cells.

Key Findings

The combined treatment of VC and SF exhibited a synergistic cytotoxic effect on CLL, Z-138 cells through enhanced mitochondrial-dependent apoptosis and inhibition of major survival pathways. VC amplified oxidative stress and apoptotic signaling, while suppressing oncogenic proteins such as MEK -1, -2, -3, -4, ERK, Akt, and EGFR. The downregulation of vimentin, MMP9, and PDL1 further suggests a reduction in metastatic potential and immune evasion. Altogether, these findings support the potential of VC as an effective adjuvant that sensitizes leukemia cells to SF, providing a foundation for future translational and preclinical investigations.

Acknowledgments

The author thanks Union University for the source and support of research funding as well as colleagues and editing tools for assistance with improving the clarity of the manuscript.

References

[1] Burger J.A., Chiorazzi N. B cell receptor signaling in chronic lymphocytic leukemia. *Blood* 2014 ; 114(2) : 3635-3644.

[2] Svanberg R., Janum S., Patten P.E.M., Ramsay A.G. Niemann CU. Targeting the Tumor microenvironment in chronic lymphocytic leukemia. *Haematologica* 2021 ; 106 : 2312-2324.

[3] Koffman B., Warwick L., Haggert P., Piers E.M., Patten M., Moura C., et al., A charter for improving care for people living with chronic lymphocytic leukemia: six principles of excellence. *Leukemia & Lymphoma* 2025 ; 66 : 2090-2096.

[4] Awan F.T., Al-Sawaf O., Fischer K., Woyach J.A. Current perspective on therapy for chronic lymphocytic leukemia. *Hematologic Malignancies* 2020 ; 40.

[5] Damle R.N., Wasil T., Fais F., Allen S.L., Budman D., Kolitz J., et al., Ig V gene mutation status and CD38 expression as novel prognostic indicators in chronic lymphocytic leukemia. *Blood* 1999 ; 94(6), 1840-1847.

[6] Mastrangelo D., Massai L., Fioritoni G., Lo Coco F., Noguera N., Testa U. High dose of vitamin C and leukemia: in vitro update. *Myeloid Leukemia* 2018; 10.5772/intechopen.71484.

[7] Mussa A., Idris R.A.M., Ahmed N., Ahmad C., Lazim N.M., Uskoković V, et al., High-dose vitamin C for cancer therapy. *Pharmaceuticals (Basel)* 2022; 15(6):711.

[8] Darwiche W., Gomila C., Ouled-Haddou H., Marolleau J.P., Ghamlouch H. Ascorbic acid (vitamin C) synergistically enhances the therapeutic effect of targeted therapy in chronic lymphocytic leukemia. *J Exp Clin Cancer Res* 2020; 39.

[9] Carr A.C., Lykkesfeldt J. Vitamin C: From bench to bedside. *Nutrients* 2021 ; 13(4) : 1102.

[10] Wilson M., Baguley B.C., Wall C., Jameson M.B., Findlay M.P. Review of high-dose intravenous vitamin C as an anticancer agent. *Asia-Pacific J Clin Oncol* 2014; 10 : 22-37.

[11] Darwiche W., Gomila C., Quled-Haddou H., Naudot M., Doualle C., Morel P, et al., Ascorbic acid (vitamin C) synergistically enhances the therapeutic effect of targeted therapy in chronic lymphocytic leukemia. *J of Exp & Clin Cancer Res* 2020 ; 39, 228.

[12] Mouchel P.L., Berard E., Tavitian S., Gadaud N., Vergez F., Rieu J.B., et al., Vitamin C and D supplementation in acute myeloid leukemia. *Blood Adv* 2023 ; 7:1-12

[13] Sun H.M., Jiang Y., Zhao Z. High-dose vitamin potently induces apoptosis in acute lymphoblastic leukemia by activating ER stress response. *Human & Exp Toxicol* 2025 ; 44 : 1177.

[14] Machado A.K.D., Machado C.B., Pessoa F.M.C.P., Barretto I.V., Gadelha R.B., Oliviera D.D.S., et al., Development and Clinical Applications of PI3K/AKT/mTOR Pathway Inhibitors as therapeutic options in leukemias. *Cancer Diag & Prog* 2024 ; 4(1) : 9-24.

[15] Bahar M.E., Kim H.J., Kim D.R. Targeting the RAS/RAF/MAPK pathway for cancer therapy: from mechanisms to clinical studies. *Signal Transduct Target Ther* 2023 : 8, 455.

[16] Gedaly R., Angulo P., Hundley J., Daily M.F., Chen C., Koch A., et al., PI-103 and Sorafenib inhibit hepatocellular carcinoma cell proliferation by blocking Ras/Raf/MAPK and PI3K/AKT/mTOR Pathways. *Anticancer Res* 2010 ; 30 (12): 4951-4958.

[17] Zhao H., Fu W., Yang X., Zhang W., Wu S., Mu J., et al., High-dose vitamin C: A promising anti-tumor agent, insight into molecular mechanisms. *Genes& Dis* 2025 ; 101742.

[18] Ye L., Mayerle Y., Ziesch A., Reiter F.P., Gerbes A.L. The PI3K inhibitor copanlisib synergizes with sorafenib to induce cell death in hepatocelular carcinoma. *Cell Death Discov* 2019 ; 5: 86.

[19] Carlo-Stella C., Locatelli S.L., Giacomini A. Sorafenib Inhibits Lymphoma Xenografts by Targeting MAPK/ERK and AKT Pathways. *PLoS One* 2013.

[20] Hadi F., Maqbool T., Aftab S., Tahir M., Ramzan S., Kiran K. Dose-dependent Effects of Vitamin C on Cancer Regulation: A Review. *J of Cancer Immunol* 2021 ; 10 : 3369.

[21] Böttger F., Vallés-Martí A., Cahn L. High-dose intravenous vitamin C, a promising multi-targeting agent in the treatment of cancer. *J Exp Clin Cancer Res* 2021 ; 40 :343.

[22] Park S. The effects of high concentrations of vitamin C on Cancer Cells. *Nutrients* 2013. 9 : 3496-3505.

[23] George S., Abrahamsen H. Redox potential of antioxidants in cancer progression and prevention. *Antioxidants* 2020 ; 11 : 1156.

[24] Talib W.H., Jum'ah D.A.A., Attallah Z.S., Jallad M.S., Al Kury L., Hadi R.W., et al., Role of vitamins A, C, D, E in cancer prevention and therapy: therapeutic potentials and mechanisms of action. *Front Nutr* 2024, 1281879.

[25] Huang A., Zeng P., LiY., Lu W., Lai Y. LY294002 Is a Promising Inhibitor to Overcome Sorafenib Resistance in FLT3-ITD mutant AML cells by interfering with PI3K/AKT Pathway. *Front Oncol* 2021, 782065.

[26] Qu B., Liu B.R., Du Y.J., Chen J., Cheng Y.Q., Xu W., et al., Wnt/β-catenin signaling pathway may regulate the expression of angiogenic growth factors in hepatocellular carcinoma. *Oncol Lett* 2014 ; 7 : 1175-1178.

[27] Fan D., Liu X., Shen Z., Wu P., Zhong L., Lin F. Cell signaling pathways based on vitamin C and their application in cancer therapy. *Biomed & Pharmacother* 2023 : 162 : 114695.

Chapter 16

Vitamin C and Sorafenib Synergy in Non-Small Cell Lung Cancer - Dual Modulation of Apoptosis and Survival Pathways

Lunawati L. Bennett*, PhD, PharmD
Union University, College of Pharmacy, Jackson, Tennessee, USA

Abstract

Lung cancer accounts for 18.4% of all cancer-related deaths, with non-small cell lung cancer comprising approximately 85% of the cases. The pathogenesis of lung cancer is driven by genetic and molecular alterations that promote uncontrolled cell proliferation, resistance to apoptosis, and tumor progression. Common mutations, such as those in the epidermal growth factor receptor along with environmental factors like tobacco smoking, contribute to the disease's mutational burden.

While targeted therapies have significantly improved outcomes for genetically selected lung cancer subpopulations, only a small proportion of patients respond to immunotherapy; therefore, continuing exploration of novel therapeutic strategies, including combination treatments and personalized medicine, to enhance patient outcomes are highly sought.

Results from SRB assays, Rhodamine 123, Hoechst 33342 staining, and Western blot analysis showed that the addition of vitamin C to sorafenib inhibits cancer cell growth by inducing Bax, increasing caspases -3, -7, -8, and -9 expressions, decreasing MEK-1,-2, -3, and -4, Bcl-2, and cell cycle proteins The combination of sorafenib and vitamin C exhibits a synergistic effect in non-small cell lung cancer cells by promoting apoptosis, inhibiting oncogenic signaling pathways, disrupting cell cycle progression, and enhancing tumor suppressor activity. These findings suggest that vitamin C may serve as a promising adjunct to sorafenib.

Keywords: non-small cell lung cancer, vitamin C, synergistic effect, NCI-H522 cells, sorafenib

* Corresponding Author's Email: llbennett@uu.edu

Abbreviations

MAPKs	Mitogen-activated protein kinases;
MEKs	Mitogen-activated protein kinase kinases;
MDM2	Mouse double minute 2 homolog;
MnSOD	Manganese superoxide dismutase;
Bax	Bcl2 Associated X-protein;
Bcl2	B cell lymphoma 2;
Cas	Caspase;
CDK7	Cyclin dependent kinase 7;
Cyt C	Cytochrome C.

Introduction

Lung cancer remains the leading cause of deaths, with poor prognosis. It Is divided into two main types, small cell lung cancer (SCLC) account for 15% and non-small cell lung cancer (NSCLC) accounts for approximately 85% of all lung cancer cases, making it the most common type of lung cancer worldwide [1]. It is especially prevalent among smokers, former smokers, and non-smokers. NSCLC incidence rates vary geographically, with the highest rates found in men over 65 years in North America, Europe, and parts of Asia [1-2]. With a steady decline in smoking rates, the incidence of NSCLC' mortality has also decreased [3].

The pathogenesis of NSCLC often involves a series of genetic and molecular alterations that lead to uncontrolled cell proliferation, resistance to cell death, and eventually cancer progression due to genetic mutations such as EGFR or tobacco smoking, which contribute to the mutational burden seen in patients with NSCLC [4-7].

Sorafenib (SF), an oral FDA-approved multi targeted tyrosine kinase inhibitor, has been shown to increase survival in renal, hepatocellular, and thyroid cancer [8]. It has also shown promise in NSCLC by targeting angiogenesis and tumor cell proliferation through inhibition of rapidly accelerated fibrosarcoma/C rat sarcoma virus/MEK/extracellular signal regulated kinase (RAF/RAS/MEK/ERK), vascular endothelial growth factor receptor (VEGFR), and platelet-derived growth factor receptor (PDGFR) signaling pathways [9-12].

High-dose intravenous vitamin C (VC) or also known as ascorbic acid to attain plasma levels of ≥ 20 mM, has recently emerged as a potential non-toxic adjuvant to standard care radio-chemotherapy-based cancer therapies across various disease sites [13-14]. The proposed anti-cancer mechanism of pharmacological of VC involves redox-active metal-mediated or auto-oxidation of ascorbate, resulting in the formation of O_2 and H_2O_2 [15-17].

This study was designed to evaluate the chemo-enhancing potential of VC in combination with low-dose SF for treating NSCLC. The findings of this investigation reveal that the use of VC with SF demonstrated greater efficacy in the treatment of NSCLC. This marks a novel discovery in the field.

To evaluate the cytotoxic potential of high-dose VC, various antineoplastic agents - including paclitaxel, doxorubicin, etoposide, temsirolimus, bortezomib, afatinib, and sorafenib - were tested on human NSCLC using the model NCI-H5222 cell line. For combination studies, the lowest concentrations of each antineoplastic and high-dose VC that yielded a synergistic reduction in cell viability were selected. General experimental procedures followed the protocols outlined in Chapter 3 (Materials and Methods), while methodological details specific to this study are described below.

Cell Culture

Non-small-cell lung carcinoma (NCI-H521, ATCC CRL 5810) exhibits epithelial morphology that was isolated from the lungs of a 58-year-old white male with adenocarcinoma, were cultured in RPMI-1640 medium. The media contains 2 mM L-glutamine, 10mM HEPES, 1 mM sodium pyruvate, 4500 mg/L glucose, and 1500 mg/L sodium bicarbonate, and supplemented with 10% fetal bovine serum and 1% penicillin/streptomycin (100 U/ml penicillin, 200 μg/ml streptomycin). The cells were maintained at 37° C in a humidified atmosphere of 5% CO_2.

Results

Cell Viability and Selection of Doses

Treatment of NCI-H522 cells with increasing concentrations of VC (0–100 mM) for 24 h resulted in a slight decrease of cell viability. A concentration of 6.25 mM was selected as a mid-range dose that produced mild cytotoxicity without excessive cell death, thereby allowing clearer assessment of potential synergistic effects when combined with SF. This concentration also falls within the pharmacologically achievable range reported in in vitro models using VC to study redox-mediated modulation of cancer signaling, without inducing non-specific oxidative damage to normal-like cells. SF alone reduced cell viability beginning at 6 μM, which was therefore chosen as the working concentration for subsequent experiments. VC was shown to sensitize NSCLC cells to SF, pushing them toward oxidative and apoptotic vulnerability - showing promise for redox-based combination therapy in lung cancer.

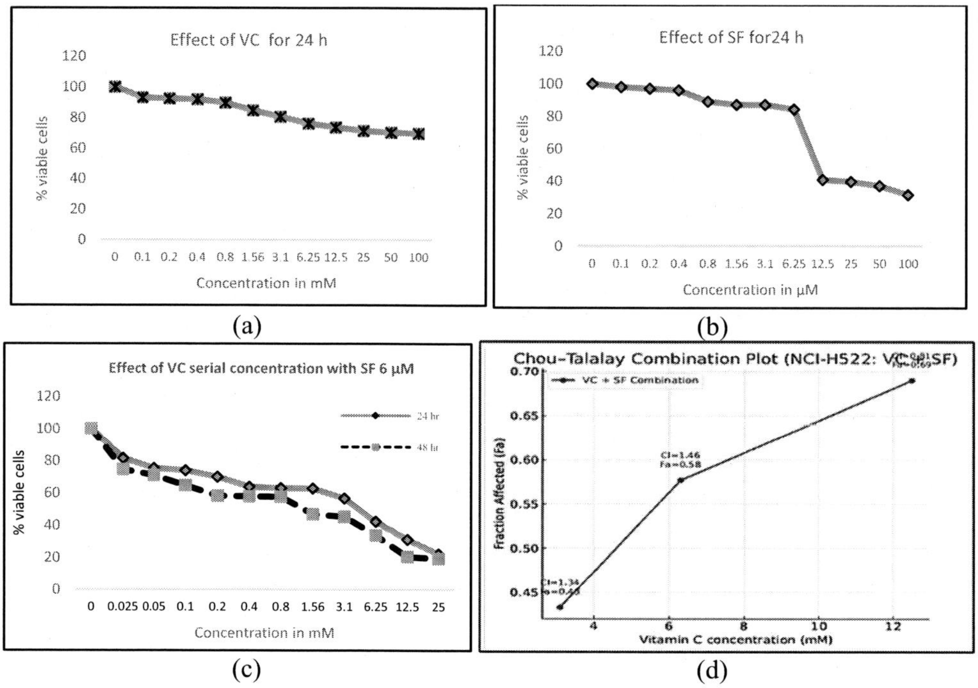

Figure 1. (a) shows that NCI-H5222 cell viability slightly decreased with VC concentrations (0 to 100 mM) after 24 h. The concentration of 6.25 mM was chosen as the mid-range concentration. (b) Indicates a reduction in cell viability starting at 6 μM of SF. (c) Indicated decreased cell viability in a time-dependent manner at 24, 48, and 72 h. Data represents SD ± 3. (d) Chou-Talalay combination plot using VC 6.25 mM and SF 6 μM showed Fa = 0.69 with CI = 0.68.

Changes in Cell Morphology

VC and SF resulted in alteration of NCI-H5222 morphologies in all treatment groups compared to the control. While control cells remained healthy, showing increased numbers and adherence after 24 h, cells treated with VC or SF alone exhibited reduced viability and morphological changes. The combination of VC and SF led to even greater cell death, with many cells appearing floating in the culture dish.

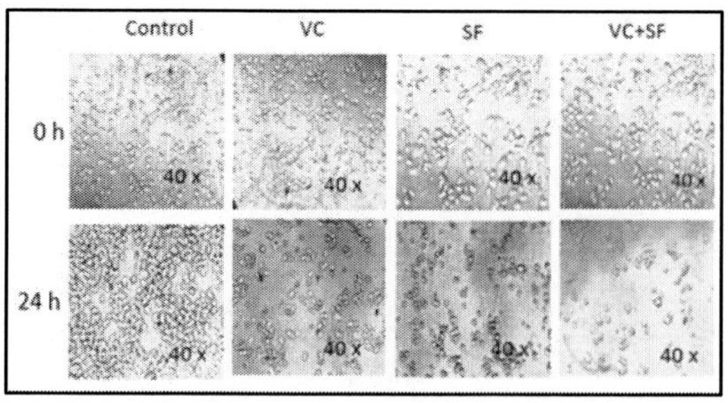

Figure 2. Inverted microscopic images of NCI-H5222 cells (40X) after 24 h treatment with VC, SF, or the combination revealed alterations in cell morphologies.

Wound-Healing

After 24 h of treatment, the combination of VC and SF led to significantly reduced migration of cells, resulting in a wider wound gap. In contrast, control cells migrated closer together, indicating early signs of invasion and potential cancer metastasis.

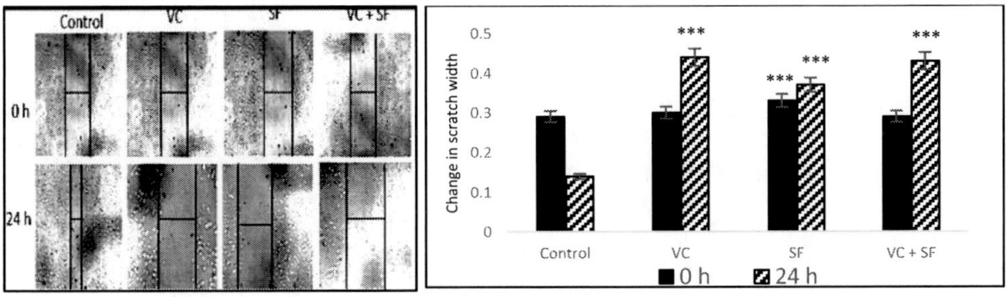

(a) (b)

Figure 3. (a) presents the results of the wound healing assay for NCI-H5222 cells treated with VC, SF, or their combination. (b) Shows a histogram comparing wound widths across different treatment groups vs. control. Data represents SD from three independent experiments. Significant difference indicated by ***p < 0.001, according to the post hoc Newman-Keuls test.

Induction of Apoptosis

The combination of VC and SF resulted in a lower rate of apoptosis in NCI-H5222 cells that confirmed by Hoechst 33342 staining and observed in fluorescence microscopy images. Control cells had lower fluorescence intensity, indicating normal, healthy nuclei. In contrast, apoptotic cells exhibited bright blue fluorescence due to nuclear condensation and fragmentation.

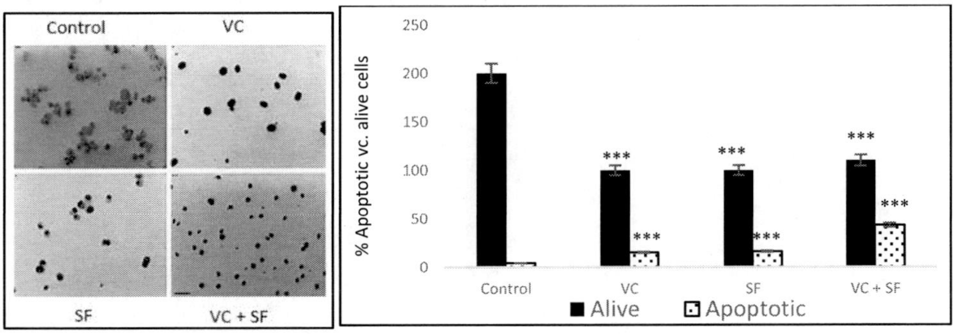

(a) (b)

Figure 4. (a) shows fluorescence microscopic images of NCI-H5222 cells treated for 24 h with VC, SF, or their combination. The scale bar represents 100 μm. (b) Presents a histogram of the percentage of apoptotic cells relative to non-apoptotic cells. Data represents SD from three independent experiments. A significant increase in the numbers of apoptotic cells was observed, with ***p < 0.001, as determined by the post hoc Newman-Keuls test.

Intracellular ROS Generation

The generation of intracellular ROS was assessed in cells following treatment with VC, SF, or their combination, using H2DCFDA staining. Variations in fluorescence intensity through microscopic images showing higher ROS generation indicated by increased fluorescence intensity. Significant ROS generation was observed in response to VC, SF, or the combination compared to the control which showed darker colors indicating lower ROS generation.

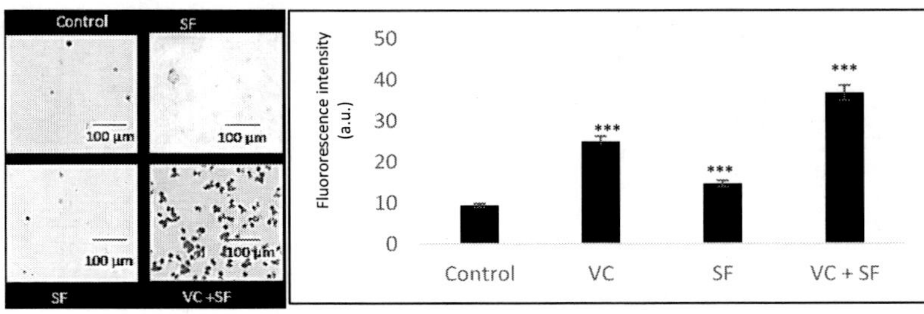

(a) (b)

Figure 5. (a) shows the results of intracellular ROS generation assessed with H2DCF staining, with a scale bar indicating 100 µm. (b) Presents a histogram illustrating the band intensity corresponding to treatments with VC, SF, or their combination versus the control. Data represents SD from three independent experiments. A significant change in ROS levels was observed, indicated by ***p < 0.001, according to the post hoc Newman-Keuls test.

Mitochondrial Membrane Potential (Ψ_m)

The generation of ROS in NCI-H5222 cells indicated cell death attributed to the depletion of mitochondrial membrane potential, as detected with Rhodamine 123 staining. Treatments with VC, SF, or the combination induced cell death. Control cells exhibited higher fluorescence intensity, indicating healthy mitochondria; however, the treatment disrupts mitochondrial $\Delta\Psi m$, impairing mitochondrial function and triggering downstream apoptotic/necrotic pathways.

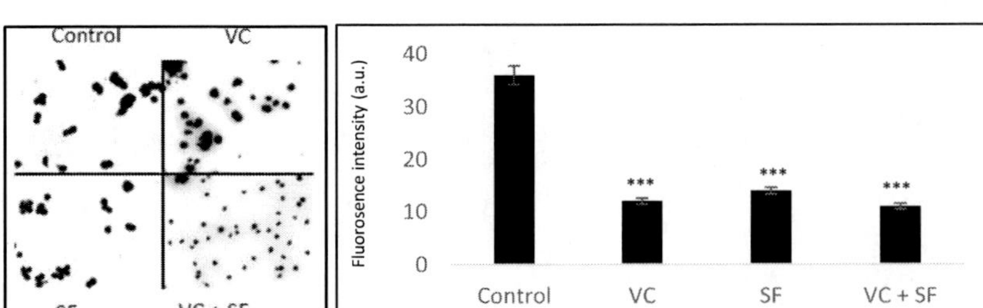

(a) (b)

Figure 6. (a) shows the results of fluorescence microscopic examination depicting changes in mitochondrial membrane depolarization in treated cells compared to control cells. The scale bar represents 100 µm. (b) Presents a histogram illustrating the fluorescence intensity corresponding to the control, VC, SF, or the combination, with a significant decrease indicated by ***p < 0.001, according to the post hoc Newman-Keuls test.

Modulation of Bax, Bcl2, AIF, and Cytochrome C

In apoptotic cells, the intracellular generation of ROS is linked to alterations in the expressions of Bax and Bcl2 proteins. The Western blot analysis shows an increase in Bax and a decrease in Bcl2 expressions in NCI-H5222 cells treated with VC, SF or the combination. ROS generation also led to a reduction in mitochondrial membrane potential. An increase in the expression of apoptosis-inducing factor (AIF) was observed in all treated cells with the combination showed the highest increase.

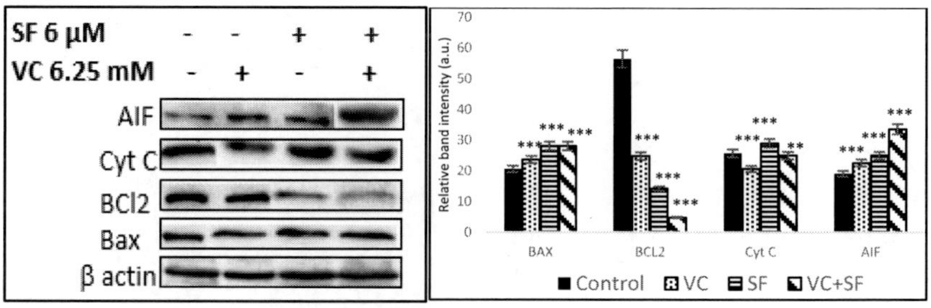

(a) (b)

Figure 7. Western blot analysis of Bax, Bcl2, AIF, and cyt C expressions in NCI-H5222 cells following treatment with VC, SF, or their combination. (a) Representative blots showing expression of these proteins. (b) Densitometric histogram compares relative protein levels normalized to β-actin. Data are expressed as mean ± SD (n = 3). Significant changes are indicated by **$p < 0.01$ and ***$p < 0.001$, according to the post hoc Newman-Keuls test.

Modulation Mitochondrial Signaling Proteins

Mitochondrial apoptosis resulting from a decline in membrane potential is linked to various crucial proteins, including caspases (Cas-9, -3, -7, and -8) and apoptotic peptidase activating factors (Apaf-1). Western blot analysis revealed elevated Apaf-1 expression in NCI-H5222 cells treated with VC. SF, or their combination. Decrease in Cas -7, -8, and -9 were observed in cells treated with VC, or SF alone, but the combination of VC and SF resulted in increases expression of these caspases.

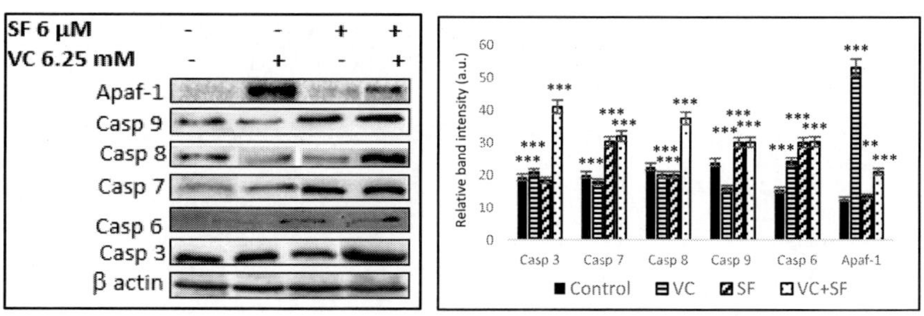

(a) (b)

Figure 8. Western blot analysis of mitochondrial signaling proteins in NCI-H5222 cells after treatment with VC SF, or the combination. (a) Representative blots showing expression of these proteins. (b) Densitometric histogram compares relative protein levels normalized to β-actin. Data are expressed as mean ± SD (n = 3). Significant changes are indicated by **$p < 0.01$ and ***$p < 0.001$, according to the post hoc Newman-Keuls test.

Modulation of MEK Kinase Pathway

To investigate the potential mechanism of VC, SF, or their combination in modulating aberrant cell signaling of mitogen-activated protein kinases (MAPKs), Western blot analysis was conducted to assess the active and phosphorylated forms of mitogen-activated protein kinase kinase (MEK). Significant decreases in MEK-1, -2, -3, and -4 expressions were observed in NCI-H5222 cells treated with the combination of VC and SF, while individual VC or SF didn't cause decrease in their expressions, highlight the advantage of combining VC and SF.

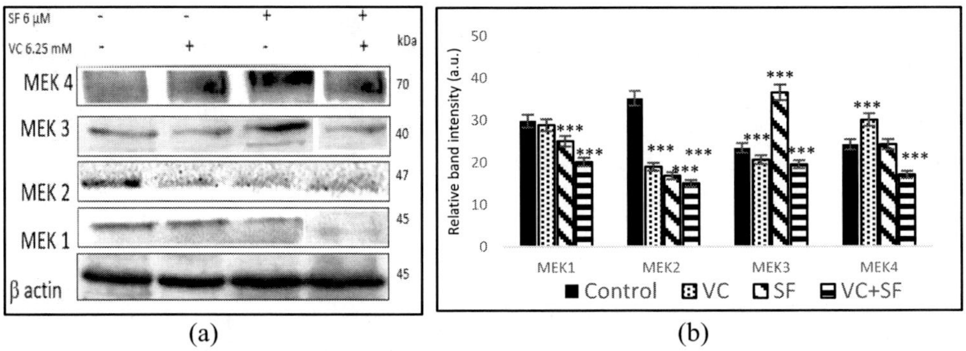

Figure 9. Western blot analysis of MEK-1, -2, -3, and -4 expressions after treating NCI-H5222 cells with VC, SF, or their combination. (a) Representative blots showing expression of these proteins. (b) Densitometric histogram compares relative protein levels normalized to β-actin. Data are expressed as mean ± SD (n = 3). Significant change indicated by ***$p < 0.001$, according to the post hoc Newman-Keuls test.

Modulation of Cell Cycle Regulatory Proteins

Inhibition of cell cycle progression is also considered an important strategy in the management of NSCLC. Decreases in proteins involved in cell cycle regulation CDk7, CDk2, cyclin B1 and cyclin D1 were observed in all treatment of NCI-H5222 with VC, SF or their combination. These proteins play critical roles in driving cell cycle progression through the G1/S and G2/M transitions; thus, their downregulation indicates inhibition of cell proliferation and induction of cell cycle arrest. The observed reductions reflect a favorable effect of VC or SF alone, further enhanced by their combination.

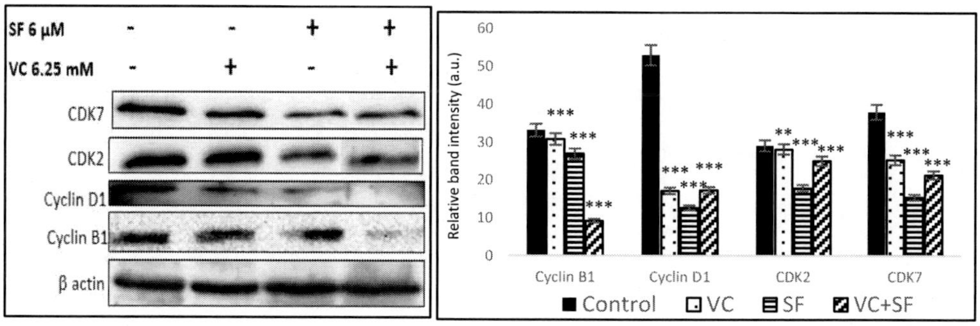

(a) (b)

Figure 10. Western blot analysis for cyclin B1, cyclin D1, CDK2, and CDK7 expressions after treating cells with VC, SF, or their combination for 24 h. (a) Representative blots showing expression of these proteins. (b) Densitometric histogram compares relative protein levels normalized to β-actin. Data are expressed as mean ± SD (n = 3). Significant increases are indicated as ***$p < 0.001$, according to the post hoc Newman-Keuls test.

Modulation of p21, p53, PTEN, and MDM2

The impact of VC, SF, and their combination on the expression of key regulatory proteins, including p21, p53, PTEN, and MDM2, was assessed in NCI-H5222 cells. Significant increase in the expression levels of p21 and PTEN indicative positive effect of tumor suppression. Conversely, the expression of MDM2 decreased, suggesting a potential inhibitory effect on the MDM2 pathway. Slight decreases in expression p53 were observed in all treatments.

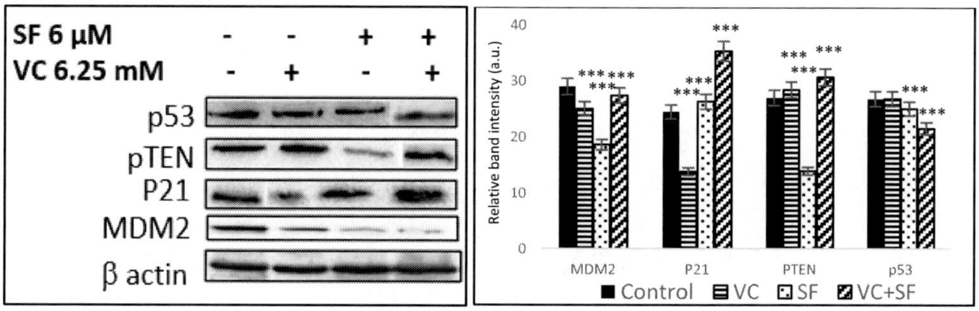

(a) (b)

Figure 11. Western blot analysis depicts the impact of VC, SF, and their combination on the expression in NCI-H5222 cells, as shown by Western blot analysis. (b). Presents the histogram of band intensities for all proteins compared to the control. Data represents SD from three independent experiments. Significant changes are marked as ***$p < 0.001$, according to the post hoc Newman-Keuls test.

Modulation of Akt/p85/mTOR

The effect of VC, SF, and their combination on Akt, p85 and mTOR was assessed on NCI-H5222 cells. While VC, SF and the combination caused decrease in the expression of Akt, mTOR and p85 expressions were increased in cells treated with SF only or the combination. VC only treatment caused decrease in Akt, mTOR and slight decrease in p85.

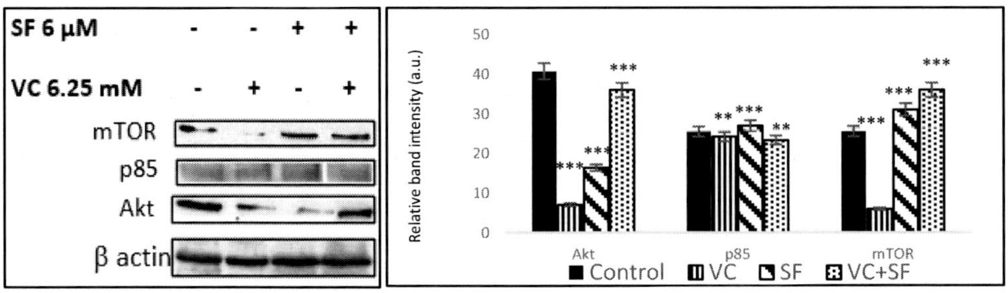

(a) (b)

Figure 12. Western blot analysis of Akt, p13, and mTOR expressions after treatment of cells with VC, SF, or their combination. (a) Representative blots showing expression of these proteins. (b) Densitometric histogram compares relative protein levels normalized to β-actin. Data are expressed as mean ± SD (n = 3). Significant changes are indicated as **p<0.01, ***p < 0.001, according to the post hoc Newman-Keuls test.

Modulation of SAPK/JNK and p38

The impact of VC, SF, and their combined treatment on SAPK/JNK and p38 proteins was evaluated in NCI-H5222 cells. Increase in p38 and SAPKK/JNK expressions in all treatments showed unfavorable effect of VC, or SF on this NSCLC model, by inducing signaling pathway associated with oxidative or mitogenic stress.

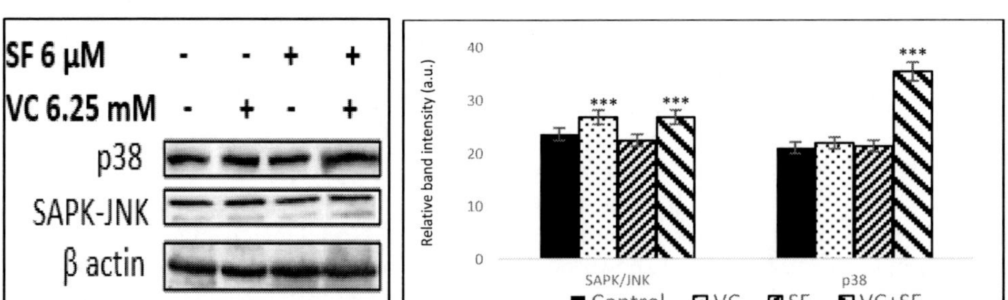

(a) (b)

Figure 13. Western blot analysis of SAPK/JNK and p38 expressions after treatment of NCI-H5222 cells with VC, SF, or their combination. (a) Representative blots showing expression of these proteins. (b) Densitometric histogram compares relative protein levels normalized to β-actin. Data are expressed as mean ± SD (n = 3). Significant changes are marked as ***p < 0.001, according to the post hoc Newman-Keuls test.

Modulation of ERK and EGFR

The impact of VC, SF, and their combined treatment on ERK and EGFR was assessed in NCI-H5222 cells. Individual VC or SF caused increase expressions of ERK and EGFR; however, the combined VC and SF showed favorable effect by causing decrease in the expression of ERK and EGFR. VC synergistically with SF inhibits proliferation and survival of NSCLC (see Fig. 14).

Modulation of Wnt, ROCK, and β-catenin

The impact of VC, SF, and their combined treatment on Wnt, ROCK, and β-catenin expressions was assessed in NCI-H5222 cells. Increased expressions of Wnt, ROCK, and β-catenin in all treatments showed unfavorable effect of VC, SF, or their combinations on NSCLS cells (see Fig. 15).

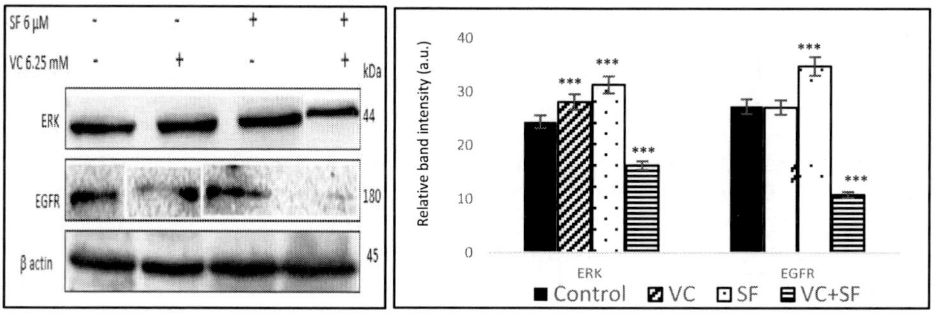

(a) (b)

Figure 14. Western blot analysis of expressions of ERK and EGFR after the treatment of cells with VC, SF, or their combination. (a) Representative blots showing expression of these proteins. (b) Densitometric histogram compares relative protein levels normalized to β-actin. Data are expressed as mean ± SD (n = 3). Significant changes are marked as ***p < 0.001, according to the post hoc Newman-Keuls test.

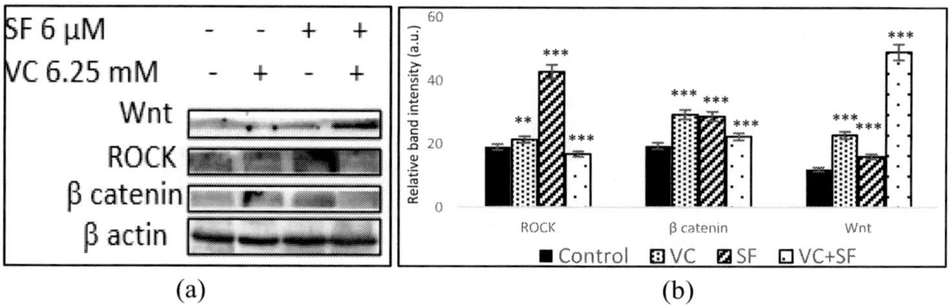

(a) (b)

Figure 15. Western blot analysis of ROCK, Wnt, and β-catenin expressions after treatment of cells with VC, SF, or their combination. (a) Representative blots showing expression of these proteins. (b) Densitometric histogram compares relative protein levels normalized to β-actin. Data are expressed as mean ± SD (n = 3). Significant changes are marked as ** p < 0.01 and ***p < 0.001, according to the post hoc Newman-Keuls test.

Modulation of MnSOD, Smac/Diablo, and Vimentin

The impact of VC, SF, and their combined treatment on MnSOD, Smac/DIABLO, and Vimentin was assessed in NCI-H5222 cells. A slight increase in Smac/DIABLO, MnSOD, and Vimentin expression were identified due to the treatment. These findings suggest that VC and SF may enhance oxidative stress defense (via MnSOD), promote pro-apoptotic signaling (via Smac/DIABLO), and influence cytoskeletal dynamics or epithelial–mesenchymal transition processes (via Vimentin).

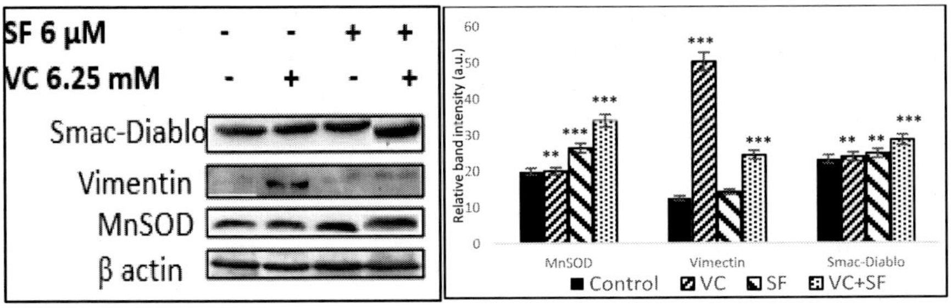

(a) (b)

Figure 16. Western blot analysis of MnSOD, Smac/Diablo, and Vimentin expressions after treatment of cells with VC, SF, or their combination. (a) Representative blots showing expression of these proteins. (b) Densitometric histogram compares relative protein levels normalized to β-actin. Data are expressed as mean ± SD (n = 3). Significant changes are marked as **p < 0.01 and ***p < 0.001, according to the post hoc Newman-Keuls test.

Modulation of MDR-ABC, Histone, and PDK1

The impact of VC, SF, and their combined treatment on MDR-ABC, PDK1, and histone proteins was assessed in NCI-H5222 cells. Decreased expressions of MDR-ABC due to VC alone or the combination of VC and SF were observed, while SF only caused increase in MDR-ABC. Histone and PDK1 expressions were increased in cells treated with VC only, while PDK1 expressions were decreased in SF only treatment.

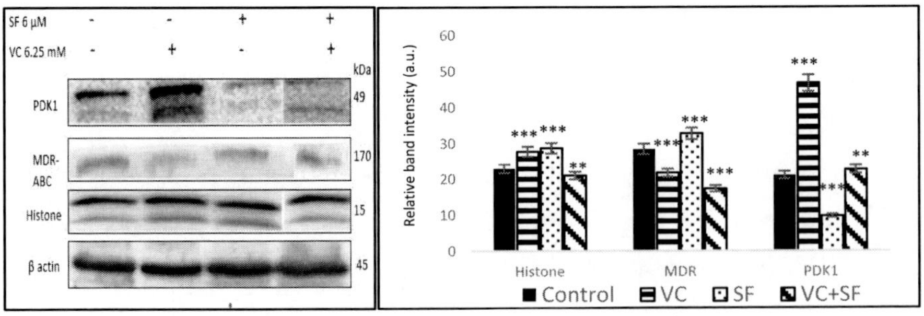

(a) (b)

Figure 17. Western blot analysis of MDR-ABC, histone, and PDK1 due to treatment of cells with VC, SF, or their combination. (a) Representative blots showing expression of these proteins. (b) Densitometric histogram compares relative protein levels normalized to β-actin. Data are expressed as me mean ± SD (n = 3). Significant changes are marked as ** p< 0.01, ***p < 0.001, according to the post hoc Newman-Keuls test.

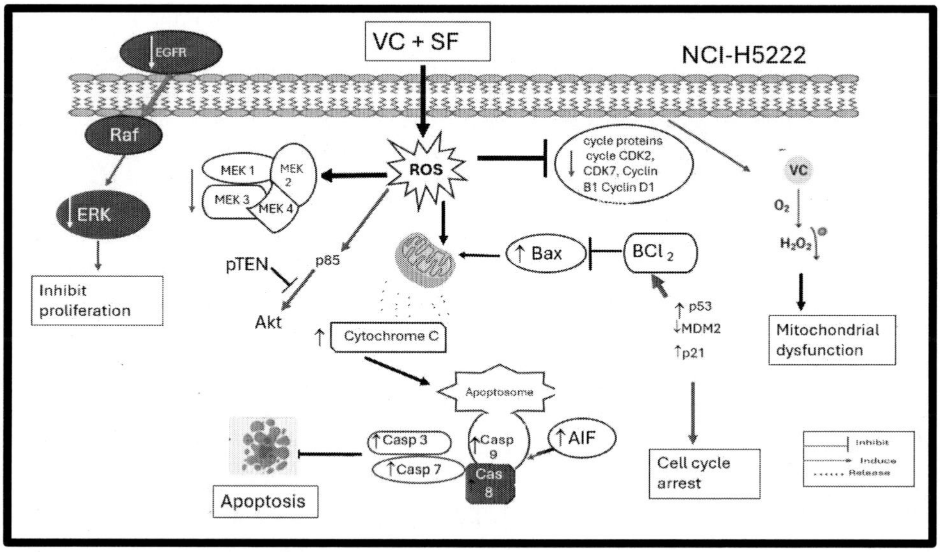

Figure 18. Proposed mechanistic model of VC and SF in NSCLC.

Discussion

As illustrated in Figure 18, VC, SF, or the combination effect on NCI-H522 cells caused consistent reductions in cells viability, greater ROS production, loss of mitochondrial membrane potential, apoptosis, and stronger nuclear condensation. At the signaling level, apoptotic markers showed increase Bax, decrease Bcl-2, increase Apaf-1 and cytochrome-c release, and increased caspase expression showing activation of the intrinsic mitochondrial apoptotic activity. These pro-death changes occurred alongside complex modulation of survival networks.

MEK isoforms were suppressed only with the combination, ERK/EGFR were downregulated by the combination but upregulated by single agents, while p38 and SAPK/JNK were upregulated broadly. Wnt/β-catenin and ROCK remained high across treatments. The net functional readout - reduced viability and increased apoptosis with combination therapy - indicates that mitochondrial death signaling predominates under the chosen conditions, although compensatory signaling modules are activated concurrently

Pharmacologic VC acts as a pro-oxidant in many cancer models by catalyzing H_2O_2 formation in extracellular fluid that diffuses into cells or via intracellular redox cycling, producing oxidative stress that preferentially damages cancer cells with limited peroxide-detoxifying capacity. The large increase in H_2DCFDA fluorescence and concordant $\Delta\Psi m$ loss in these experiments support ROS as an early mediator of cytotoxicity. ROS-induced mitochondrial injury drives MOMP (mitochondrial outer membrane permeabilization), releasing cytochrome-c and Smac/DIABLO, which in turn activate Apaf-1 and caspase-9, culminating in caspase-3/7 executioner activity and apoptotic morphology - precisely the sequence observed in the blots and staining. This mechanism is well described in preclinical pharmacologic VC literature and is consistent with multiple NSCLC models showing P-AscH$^-$ mediated oxidative distress and apoptosis [18-19].

Notably, suppression of MEK1–4 occurred predominantly when VC and SF were combined, whereas single-agent exposures did not achieve the same effect. Sorafenib is a multi-kinase inhibitor with activity against Raf kinases and several receptor tyrosine kinases; however, feedback activation and incomplete pathway suppression commonly limit its efficacy. The addition of VC appears to enhance Raf/MEK/ERK downregulation, possibly by promoting oxidative modification of signaling proteins or by altering upstream RTK activity [18, 20]. The resultant dual pressure - oxidative mitochondrial injury plus blockade of mitogenic signaling - provides a plausible mechanistic basis for the stronger apoptotic response with combination therapy. This concept parallels prior preclinical reports in which VC potentiated SF's anticancer effects in other cancer types [21].

Increased p38 and SAPK/JNK across treatments was observed. JNK activation is a recognized sensor of oxidative stress and can promote apoptotic signaling by phosphorylating and promoting Bax translocation; however, p38 and JNK family responses are context dependent and can support either death or survival depending on duration and crosstalk with other pathways. The persistent elevation of p38/SAPK in this study likely reflects sustained oxidative stress; whether their net contribution is pro-apoptotic or compensatory requires kinetic and inhibition experiments. Importantly, some survival mediators (ERK/EGFR) were decreased only with combination therapy, reinforcing the hypothesis that simultaneous ROS overload plus mitogenic blockade tips signaling balance toward death [22].

Combination treatments decreased CDK7, CDK2, cyclin B1, and cyclin D1 - changes consistently with repression of proliferative drive [18]. Upregulation of p21 and PTEN and downregulation of MDM2 further indicate activation of checkpoint control and dampening of oncogenic PI3K/Akt signaling. Although Akt and mTOR showed mixed regulation (some studies show single-agent SF can paradoxically increase upstream signals through feedback loops), this data suggests that combination treatment tends to reduce Akt pathway activity. This dual suppression of cell-cycle drivers alongside stabilization of tumor suppressor signals likely contributes to growth arrest and enhanced susceptibility to apoptosis. These observations align with reports that co-targeting metabolic/redox stress with kinase inhibitors can suppress both proliferative and survival signaling in lung cancer models [23].

Wnt, ROCK, and β-catenin levels remained elevated across treatments in this NSCLC model, which is an unfavorable signature with respect to motility and stem-like behavior. However, decreases in MDR-ABC with VC or combination treatment and mixed regulation of PDK1 and histone proteins showed favorable effect of VC in treatment of NSCLC. The persistent Wnt/ROCK activation suggests that, while mitochondria-driven apoptosis reduces viability, subpopulations may retain or even increase pro-survival/EMT features that confer resistance or contribute to residual disease. These data argue for a combination strategy that includes inhibitors of Wnt/ROCK signaling in models where these pathways are dominant. Prior literature documents that SF can modulate MMPs and invasiveness in some cancer types, and that VC can influence EMT markers, but context and dose are critical determinants [23].

Although several unfavorable markers (Wnt/β-catenin, ROCK, some stress kinases) increased, the phenotypic outcome - reduced viability and increased apoptotic nuclei - indicates that mitochondrial injury and MEK/ERK suppression are dominant under the experimental conditions. This is consistent with the concept that a sufficiently strong proximal insult (ROS, MOMP) can override downstream compensatory signaling temporarily. However, the activation of survival pathways in portions of the signaling network cautions that such responses could facilitate rebound growth if not durably suppressed, especially in vivo where microenvironmental support and antioxidant systems differ from culture. The translational implication is that VC and SF may offer therapeutic benefit in NSCLC, especially in cancer contexts with limited antioxidant buffering, but durable responses will likely require strategies to prevent feedback activation (e.g., combined PI3K/mTOR or Wnt pathway inhibition). Clinical trials combining pharmacologic VC with standard therapies in lung cancer are ongoing and underscore the translational interest in this approach [20].

Several limitations temper interpretation. First, the data are from a single cell line (NCI-H522) and a limited set of time points; signaling kinetics and dose dependence could reveal different dynamics (e.g., transient ERK activation followed by suppression). Second, ROS measurements using H_2DCFDA are general and do not distinguish species (H_2O_2 vs. superoxide); catalase/PEG-catalase or NAC rescue experiments are needed to confirm ROS dependency. Third, bulk biochemical assays cannot resolve cell-to-cell heterogeneity; single-cell or flow cytometry studies for annexin V/PI, $\Delta\Psi m$, and cell-cycle distribution would strengthen conclusions. Finally, SF's pharmacodynamics *in vitro* do not fully model *in vivo* exposure - thus, xenograft or orthotopic models using intravenous VC will be required to assess translational potential. These limitations are common to preclinical combination studies but can be addressed with the follow-up work.

Conclusion

VC enhances SF-induced cytotoxicity primarily by increasing oxidative stress and promoting mitochondrial apoptosis, while combination treatment uniquely suppresses MEK isoforms and ERK/EGFR signaling. Although some pro-survival and EMT-associated signals remain elevated, the net effect is increased apoptosis and reduced viability under the tested conditions. These results support further preclinical evaluation of VC and SF combinations in NSCLC, ideally with additional pathway inhibitors to block adaptive resistance mechanisms.

Key Findings

VC and SF in NSCLC cells produced a complex interplay between pro-apoptotic activation and selective survival signaling. Morphological analyses and nuclear staining confirmed enhanced cell death following VC and SF treatment compared to either agent alone, consistent with mitochondrial dysfunction or elevated ROS generation. Western blot results demonstrated increased Bax/Bcl2 ratio, cytochrome c release, and Apaf-1 expression, supporting mitochondrial apoptosis activation. Concomitant decreases in MEK isoforms, Akt, and ERK1/2 suggest suppression of proliferative and survival pathways, while upregulation of p21 and PTEN indicates restored tumor suppressive signaling. However, elevated β-catenin, Wnt, and ROCK in all treatment groups highlight partial pro-oncogenic feedback, suggesting differential regulation within the MAPK and Wnt axes. therapy.

Acknowledgments

The author thanks Union University for providing source and research funding and colleagues and editing tools for assistance with improving the clarity of the manuscript.

References

[1] National Cancer Institute ; 2025. Available from: *https://www.cancer.gov/policies/linking*.

[2] Bray F., Ferlay J., Soerjomataram I., Siegel R.L., Torre L.A., Jemal A. Global cancer statistics 2018: GLOBOCAN estimates of incidence and mortality worldwide for 36 cancers in 185 countries. C*A Cancer J Clin 2*018 ; 68 : 394-424.

[3] Cleveland Clinic. 2025. "Non-Small Cell Lung Cancer." *Cleveland Clinic*. Accessed January 9, 2026. https://my.clevelandclinic.org/health/diseases/6203-non-small-cell-lung-cancer.

[4] Jeon H., Wang S., Song J., Gill H., Cheng H. Update 2025: Management of non-small-cell lung cancer. *Lung* 2025 ; 203 : 23.

[5] Huang Q., Li Y., Huang Y., Wu J., Bao W., Xue C., et al., Advances in molecular pathology and therapy of non-small cell lung cancer. *Signal Transduct Target Ther* 2025 ; 10 : 186.

[6] Herbst R.S., Morgensztern D., Boshoff C. The biology and management of non-small cell lung cancer. *Nature* 2018 ; 553 : 446-454.

[7] Cheng T.Y., Cramb S.M., Baade P.D., Youlden D.R., Nwogu C., Reid M.E. The international epidemiology of lung cancer : Latest trends, disparities, and tumor characteristics. *J Thorac Oncol* 2016 ; 11 : 1653-1671.

[8] Liu L., Soler J., Reckamp K.L., Sankar K. Emerging targets in non-small cell lung cancer. *Int J Mol Sci* 2024 ; 25 : 10046.

[9] Hendrixson M., Gladkiy Y., Thyagarajan A., Sahu R.P. Efficacy of sorafenib-based therapies for non-small cell lung cancer. *Med Sci* 2024 ; 12 : 20.

[10] Wilhelm S.M., Carter C., Tang L., Wilkie D., McNabola A., Rong H., et al., BAY 43-9006 exhibits broad spectrum oral antitumor activity and targets the RAF/MEK/ERK pathway and receptor tyrosine kinases involved in tumor progression and angiogenesis. *Cancer Res* 2004 ; 64 : 7099-7109.

[11] Carlomagno F., Anaganti S., Guida T., Salvatore G., Troncone G., Wilhelm S.M., et al., BAY 43-9006 inhibition of oncogenic RET mutants. *J Natl Cancer Inst Monogr* 2006 ; 98 : 326-334.

[12] Tsukumo Y., Naito M., Suzuki T. Influence of EGFR-activating mutations on sensitivity to tyrosine kinase inhibitors in a KRAS mutant non-small cell lung cancer cell line. *PLoS One* 2020 ; 15 : e0229712.

[13] Schoenfeld J.D., Sibenaller Z.A., Wagner B.A., Spitz D.R., Allen B.G. Redox active metals and H2O2 mediate the increased efficacy of pharmacological ascorbate in combination with gemcitabine or radiation in pre-clinical sarcoma models. *Redox Biology* 2018 ; 14 : 417-422.

[14] Du J., Martin S.M., Levine B.A., Wang S., Knudsen C.M., Cullen J.J. Mechanism of ascorbate-induced cytotoxicity in pancreatic cancer. *J Am Assoc Cancer Res* 2010 ; 16 :509-520.

[15] Chen Q., Espey M.G., Krishna M.C., Mitchell J.B., Corpe C.P., Buettner G.R., et al., Pharmacological ascorbic acid concentrations selectively kill cancer cells : action as a pro-drug to deliver hydrogen peroxide to tissues. *PNAS* 2005 ; 102 : 13604-13609.

[16] Chen Q., Espey M.G., Sun A.Y., Lee J.H., Buettner G.R., Levine M. Ascorbate in pharmacologic concentration selectively generate ascorbate radical and hydrogen peroxide in extracellular fluid *in vivo*. *PNAS* 2007 ; 104 : 8749-8754.

[17] Olney K.E., Du J., Van Erve T.J., Witmer J.R., Wagner B.A., Buettner G.R., et al., Inhibitors of hydroperoxide metabolism enhance ascorbate-induce cytotoxicity. *Free Radic Res* 2013 ; 47 :154-163.

[18] Bennett L.L. Potential synergistic interaction between curcumin and sorafenib enhances cytotoxicity in NCI-H5222 lung cancer cells. *OBM Genetics* 2025 ; 9, 4.

[19] Sanookpan K., Chantaravisoot N., Kalpongnukul N., Chuenjit C., Wattanathamsan O., Shoaib S., et al., Pharmacological Ascorbate Elicits Anti-Cancer Activities against NSCLC through Hydrogen Peroxide-Induced DNA Damage. *Antioxidants* 2023 ; 12 :9.

[20] Paz-Ares L., Hirsh V., Zhang L., Marinis F., Yang Y.C.H., Wakelee H., et al., LBA33_PR-Monotherapy administration of Sorafenib in patients with NSCLC : phase III, randomized, double-blind, placebo-controlled mission trial. *Annals of Oncol* 2012 ; 23, suppl 9, ixe23.

[21] Rouleau L., Antony A.N., Bisetto S., Newberg A., Doria C., Levine M., et al., Synergistic effects of ascorbate and sorafenib in cancer models. *Free Radic Biol Med* 2016 ; 95 : 308-322.

[22] Böttger F., Valles-Marti A., Cahn L., Jimenez C.R. High-dose intravenous vitamin C, a promising multi-targeting agent in the treatment of cancer. *J Exp Clin Cancer Res* 2021 ; 40 : 343.

[23] Glorieux C., Calderon P.B. Vitamin C (Ascorbate) and redox topics in cancer. *Antioxidants & Redox Signal* 2021 ; 35, 14.

Chapter 17

The Synergistic Anticancer Effects of Temsirolimus and Vitamin C on Renal Carcinoma Cells

Lunawati L. Bennett*, **PhD, PharmD**
Union University, College of Pharmacy, Jackson, Tennessee, USA

Abstract

Renal cancer incidence continues to rise globally, and therapeutic responses remain limited by resistance and compensatory survival signaling. Temsirolimus, an mTOR inhibitor, is used clinically for advanced renal cell carcinoma, yet its efficacy is frequently reduced by feedback activation within the PI3K/Akt/mTOR axis.

This study examined whether high-dose vitamin C, a redox-modulating agent, enhances the anticancer effects of temsirolimus in A-498 renal carcinoma cells. SRB viability assays, Rhodamine 123 mitochondrial membrane potential analysis, Hoechst 33342 nuclear staining, and Western blot profiling demonstrated that vitamin C and temsirolimus together increased oxidative stress, disrupted mitochondrial function, and elevated pro-apoptotic markers including Bax, AIF, Smac/DIABLO, and caspases-3, -7, -8, and -9, while reducing Bcl-2 expression. Importantly, the interaction was time dependent. At 24 h, the combination displayed a less-than-additive effect, associated with compensatory mTOR upregulation. However, with prolonged exposure (48–72 h), the combination produced synergistic and strongly synergistic cytotoxicity, coinciding with sustained ROS accumulation and irreversible mitochondrial-dependent apoptosis. These findings indicate that vitamin C can enhance temsirolimus efficacy when treatment duration and sequencing are optimized, highlighting the importance of timing in modulating apoptotic sensitivity and overcoming mTOR feedback resistance in renal cancer therapy.

Keywords: renal cancer, kidney, vitamin C, mTOR inhibitor, papillary renal cell cancer

Abbreviations

APAF	Apoptotic peptidase activating factor;
Bax	Bcl2 Associated X-protein;
Bcl2	B cell lymphoma 2;

* Corresponding Author's Email: llbennett@uu.edu

Cas	Caspase;
CDK7	Cyclin dependent kinase 7;
Cyt C	Cytochrome C;
PTEN	Phosphatase and tensin homolog;
ROCK	Rho-associated kinase;
ROS	Reactive oxygen species.

Introduction

In recent decades, renal cancer, which was relatively rare compared to other cancers, has been on the rise. According to the Global Cancer Observatory, renal cancer was estimated to cause approximately 431,288 new cases and 179,368 deaths worldwide in the next decade, emphasizing the urgency of addressing this significant global health trend [1-2]. The highest incidence rates are observed in North America and Europe, while lower rates are reported in Asia and Africa. Risk factors for developing renal cancer include smoking, obesity, hypertension, and genetic syndromes, such as von Hippel-Lindau (VHL) disease and hereditary papillary renal cell carcinoma.

The most common subtype of this cancer is renal cell carcinoma (RCC) that accounts for 90% of cases. RCC are further divided into clear cell (ccRCC) account for 70% of the cases, papillary (pRCC-type 1 and 2) account for 10–15%, and chromophobe (chRCC) account for 5% [3]. Each has distinct genetic alterations and clinical manifestations. Histological subtypes are linked to overall survival and cancer specific survival, with a better prognosis is usually with chRCC subtype [4].

RCC is characterized by several identified biomarkers such as VHL, HIF-1α, HIf-2α, MET, FH, BHD, HRPT2. Heredity forms of chromosome 3 alteration leading to loss of silencing von-Hippel-Lindau (VHL) gene, a tumor suppressor protein [5-6]. This inactivation leads to the accumulation of hypoxia-inducible factors (HIFs), which cause angiogenesis and promote cancer growth [7-9]. Overexpression of MET gene, an oncogene on chromosome 7q31 is among others identified genetic alterations in RCC [10].

The prognosis for renal cancer depends on several factors such as cancer stage, histological subtype, and patient health. The 5-year survival rate for localized renal cancer can be as high as 90%, while advanced stages show a decline in survival rate. The overall 5-year survival rate for kidney cancer is approximately 75% [11].

The pathophysiology of renal cancer is complex and often involves multiple pathways such as mammalian target of rapamycin (mTOR), mitogen-activated protein kinase/extracellular signal-regulated kinase (MAPK/ERK*)*, and the phosphatidylinositol 3-kinase/protein kinase B (PI3K/AKT*)* signaling pathway implicated in cancer progression and metastasis. In advanced stages, this cancer can metastasize to various organs, including the lungs, liver, bones and adrenal gland [12-13].

Treatment of renal cancer varies based on the stage of the disease and individual patient factors. The treatment modalities include chemotherapy, surgical, radiofrequency ablation (RFA), targeted therapy and immunotherapy [14-16]. Chemotherapy is generally not effective for RCC and is rarely used, except in specific cases of advanced or metastatic disease [17].

Tyrosine kinase inhibitors (TKIs) such as sunitinib, pazopanib, cabozantinib, axitinib, sorafenib have been approved to treat advanced RCC. These agents target specific pathways involved in cancer growth and angiogenesis [18-19]. Besides TKIs, another targeted therapy such as immune checkpoint inhibitors (ICIs), such as nivolumab and pembrolizumab, have also revolutionized the treatment landscape for RCC and metastatic RCC by enhancing the body's immune response against cancer cells. In addition, various combinations of TKIs and ICIs have been assessed and are currently considered the preferred regimens for all metastatic RCC patients [20-21]. Other treatment options for renal cancer includes mTOR inhibitors such as temsirolimus (TM).

Pharmacological ascorbate, achieved through high-dose intravenous vitamin C (VC) to attain plasma levels of $\geq$20 mM, has recently emerged as a potential non-toxic adjuvant to standard care radio-chemotherapy-based cancer therapies across various disease sites [22-23]. The proposed anti-cancer mechanism of pharmacological VC involves redox-active metal-mediated or auto-oxidation of ascorbate, resulting in the formation of O_2 and H_2O_2 [23-24].

This study was designed to evaluate the chemo-enhancing potential of VC in combination with MT for treating renal carcinoma, utilizing A-498 cells as the model. The findings of this investigation reveal that the use of VC with TM demonstrated greater efficacy in the treatment of renal carcinoma. This marks a novel discovery in the field.

To evaluate the cytotoxic potential of high-dose VC, various antineoplastic agents - including paclitaxel, doxorubicin, etoposide, temsirolimus, bortezomib, afatinib, and sorafenib - were tested on renal cancer using the model A-498 cell line. For combination studies, the lowest concentrations of each antineoplastic and high-dose VC that yielded a synergistic reduction in cell viability were selected. General experimental procedures followed the protocols outlined in Chapter 3 (Materials and Methods), while methodological details specific to this study are described below.

Cell Culture

The renal cell (A-498, ATCC HTB-44) exhibits epithelial morphology. This cell was isolated from kidney of 52-year-old white female which cultured in EMEM supplemented with 10% fetal bovine serum (FBS) and 1% streptomycin/penicillin. The cells were cultured in T75 dishes and maintained in an incubator at 37°C in a 5% CO_2 humidified environment.

Results

Cell Viability and Selection of Doses

Treatment of A-498 renal carcinoma cells with the combination of VC and TM demonstrated a clear time-dependent decrease in cell viability. At a fixed concentration TM 12.5 μM, co-treatment with VC at 2.5 mM resulted in viability values of 63.8%, 53.6%, and 39.2% at 24, 48, and 72 h, respectively, whereas VC at 5 mM yielded 79.8%, 62.5%, and 49.1% viability over the same period. The corresponding fractions affected (Fa) increased progressively from 0.36 to 0.61 (VC 2.5 mM) and from 0.20 to 0.51 (VC 5 mM), confirming that cytotoxicity intensified with prolonged exposure. These findings indicate a time-dependent additive to synergistic interaction between VC and TM, particularly evident after 48 h, suggesting that oxidative stress enhancement and sustained mTOR inhibition act cooperatively to promote apoptotic cell death.

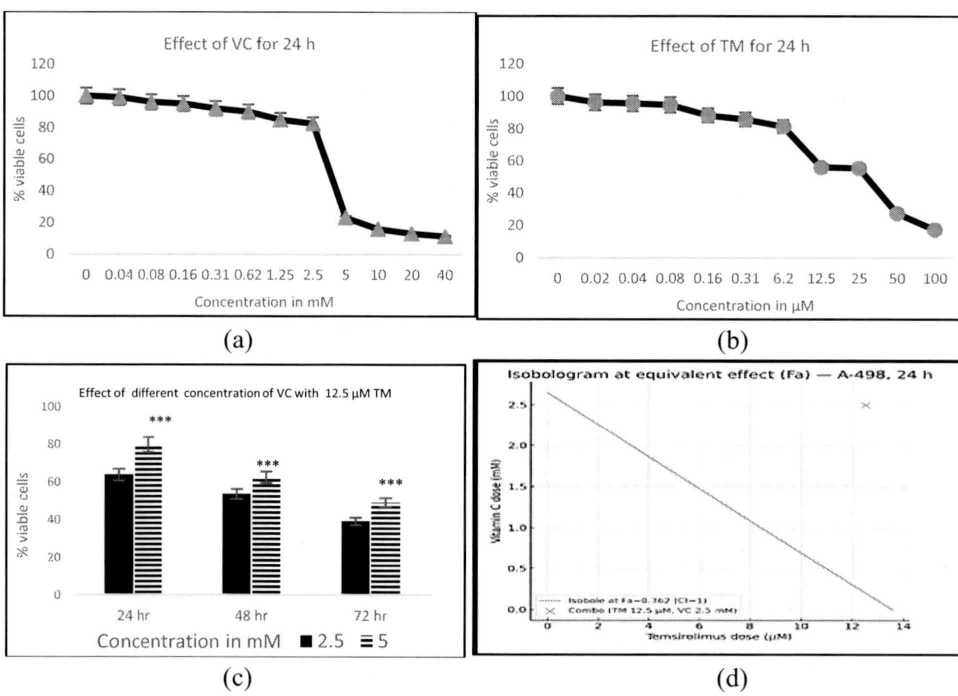

Figure 1. (a) Shows A-498 cell viability decreased with increasing VC concentrations (0 to 40 mM) after 24 h. (b) Indicates a reduction in cell viability starting at 12.5 μM of TM. (c) Demonstrates a further decrease in cell viability with a 72-h treatment of 2.5 mM VC and 12.5 μM TM, highlighting a combined effect. (d) The combination of VC 2.5 mM and TM 12.5 μM lies above the isobole (Fa = 0.36, CI = 1.87) indicating antagonism at 24 h.

Changes in Cell Morphology

VC and TM resulted in alteration of A-498 morphologies in all treatment groups compared to the control. While control cells remained healthy, showing increased numbers and adherence after 24 h, cells treated with VC or TM alone exhibited reduced viability and morphological changes. The combination of VC and TM led to even greater cell death, with many cells appearing floating in the culture dish.

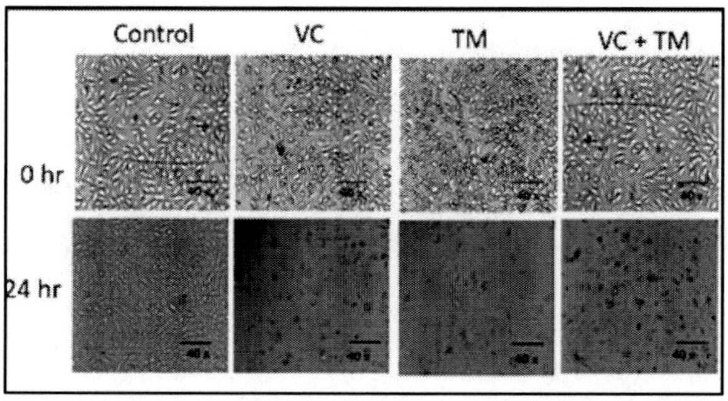

Figure 2. Inverted microscopic images of A-498 cells (40X) after 24 h treatment with VC, TM, or the combination revealed alterations in cell morphologies. Cells treated with VC or TM exhibited some changes in morphology, while in the combo treatment, most cells were detached from the dish, with only a few remaining attached.

Wound-Healing

After 24 h of treatment, the combination of VC and TM led to significantly reduced migration of A-498 cells, resulting in a wider wound gap compared to treatments with VC or TM alone. In contrast, control cells migrated closer together, indicating early signs of invasion and potential cancer metastasis. The histogram compares the wound widths across control, VC, TM, and combination treatments.

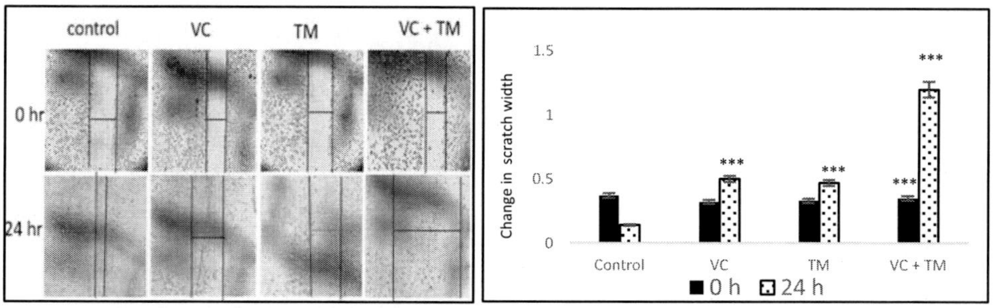

(a) (b)

Figure 3. (a) Presents the results of wound healing for A-498 cells treated with VC, TM, or the combination, compared to the control at 0 and 24 h. (b) Shows a histogram comparing wound widths across different treatment groups. Data are presented as mean ± SD (n = 3); ***p < 0.001, according to the post hoc Newman-Keuls test.

Induction of Apoptosis

Cells treated with VC, TM, or the combo, resulted in a lower rate of apoptosis in A-498 cells compared to control staining with Hoechst 33342 and observed in fluorescence microscopy. Control cells had lower fluorescence intensity, indicating normal, healthy nuclei. In contrast, apoptotic cells exhibited bright blue fluorescence due to nuclear condensation and fragmentation.

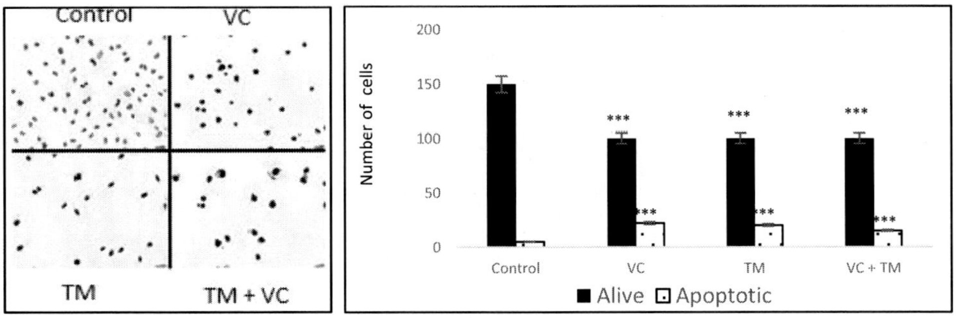

(a) (b)

Figure 4. (a) Shows fluorescence microscopic images of A-498 cells treated for 24 h with VC, TM, or their combination. The images reveal a significantly higher number of apoptotic cells, indicated by bright nuclei, in the individual VC, TM, or the combo. The scale bar represents 100 μm. 4(b) Histogram showing the percentage of apoptotic versus viable cells across treatment groups. Data are presented as mean ± SD (n = 3); ***$p < 0.001$ vs control (post hoc Newman–Keuls test.

Intracellular ROS Generation

The generation of intracellular ROS was assessed in A-498 cells following treatment with VC, TM, or their combination, using H2DCFDA staining. Variations in fluorescence intensity through microscopic images, with higher ROS generation indicated by increased fluorescence intensity. Significant ROS generation was observed in response to VC or combo compared to the control, with darker colors indicating lower ROS generation. Histogram of fluorescence intensity corresponding to the VC, TM, and combined treatments (see Fig. 5).

Mitochondrial Membrane Potential (Ψ_m)

The generation of ROS in A-498 cells indicated cell death attributed to the depletion of mitochondrial membrane potential, as detected with Rhodamine 123 staining. Treatments with VC, TM, or the combo induced cell death, as shown in the fluorescence microscopic images. Control cells exhibited higher fluorescence intensity, indicating healthy mitochondria, compared to treated cells (see Fig. 6).

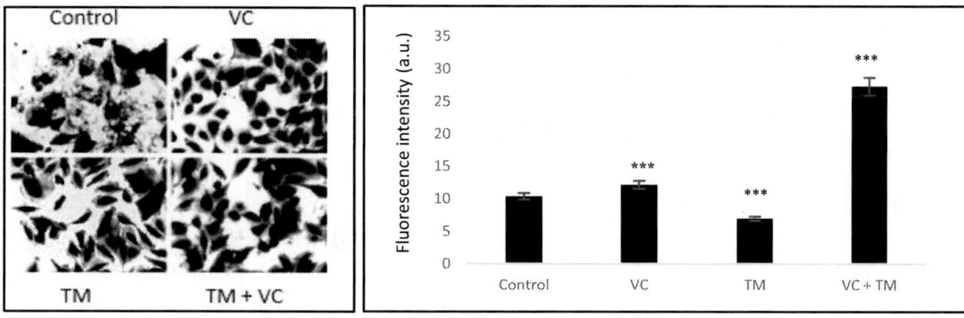

(a) (b)

Figure 5. Intracellular ROS generation was assessed with H2DCF staining. (a) Increased fluorescence intensity corresponds to higher ROS levels. (b) Presents a histogram illustrating the band intensity corresponding to treatments with VC, TM, or their combination. Data are expressed as mean ± SD (n = 3). Significant indicated by ***p < 0.001, according to the post hoc Newman-Keuls test. The scale bar indicates100 μm.

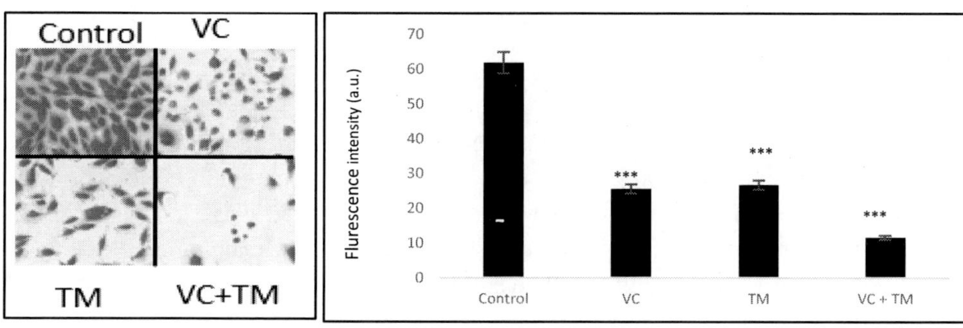

(a) (b)

Figure 6. (a) Shows the results of fluorescence microscopic examination depicting changes in mitochondrial membrane depolarization in treated A-498 cells. (b) Presents a histogram illustrating fluorescence.

Modulation of Bax, Bcl2, AIF, Cytochrome C

In apoptotic cells, elevated intracellular ROS levels were associated with marked alterations in mitochondrial apoptotic regulators. Combination treatment with VC and TM increased Bax expression and decreased Bcl-2 levels, thereby promoting Cyt C release into the cytosol of A-498 cells. The enhanced ROS production also contributed to a significant loss of mitochondrial membrane potential, further facilitating apoptotic progression. In addition, upregulation of apoptosis-inducing factor (AIF) was evident in all treatment groups, supporting the activation of both caspase-dependent and caspase-independent cell death pathways.

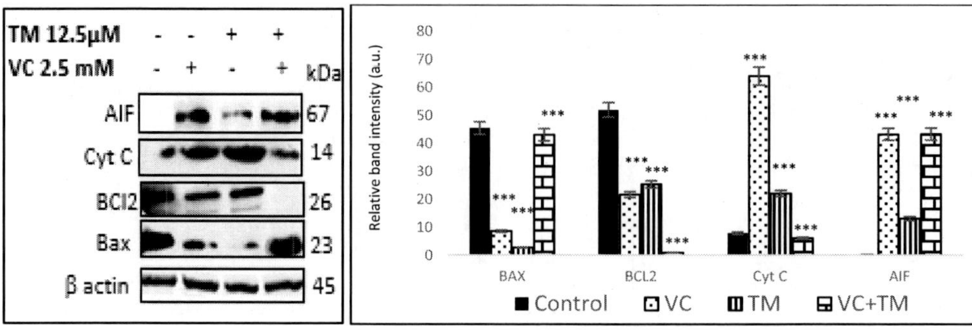

(a) (b)

Figure 7. Western blot analysis of mitochondrial apoptotic signaling expressions after treatment of A-498 with VC, TM, and their combination. (a) Representative blots showing expression of these proteins. (b) Densitometric histogram compares relative protein levels normalized to β-actin. Data are expressed as mean ± SD ($n = 3$). Significant changes are indicated by $^{***}p < 0.001$, according to the post hoc Newman-Keuls test.

Modulation Mitochondrial Signaling Proteins

Mitochondrial apoptosis resulting from a decline in membrane potential is linked to various crucial proteins, including caspases (-3, -7, -8, and -9) and apoptotic peptidase activating factor (Apaf). Western blot analysis revealed elevated Apaf and caspases -3, -7, -8, -9, in all treatment groups as compared to the control, with slight decrease in cas -3 expression with VC only treatment. The band intensity histogram is illustrated.

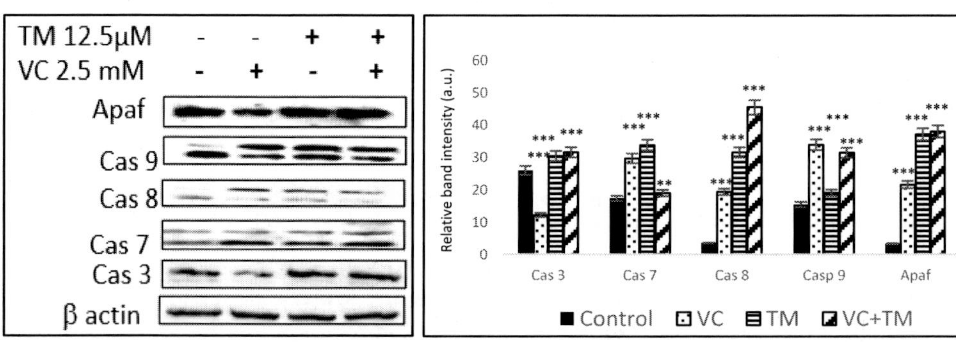

(a) (b)

Figure 8. Western blot analysis of various mitochondrial signaling proteins in A-498 cells after treatment with VC, TM, or combination. a) Representative blots showing expression of these proteins. (b) Densitometric histogram compares relative protein levels normalized to β-actin. Data are expressed as mean ± SD ($n = 3$). Significant changes are indicated by $^{**}p < 0.01$ and $^{***}p < 0.001$, according to the post hoc Newman-Keuls test.

Modulation of MEK Kinase Pathway

To investigate the potential mechanism of VC, TM, or their combo in modulating aberrant cell signaling of mitogen-activated protein kinases (MAPKs), Western blot analysis was conducted to assess the active and phosphorylated forms of mitogen-activated protein kinase (MEK). Significant decreases in MEK-1, -2, -3, and -4 expressions were observed in A-498 cells treated with VC, TM, or their combo as illustrated.

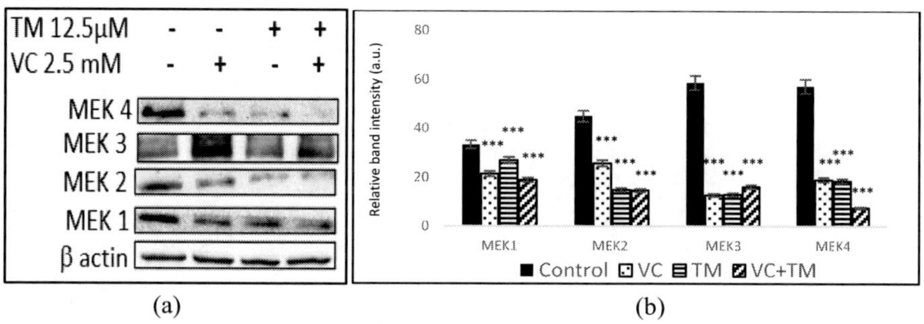

Figure 9. Western blot analysis of MEK-1, -2, -3, and -4 after treating A-498 cells with VC, TM, or the combo. (a) Representative blots showing expression of these proteins. (b) Densitometric histogram compares relative protein levels normalized to β-actin. Data are expressed as mean ± SD (n = 3). Significant change indicated by ***p < 0.001, according to the post hoc Newman-Keuls test.

Modulation of Cell Cycle Regulatory

The inhibition of cell cycle progression is also considered an important strategy in the management of renal carcinoma. Decrease in proteins involved in cell cycle regulation CDK2, and cyclin B1 were observed in all treatments of A-498 with VC, TM or the combo, with slight increase in CDK7. Cyclin D1 wasn't detected in the cells. The band intensity histogram showed different expressions of proteins compared to the control.

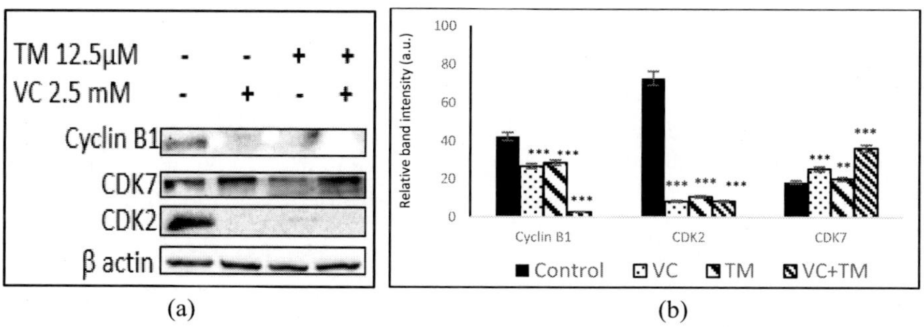

Figure 10. Western blot analysis of cyclin B1, CDK2, and CDK7 after treating A-498 cells with VC, TM, or the combo. (a) Representative blots showing expression of these proteins. (b) Densitometric histogram compares relative protein levels normalized to β-actin. Data are expressed as mean ± SD (n = 3). Significant increases are indicated as **p < 0.01 and ***p < 0.001, according to the post hoc Newman-Keuls test.

Modulation of p21, PTEN, and MDM2

The impact of VC, TM, and the combo on the expression of key regulatory proteins, including p21, PTEN, and MDM2, was assessed in A-498 cells. There was significant increase in the expression levels of p21 and PTEN indicative a positive regulatory effect on cell cycle control and tumor suppression. Conversely, the expression of MDM2 decreased, suggesting a potential inhibitory effect on the MDM2 pathway. The p53 expression was not detected in this cell.

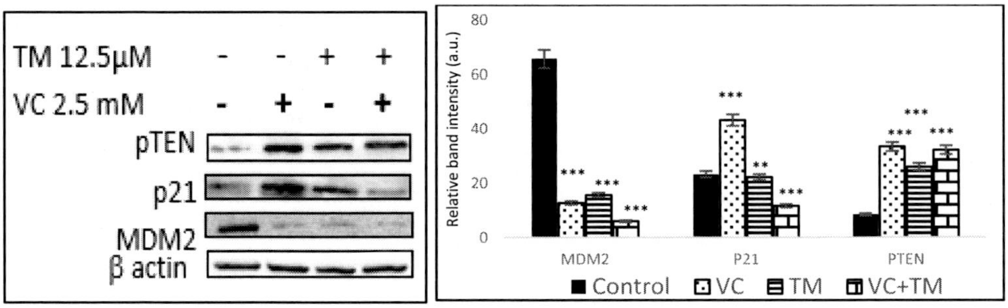

(a) (b)

Figure 11. Western blot analysis of p21, MDM2, and PTEN expressions A-498 after treatment with VC, TM, or the combination. (a) Representative blots showing expression of these proteins. (b) Densitometric histogram compares relative protein levels normalized to β-actin. Data are expressed as mean ± SD (n = 3). Significant changes are marked as $^{**}p < 0.01$, $^{***}p < 0.001$ according to the post hoc Newman-Keuls test.

Modulation of Akt/p85/mTOR

The effects of VC, TM, and their combination on the expression of Akt, p85 (a regulatory subunit of PI3K), and mTOR (mammalian target of rapamycin) proteins were evaluated in A-498 cells. A noticeable reduction in the expression levels of Akt, p85, and mTOR was observed across all treatment groups compared to the control, indicating a potentially favorable anti-cancer effect. Among the treatments, VC alone produced a more pronounced inhibitory effect than TM alone. Interestingly, TM treatment alone led to a slight increase in mTOR expression, suggesting a possible unfavorable feedback response. In contrast, VC alone effectively reduced mTOR expression. These findings suggest that VC, particularly when used alone or in combination with TM, may exert greater inhibitory effects on the PI3K/Akt/mTOR pathway in A-498 cells (see Fig.12).

Modulation of SAPK/JNK and p38

The impact of VC, TM, and their combined treatment on SAPK/JNK and p38 proteins was evaluated in A-498 cells. A decrease in p38 and SAPK/JNK expression was observed showing VC and TM effectively suppresses stress-induced signaling pathways, potentially contributing to enhanced apoptotic sensitivity (see Fig.13).

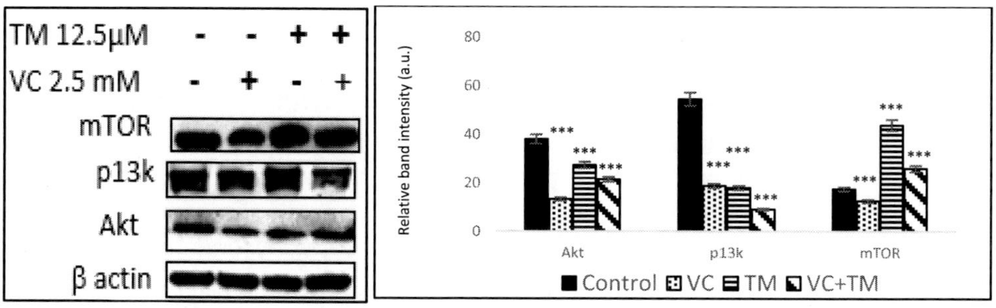

(a) (b)

Figure 12. Western blot analysis of Akt, p85 and mTOR expressions after treatment of A-498 cells with VC, TM, or the combination. (a) Representative blots showing expression of these proteins. (b) Densitometric histogram compares relative protein levels normalized to β-actin. Data are expressed as mean ± SD (n = 3). Statistical significance was determined as ***$p < 0.001$, according to the post hoc Newman-Keuls test.

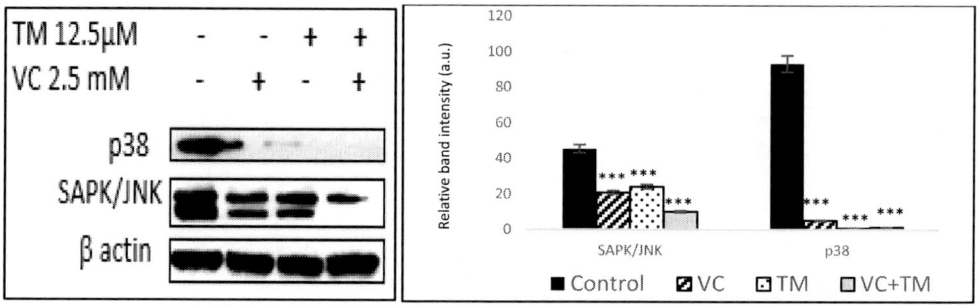

(a) (b)

Figure 13. Western blot analysis of SAPK/JNK and p38 expressions after treatment of cells with VC, TM, or their combination. (a) Representative blots showing expression of these proteins. (b) Densitometric histogram compares relative protein levels normalized to β-actin. Data are expressed as mean ± SD (n = 3). Statistical significance determines with ***$p < 0.001$, according to the post hoc Newman-Keuls test.

Modulation of ERK 1/2, Raf, and EGFR

The impact of VC, TM, and their combined treatment on ERK, Raf, and EGFR proteins was assessed in A-498 cells. Increase expressions of ERK, Raf, and EGFR in all treatments indicate unfavorable effect of VC, TM, or the combo in A-498 cells. Activation of the ERK1/2 and EGFR signaling suggests a compensatory response.

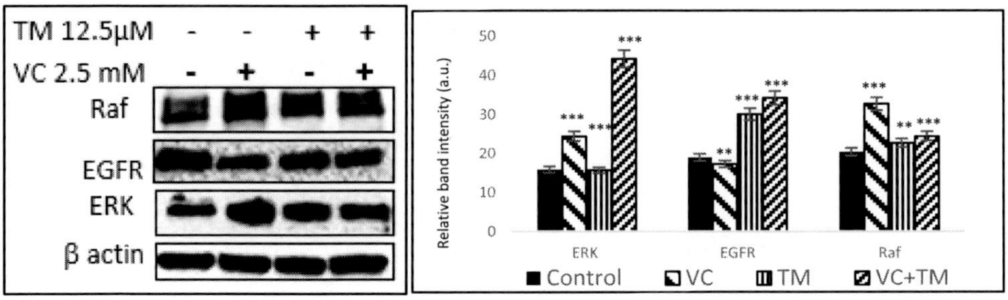

(a) (b)

Figure 14. Western blot analysis of ERK 1/2, Raf, and EGFR expressions after the treatment of A-498 cells with VC, TM, or the combination. (a) Representative blots showing expression of these proteins. (b) Dcnsitometric histogram compares relative protein levels normalized to β-actin. Data are expressed as mean ± SD (n = 3). Significant changes are marked as $**p < 0.01$, $***p < 0.001$, according to the post hoc Newman-Keuls test.

Modulation of Wnt, β catenin, and ROCK

The impact of VC, TM, and their combined treatment on Wnt, β catenin, and ROCK proteins was assessed in A-498 cells showing their increase expressions were in all treatments as compared to control. This increase signifies an unfavorable effect of using VC, TM, or the combination of renal cancer. These proteins are key components of signaling systems that regulate cell polarity, cytoskeletal organization, and epithelial–mesenchymal transition.

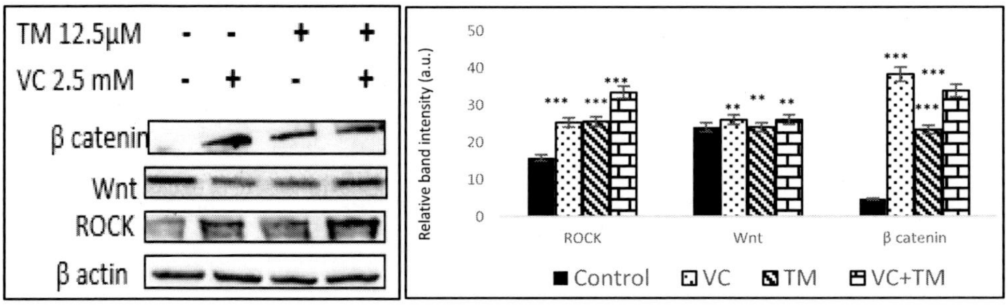

(a) (b)

Figure 15. Western blot analysis of ROCK, β catenin, and Wnt expressions after treatment of A-498 cells with VC, TM, or their combination. (a) Representative blots showing expression of these proteins. (b) Densitometric histogram compares relative protein levels normalized to β-actin. Data are expressed as mean ± SD (n = 3). Significant changes are marked as $**p < 0.01$, $***p < 0.001$, according to the post hoc Newman-Keuls test.

Modulation of MnSOD, Vimentin, PDL-1, Smac/DIABLO

The impact of VC, TM, and their combined treatment on MnSOD and Vimentin proteins was assessed in A-498 cells. An increase in MnSOD and Vimentin expressions in VC, while slight increase in TM or the combo treatment are observed. VC can increase intracellular ROS. Vimentin may be upregulated during oxidative stress, causing a slight increase in TM or the combination.

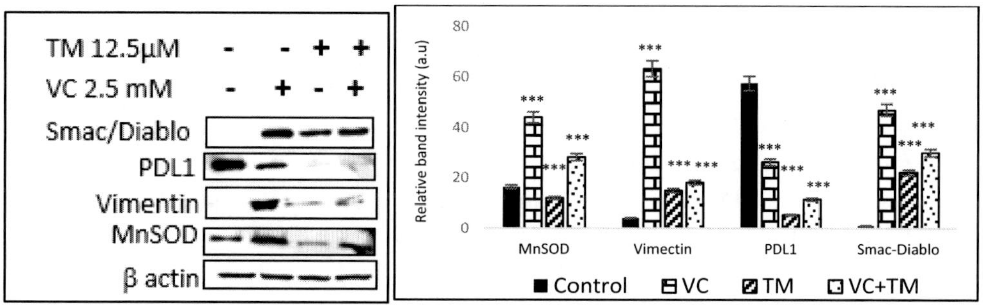

(a) (b)

Figure 16. Western blot analysis of MnSOD and Vimentin expressions after treatment of cells with VC, TM, or their combination. (a) Representative blots showing expression of these proteins. (b) Densitometric histogram compares relative protein levels normalized to β-actin. Data are expressed as mean ± SD (n = 3). Significant changes are marked as ***$p < 0.001$, according to the post hoc Newman-Keuls test.

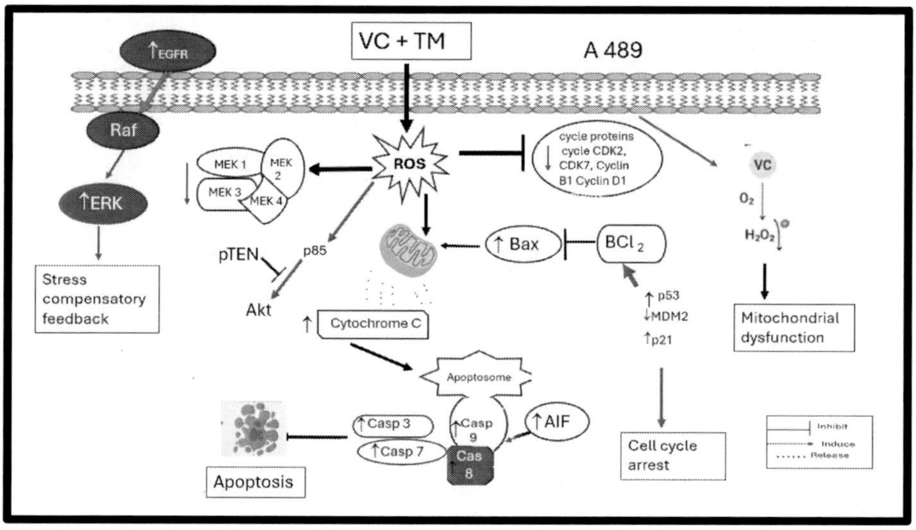

Figure 17. Proposed mechanistic model of VC and SF in Renal cancer.

Discussion

As illustrated on Figure 17, treatment of A-498 cells with VC, TM, or their combination induced mitochondrial stress, cell cycle disruption, and apoptotic signaling. However, the overall cytotoxic effect at 24 h did not reflect synergy, as the combination treatment yielded Fa = 0.362 and CI = 1.87, indicating an antagonistic interaction at 24 h. This finding is especially relevant in the context of RCC, a cancer known for its signaling plasticity, intrinsic resistance to apoptosis, and strong dependence on mTOR-driven survival pathways.

Temsirolimus, while clinically approved for advanced RCC, has limited effect on cancer cells due to compensatory pathway reactivation, particularly mTORC1 and mTORC2. In the current study, while VC and TM together increased ROS generation, disrupted mitochondrial membrane potential, and elevated several pro-apoptotic markers (caspases-3, -7, -8, -9, Bax, Smac/DIABLO, and AIF), a concurrent increase in total mTOR expression suggests activation of a feedback survival response that may have temporarily blunted full apoptotic execution [22-26].

Importantly, the interaction between VC and TM was time dependent. At 24 h, the combination produced a less-than-additive effect (Fa = 0.362; CI = 1.87), coinciding with compensatory mTOR upregulation despite suppression of PI3K and Akt, suggesting an early survival feedback response. However, as exposure continued to 48 and 72 h, cell viability declined more rapidly in the combination groups than with either agent alone, and the interaction shifted to synergistic and then strongly synergistic, respectively. This transition aligns with the delayed collapse of mitochondrial integrity, sustained ROS accumulation, and commitment to caspase-dependent apoptosis, indicating that VC enhances TM efficacy once feedback resistance mechanisms are overcome. Thus, the VC and TM response in RCC is not instantaneous but rather emerges over time as apoptotic signaling surpasses adaptive survival pathways.

VC and TM co-treatment suppressed PI3K and Akt, yet the observed upregulation of total mTOR indicates a compensatory signaling loop, consistent with known limitations of mTOR inhibitors [27-29]. This helps explain why the biochemical signature of apoptosis was present, but the measured cytotoxicity did not reach synergistic thresholds at 24 hours. Additionally, decreases in Cyclin B1 and CDK2 and increased p21 and PTEN expression indicate cell cycle checkpoint stress, while undetectable Cyclin D1 suggests early-phase arrest consistent with metabolic strain. The observed modulation of MEK 1–4, SAPK/JNK, and p38 MAPK pathways further supports broad stress signaling reprogramming [30-33]. Interestingly, upregulation of EGFR, ERK, Wnt/β-catenin, and vimentin across treatment groups may reflect a compensatory attempt toward survival or phenotypic adaptation, underscoring the dynamic balance between apoptosis induction and stress adaptation in RCC cells [34-37].

Conclusion

While VC and TM activated pro-apoptotic and cell cycle inhibitory pathways, the net cytotoxic outcome at 24 h was antagonistic, likely due to early compensatory mTOR feedback and redox-buffering responses. These results highlight that the therapeutic efficacy of VC in RCC is timing-dependent, and that dosing sequence or extended exposure may be required to shift this interaction toward synergy.

Key Findings

VC and TM treatment resulted in mitochondrial stress and activation of apoptotic signaling markers, including Bax, caspases-3, -7, -8, -9, Smac/DIABLO, and AIF, along with reduced Bcl-2 and cytochrome c release, indicating engagement of intrinsic apoptotic pathways. VC and TM jointly suppressed PI3K and Akt, but mTOR levels increased, suggesting a compensatory feedback response that may have temporarily protected cells from full apoptotic execution. The overall cytotoxic response at 24 h reflects antagonistic (Fa = 0.362, CI= 1.87). However, by 48 and 72 h treatments, the response shifted to synergistic and strongly synergistic cytotoxicity as mitochondrial apoptosis fully engaged. The effects of VC and TM were highly time-dependent that early co-administration may produce antagonism, whereas optimized sequencing or longer exposure may be required to achieve therapeutic benefit. This model highlights that VC is not universally synergistic, and its therapeutic benefit depends on timing, redox state, and pathway adaptability, underscoring the importance of treatment scheduling in RCC.

Acknowledgments

The author thanks Union University for the source and support of research funding as well as colleagues and editing tools for assistance with improving the clarity of the manuscript.

References

[1] Cirillo L., Innocenti S., Becherucci F. Global epidemiology of kidney cancer. *Nephrol Dial Transplant* 2024 ; 39 :920-928.

[2] Sung H., Ferlay J., Siegel R.L., Laversanne M., Soerjomataram I., Jemal A., et al., Global Cancer Statistics 2020: GLOBOCAN Estimates of Incidence and Mortality Worldwide for 36 Cancers in 185 Countries. *CA Cancer J Clin* 2021 ; 71(3) : 209-249.

[3] Mancini M., Righetto M., Baggio G .Gender-related approach to kidney cancer management: Moving forward. *Int J Mol Sci* 2020 ; 21(9) :3378.

[4] Patard J.J., Leray E., Rioux L.N., Cindolo L., Ficarra V., Zisman A., et al., Prognostic Value of Histologic Subtypes in Renal Cell Carcinoma: A Multicenter Experience. *J Clin Oncol* 2005 ; 23 :2763–2771.

[5] Pontes O., Oliveira-Pinto S., Baltazar F., Costa M. Renal cell carcinoma therapy: current and new drug candidates. *Drug Discov Today* 2022; 27:1.

[6] Pena-Llopis S., Christie X., Xie J., Brugarolas J. Cooperation and antagonism among cancer genes: the renal cancer paradigm. *Cancer Res* 2013 ; 73 : 4173-4179.

[7] Kaelin W.G. The von-Hippel-Lindau tumor suppressor protein: O2 sensing and cancer. *Nat Rev Cancer* 2008 ; 8 : 865-873.

[8] Kaelin W.G., Ratcliffe P.J. Oxygen sensing by metazoans: the central role of the HIF hydroxylase pathway. *Mol Cell* 2008; 30: 393-402.

[9] Gkagkalidis K., S Kampantais S., Dimitriadis G., Mironidou-Tzouveleki M. Expression of HIF-2a in clear-cell renal cell carcinoma independently predicts overall survival. *Med Mol Morph* 2020; 53: 229-237.

[10] Bahadoram S., Davoodi M., Hassanzadeh S., Bahadoram M., Barahman M., Mafakher L. Renal cell carcinoma: an overview of the epidemiology, diagnosis, and treatment. *G Ital Nephrol* 2022 ; 39.

[11] American Cancer Society. *Cancer Facts & Figures*. Atlanta : American Cancer Society. 2022.

[12] Capitanio U., Montorsi F. Renal cancer. *Lancet* 2016 ; 387 : 894-906.

[13] Bianchi M., Sun M., Jedres C. Distribution of metastatic sites in renal cell carcinoma: a population-based analysis. *Ann Oncol* 2012 ; 23 :973-980.

[14] Huang W.C., Elkin E.B., Levey A.S., Jang T.L., Russo P. Partial nephrectomy versus radical nephrectomy in patients with small renal tumors-is there a difference in mortality and cardiovascular outcomes? *J Urol* 2009; 181: 55-61.

[15] Ziglioli F. , De Filippo M., Cavalieri D.M., Pagnini F., Campobasso D., Guarino G. , et al., Percutaneous radiofrequency ablation (RFA) in renal cancer. How to manage challenging masses. A narrative review. *Acta Biomed* 2022; 26: 2022220.

[16] Lee J.H., You C.H., Min G.E. Comparison of the surgical outcome and functional outcome between radical and nephron-sparing surgery for renal cell carcinoma. *Korean J Urol* 2007 ; 48 :671-676.

[17] Wolf M.M., Rathmell W.K., Beckermann K.E. Modeling clear cell renal cell carcinoma and therapeutic implications. *Oncogene* 2020; 39 (17): 3413-3426.

[18] Catalano M., Procopio G., Sepe P., Santoni M., Sessa F., Villari D., et al., Tyrosine kinase and immune checkpoints. Tyrosine kinase and immune checkpoints inhibitors in favorable risk metastatic renal cell carcinoma: trick or treat? *Pharmacol Ther* 2023; 249:108499.

[19] Aparicio L.M.A., Fernandez I.P., Cassinello J. Tyrosine kinase inhibitors reprogramming immunity in renal cell carcinoma: rethinking cancer immunotherapy. *Clin Trans Oncol* 2017 ; 19(10) :1175-1182.

[20] Uzzo R.G., Novick A.C. Nephron-sparing surgery for renal tumors: indications, techniques and outcomes. *J Urol* 2001 ; 166 :6–18.

[21] Robert J., Motzer R.J., Penkov K.K., Rini A. Avelumab plus Axitinib versus Sunitinib for Advanced Renal-Cell Carcinoma. *N Eng J Med* 2019 ; 380 : 1103-1115.

[22] Chen Q., Espey M.G., Krishna M.C., Mitchell J.B., Corpe C.P., Buettner G.R., et al., Pharmacological ascorbic acid concentrations selectively kill cancer cells: action as a pro-drug to deliver hydrogen peroxide to tissues. *PNAS* 2005 ; 102 : 13604-13609.

[23] Chen Q., Espey M.G., Sun A.Y., Lee J.H., Buettner G.R., Levine M. Ascorbate in pharmacologic concentration selectively generate ascorbate radical and hydrogen peroxide in extracellular fluid *in vivo*. *PNAS* 2007 ; 104 : 8749-8754.

[24] Olney K.E., Du J., Van-Erve T.J., Witmer J.R., Wagner B.A., Buettner G.R., et al., Inhibitors of hydroperoxide metabolism enhance ascorbate-induce cytotoxicity. *Free Radic Res* 2013 ; 47 :154-163.

[25] Doskey C.M., Buranasudja V., Wagner B. A., Wilkes J.G., Du J., Cullen J.J., et al., Tumor cells have decreased ability to metabolize H2O2: implications for pharmacological ascorbate in cancer therapy. *Redox Biol* 2016 ; 10 : 274–284.

[26] Hudes G., Carducci M., Dutcher J., Figlin R., Kapoor A., Staroslawska E. Temsirolimus, interferon alfa, or both for advanced renal-cell carcinoma. *NEJM* 2007 ; 356(22) : 2271–2281.

[27] Aguilera O., Muñoz-Muela E., Gallego-Ortega D. Vitamin C uncouples the Warburg effect in KRAS mutant colon cancer. *Oncotarget* 2021 ; 7(30): 47954–47965.

[28] O'Reilly K.E., Rojo F., She Q.B., Solit D., Mills G.B., Smith D., et al., mTOR inhibition induces upstream receptor tyrosine kinase signaling and activates Akt. *Cancer Res* 2006 ; 66(3) :1500–1508.

[29] Yi J., Luo J., Liu L., Han R. Vitamin C suppresses cell proliferation in hepatocellular carcinoma cells via the inhibition of the PI3K/Akt pathway. *Oncol Lett* 2020 ; 19(3) : 1555–1562.

[30] Qie S., Diehl A. Cyclin D1, cancer progression, and opportunities in cancer treatment. *J Mol Med* 2016 ; 94 : 1313–1326.

[31] Song M.S., Salmena L., Pandolfi P.P. The functions and regulation of the PTEN tumor suppressor. *Nature Rev Mol Cell Biol* 2012 ; 13(5) : 283–296.

[32] MacDonald B.T., Tamai K., He X. Wnt/β-catenin signaling components, mechanisms, and diseases. *Dev Cell* 2009 ; 17(1) : 9–26.

[33] Kalluri R., Weinberg R.A. The basics of epithelial-mesenchymal transition. *J Clin Invest* 2009 ; 119(6): 1420–1428.

[34] [34] Choueiri T.K., Fay A.P., Gray K.P., Ho T.H., Albiges L., Carvo I., et al., PD-L1 expression in nonclear- cell renal carcinoma. *Ann Oncol* 2014 ; 25 (11): 2178-2184.

[35] Zhang Y., Wang L., Li Y., Pan Y., Wang R. PD-L1 expression in renal cell carcinoma and its correlation with tumor-infiltrating lymphocytes and clinicopathological parameters. *Sci Reports* 2018 ; 8(1), 11245.

[36] Doskey C.M. Redox control of the cell cycle in health and disease. *Free Radic Biol Med* 2016 ; 107 : 148–167.

[37] Liu M.F., Sun X., Chen B., Dai R., Xi Z., Xu H. Insight into manganese superoxide dismutase and human diseases. *Int J Mol Sci* 2022 ; 23 (24) : 15893.

Conclusion

Revisiting Vitamin C in Cancer - From Bench Mechanisms to Translational of Hope

Lunawati L. Bennett*, PhD, PharmD
Union University, College of Pharmacy, Jackson, Tennessee, USA

Abstract

This last chapter integrates the mechanistic and therapeutic insights gained from the investigation of vitamin C across diverse cancer models. By examining its dual antioxidant and pro-oxidant roles, this book highlights how vitamin C may enhance anticancer efficacy when combined with selected antineoplastic agents. The collective findings emphasize the importance of dose, cellular context, and drug pairing in determining therapeutic outcomes. This final chapter reflects translational implications, future research directions, and the potential role of vitamin C as a complementary strategy in oncology.

Keywords: vitamin C, combination therapy, oxidative stress, apoptosis, translational oncology

Completing the Vitamin C Journey

The journey through this book has explored the multifaceted role of VC in the context of cancer biology and therapeutic synergy. This book began with a humble but powerful molecule: vitamin C, also known as ascorbate, known globally as a dietary antioxidant, but rediscovered in the context of cancer metabolism and redox regulation by Linus Pauling, the Nobel prize winner in Chemistry.

Across the preceding chapters, VC was examined in multiple cellular landscapes - from hepatocellular carcinoma (HepG2), osteosarcoma (Saos-2), pancreatic (BxPC3), brain cancer (SK-N-SH and SH-SY5Y), colorectal (Caco-2), breast (MCF7), triple negative breast cancer (MB-MDA 231), renal (A-498), malignant pleural mesothelioma (MSTO), non-small cell lung cancer (NCI-H5222), prostate (LnCaP clone FGC) to hematologic malignancies such as chronic myelogenous leukemia (K562) and chronic lymphocytic leukemia (Z-1380).

* Corresponding Author's Email: llbennett@uu.edu

In each system, VC are partnered with a defined chemotherapeutic or targeted agent: sorafenib, paclitaxel, afatinib, doxorubicin, bortezomib, temsirolimus, and others.

What emerged from these models is more than a sequence of experiments - it is a portrait of *contextual activity*. VC rarely behaves as a one-dimensional antioxidant. Rather, it acts as a *redox modulator,* capable of both protecting normal cells and stressing malignant ones beyond their oxidative tolerance. This redox duality underlies much of its therapeutic potential.

Across all chapters, a consistent theme emerged: *VC alters cancer cell fate by modulating oxidative stress, mitochondrial function, apoptotic signaling, and survival pathways.* This multidimensional influence challenges the historical skepticism surrounding VC's role in oncology and invites its reconsideration within modern molecular frameworks.

At the start of this work, the field of oncology still regarded VC with a divided lens - some viewing it as complementary, others as scientifically unsupported. Yet through systematic laboratory exploration, this book contributes to redefining VC's biological space, positioning it not as a supplement, but as a *bioactive small molecule* with pharmacologic properties when administered at high concentrations.

Mechanistic Integration Across Cancers

Despite differences in cell origin and genetic background, a striking unity of mechanism unfolded. VC consistently disrupted mitochondrial integrity, leading to cytochrome c release, activation of caspase cascades, and suppression of anti-apoptotic proteins like Bcl-2. Upregulation of pro-apoptotic factors such as Bax, PTEN, and p21 often paralleled these events. These molecular hallmarks suggest that VC exerts a central role in *amplifying mitochondrial-dependent apoptosis.*

Moreover, VC's interaction with reactive oxygen species (ROS) proved central. Cancer cells, characterized by elevated basal ROS and weakened antioxidant capacity, are vulnerable to further oxidative pressure. VC amplified this imbalance - not as a mere donor or scavenger of electrons, but as a catalyst of oxidative stress when exposed to transition metals like iron or copper. In this pro-oxidant mode, VC converted hydrogen peroxide and hydroxyl radicals into cytotoxic species capable of selectively damaging cancer cell membranes and DNA.

Additionally, VC influenced multiple signaling pathways:

- *MEK/ERK downregulation*, observed prominently in HepG2, NSCLC, and prostate models, indicating suppression of proliferative and survival signaling.
- *p21 and PTEN upregulation,* reinforcing tumor-suppressive activity and potential restoration of cell cycle control.
- *MDM2 reduction,* possibly enhancing p53 stability and apoptotic competence.
- *Cyclins (D1, B1) and CDKs (2, 7) downregulation*, pointing toward cell cycle arrest mechanisms that complement apoptotic induction.

These findings collectively establish VC as a *broad-spectrum modulator of stress and death signaling*, not limited to oxidative chemistry but extending into regulatory networks that govern proliferation, differentiation, and repair.

In the context of drug synergy, VC enhanced the efficacy of agents with distinct mechanisms:

- *Sorafenib (multi-kinase inhibitor):* VC amplified mitochondrial dysfunction and MEK/ERK downregulation, enhancing apoptosis in liver, breast, renal, and prostate cancers.
- *Paclitaxel (microtubule stabilizer):* VC increased oxidative load and DNA fragmentation, and promoting greater mitotic arrest in mesothelioma.
- *Afatinib (EGFR/HER2 inhibitor):* VC augmented ER stress and Bax expression, suppressing survival signaling in osteosarcoma cells.
- *Doxorubicin and bortezomib:* VC appeared to mitigate drug-induced toxicity in normal cells while preserving cytotoxicity in malignant ones - suggesting a selective redox protective role.

These patterns reinforce VC's identity as a *context-dependent modulator,* bridging oxidative biochemistry with signaling and metabolic control.

The Redox Balance as a Therapeutic Options

The concept that VC functions only as an antioxidant is now obsolete. The data presented across these chapters align with the newer model of VC as a *pro-oxidant under pharmacologic conditions.* At high concentrations (achieved only via intravenous administration), VC drives Fenton-type reactions that generate extracellular hydrogen peroxide, diffusing into nearby cancer cells. Normal cells, equipped with catalase and glutathione peroxidase systems, neutralize this hydrogen peroxide, while many malignant cells fail to do so - resulting in *selective cytotoxicity.*

This redox selectivity underlies one of the most compelling translational implications: *high-dose VC can differentially affect malignant versus normal tissues*, an effect that could be therapeutically exploited to enhance drug response while reducing collateral damage.

Furthermore, VC's influence extends beyond ROS generation. It affects epigenetic regulation through its role as a cofactor for Fe^{2+}/2-oxoglutarate–dependent dioxygenases, including TET enzymes that demethylate DNA and histones. Such actions may restore tumor-suppressive gene expression patterns, as observed in studies where VC reversed hypermethylation of key promoters (e.g., BRCA1, PTEN). The ability of VC to affect both redox balance and epigenetic status positions it as a *unique metabolic–epigenetic bridge* in cancer biology.

Integrating Evidence: Vitamin C as a Systems Modulator

Taken together, the experimental results and current literature suggest that VC should not be categorized solely as a chemotherapeutic adjunct or metabolic supplement. Instead, it acts as a *systems modulator* -influencing redox balance, mitochondrial dynamics, signal transduction, gene expression, and even the tumor microenvironment.

This system's view aligns with the growing field of metabolic oncology, which recognizes cancer not merely as a genetic disorder, but as a metabolic disease with redox dysregulation at its core. VC's ability to tilt redox balance selectively against malignant cells makes it an intriguing therapeutic candidate, especially when combined with drugs that rely on oxidative signaling or mitochondrial dysfunction.

For instance, the combination of VC with SF across several cancer types illustrates this principle clearly. SF targets multiple kinases within the RAF/MEK/ERK pathway and disrupts mitochondrial respiration. VC's pro-oxidant action amplifies this stress, promoting cytochrome c release and cell death. Meanwhile, normal cells remain largely protected - a dual action that exemplifies the potential for *therapeutic selectivity through redox modulation.*

Across all models, a unifying pattern emerges *VC acts as a redox modulator,* capable of tipping the intracellular oxidative balance toward apoptosis in malignant cells while sparing non-cancerous ones. The consistent observation of *ROS elevation, Bax/Bcl2 ratio shift,* and *cytochrome c release* across diverse cancer types suggests that VC enhances intrinsic mitochondrial apoptosis regardless of tissue origin.

The synergistic combinations, particularly in *HepG2, MCF7, BxPC3, K562, and NCI-H5222,* underscore the mechanistic overlap between VC's pro-oxidant behavior and the stress responses triggered by targeted agents. These observations align clinical hypotheses that VC's pharmacologic concentration achieved via *intravenous (IV) administration* may potentiate drug efficacy by creating a localized pro-oxidant microenvironment lethal to tumor cells but tolerable to normal tissue.

However, certain pathways showed *context-specific variability*. For instance, in NSCLC and mesothelioma models, despite strong apoptotic signaling, upregulation of *JNK/p38* or *Wnt/β-catenin* indicated adaptive stress responses, hinting at potential resistance mechanisms that could emerge under prolonged exposure. Similarly, in some combinations, VC modestly affected *mTOR* and *Akt* signaling, suggesting selective sensitivity dependent on the cancer's metabolic phenotype.

Collectively, these data reinforce VC's versatility as both *a sensitizer and a stress amplifier.* Its ability to modulate multiple signaling axes - MEK/ERK, PI3K/mTOR, EGFR, and apoptotic cascades - supports its candidacy for integration into low-dose combination regimens. Yet, while *in vitro* results are compelling, translation into clinical protocols remains contingent upon pharmacokinetics, tumor selectivity, and timing of administration.

Vitamin C and Sorafenib Synergy Across Models

Among all drug combinations tested, VC with *SF* displayed particularly consistent synergy such as in liver, breast, renal, prostate, and lung models. The combination resulted in enhanced apoptosis and suppression of MAPK and PI3K/Akt pathways.

Sorafenib inhibits multiple kinases, including RAF and VEGFR, thereby blocking cancer cell proliferation and angiogenesis. VC's oxidative stress amplified SF's mitochondrial disruption, leading to *greater cytochrome release and caspase activation.* Furthermore, the combination suppressed *MEK-1, -2, -3, -4 and ERK1/2,* implicating downstream effects on cell cycle regulators (CDK2, cyclin D1) and survival mediators (Bcl-2, MDM2).

In the prostate (LnCaP Clone FGC) and NSCLC (NCI-H5222) models, the VC and SF pairing demonstrated reductions in cell viability, increased ROS generation, and modulation of mitochondrial proteins including Smac/DIABLO and MnSOD. These converging data support the hypothesis that *VC enhances SF efficacy by targeting mitochondrial resilience and survival signaling simultaneously.*

Vitamin C in Hematologic Malignancy-and Beyond

The CLL model (Z-138 cells) highlighted another layer of VC biology - its ability to influence apoptosis regulators such *as Smac/DIABLO, MnSOD,* and *vimentin.* The increase in Smac/DIABLO suggests activation of mitochondrial-mediated apoptotic machinery, while MnSOD upregulation may represent a compensatory antioxidant defense. Interestingly, vimentin reduction suggests a possible interference with cellular plasticity and metastatic potential.

Together, these changes indicate that VC and SF disrupt both metabolic and structural stability in leukemic cells. This observation resonates with clinical findings suggesting that VC can sensitize hematologic malignancies to chemotherapy and reduce resistance mediated by anti-apoptotic proteins.

Vitamin C Beyond Redox - Epigenetic and Immunologic Horizons

Emerging research suggests that VC's influence extends beyond oxidative modulation. As a cofactor for Fe^{2+}/2-oxoglutarate–dependent dioxygenases, VC supports *TET-mediated DNA demethylation and Jumonji histone demethylase* activity. This enables reactivation of silenced tumor suppressor genes and correction of aberrant methylation patterns - epigenetic reprogramming that could complement classical cytotoxic therapies.

Moreover, VC may enhance anti-cancer immunity. It stabilizes HIF-1α and modulates T-cell differentiation, suggesting potential synergy with *immune checkpoint inhibitors* and other immunotherapeutic modalities. This broadens VC's potential role from redox cofactor to *epigenetic–immune metabolic regulator,* a promising concept for next-generation integrative oncology.

Mechanism and Key Signaling Pathways from Previous Chapters

For clinical oncology, the implication is clear: the era of monotherapy dominance is fading. Modern cancer treatment increasingly relies on *combination strategies* that exploit multiple vulnerabilities simultaneously. VC fits this paradigm perfectly - inexpensive, well-tolerated, mechanistically rich, and potentially synergistic with standard drugs.

Several clinical trials are now testing VC alongside immune checkpoint inhibitors, radiotherapy, or targeted kinase inhibitors. The future will depend not only on outcomes but also on the ability to *standardize VC pharmacology*, ensuring reproducibility across institutions.

Table 1. Consolidated summary of the modulatory actions of VC alone and in combination with selected antineoplastic agents across diverse human cancer cell models, as previously described in the respective experimental chapters of this book.

To further substantiate the mechanistic observations summarized in Table 1, a comparative quantitative analysis was conducted using the Chou–Talalay method to determine the degree of interaction between VC and various antineoplastic agents. Table 2 presents the concentration ranges of both agents used in each cancer model, the corresponding cell viability outcomes, and the calculated Combination Index (CI) values. The concentrations of VC and respective antineoplastic agents used in each combination were selected to achieve approximately 40–70% cell viability in monotherapy, enabling valid combination index (CI) calculations. CI values ranged from 0.61 to 0.83, confirming synergism in nearly all models tested. The most pronounced synergy was observed in *CLL Z-138,* followed by *K562* and *NCI-H522* cells, while *A-498* demonstrated a *time-dependent additive to synergistic* response. These results provide quantitative validation for the cooperative cytotoxic effects of VC with diverse chemotherapeutics, reinforcing the redox–signaling axis as a unifying mechanism for enhanced anticancer efficacy. These data provide numerical confirmation of the synergistic trends observed experimentally and highlight the reproducible enhancement of cytotoxic efficacy across multiple cancer types. The inclusion of both mechanistic and quantitative datasets strengthens the overall translational value of this work, bridging the gap between biochemical insight and therapeutic applicability. The detailed dose–response relationships and CI values are summarized in Table 2.

Table 1. Mechanisms, pathways and biological analysis

Cancer Type	Drug Combined with VC	Major Mechanisms Observed	Key Signaling Pathways	Outcome Viability/Apoptosis	Translational Implication of VC
HepG2 (Liver)	Sorafenib	↑ROS, ↑Bax/Bcl2 ratio, ↓ MEK	MEK ERK	Intrinsic apoptosis activation	Suppress cell proliferation
MSTO (MPM)*	Paclitaxel	↑ Cytochrome, ↑ AIF, ↓ Bcl2	Caspase cascade	Enhance apoptosis	Enhance microtubule stress
SaOS-2 (Bone)	Afatinib	↑ PTEN, ↓p85/AKT/ ↓mTOR	P85/Akt/ mTOR	Caspase activation	Block EGFR
BxPC3 (Pancreas)	Doxorubicin	↑ROS, ↓MMP, ↑Smac/Diablo	Tumor suppressor gene	Enhanced apoptosis	Enhances mitochondrial stress
Caco-2 (Colorectal)	Bortezomib	↑ p53, ↓ MEK 1-4, ↑p21	Proteasome	Apoptosis of mitochondria	Modulate proteasome
MCF7 (Breast)	Sorafenib	↓MEK/ERK, ↑ p21, ↓MMP-2, -9	MAPK, Cell cycle	Enhanced ROS	Targeting dual pathways
MDA-MB-231 (TNBC)*	Mono-therapy	↓oxidative stress, ↑apoptosis	↑ Bax, ↓ Bcl-2, ↑ Cas 3	↓ cell cycle ↑PTEN, ↑p53	↓Initiation of carcinogenesis
A-498 (Renal)	Temsiro-limus	↓ mTOR, ↑ PTEN, ↓p85	Caspases	Not synergy	Adaptive compensatory pro-survival
K562 (CML)*	Sorafenib	↑ROS, ↑ Cytochrome	Intrinsic apoptosis	Enhanced oxidative	ROS-mediated mitochondrial apoptosis
Z-138 (CLL)*	Sorafenib	↑ROS, ↓Vimentin, ↑ p21, ↑PTEN	↓EMT ↓efflux ↓immune	ROS driven	Mitochondrial apoptosis, ↓EMT
SK-N-SH (Brain)	Etoposide	↓ PDK-1, ↓ MDR-ABC	↑intrinsic apoptotic cascade	↓ EGFR ↓ ERK ↓MEK 1-4	ROS-mediated mitochondrial apoptosis
SH-SY5Y (Brain)	Etoposide	↓ BRCA1/2, ↓ MDR-ABC	Redox potential	Adaptive to oxidative tress	↓DNA repair mechanism
NCI-H5222 (NSCLC)*	Sorafenib	↓MEK, ↓EGFR, ↑ Bax, ↓ Bcl2	MAPK EGFR	↓MEK 1-4 ↓ERK, ↓Akt/P85	ROS-mediated mitochondrial apoptosis
LnCaP FGC) (Prostate)	Sorafenib	↑Cas 3, 7, 8, 9, ↑Akt/MEK, ↑ERK 1/2	Caspases	Not synergy	Redox modulator

Abbreviation: TNBC- triple negative breast cancer; MPM- malignant pleural mesothelioma; CLL- chronic lymphocytic leukemia; CML-chronic myelogenous leukemia; NSCLC- Non small cell lung carcinoma; ROS-reactive oxygen species; MAPK- Mitogen-activated protein kinase; mTOR-mammalian target of rapamycin; EGFR- epidermal growth factor; MEK-Mitogen-activated protein kinase; ERK- epidermal growth factor; MDR-multi drug resistance; Cas- caspase; PTEN- phosphatase and tensin homolog.

The collective Chou–Talalay analyses presented in Tables 1 and 2 illustrate that *VC–drug interactions are context-dependent rather than universally synergistic.* Many cancer models demonstrated *clear synergistic cytotoxicity,* characterized by enhanced oxidative stress, mitochondrial membrane destabilization, and activation of caspase-dependent apoptosis. However, in other models, such *as A-498 renal carcinoma and LNCaP prostate cancer*, synergy was *conditional* - emerging only under prolonged exposure or attenuated by *compensatory survival signaling* involving the MAPK, PI3K/Akt, and Wnt/β-catenin networks. These results indicate that VC functions as a *redox based signaling modulator*, whose therapeutic impact depends on *intracellular signaling state, redox capacity, and treatment timing,* rather than as a uniformly additive agent.

Table 2. Quantitative synergy parameters for all cell lines being tested

Cell Line/Cancer	VC (mM)	Antineoplastic (μM or nM)	% Viability (Combination)	Average CI	Interaction
Caco-2	5	BZ 62.5 nM	75.8–48.2	0.76	Synergistic
MCF7	3	SF 3 μM	39.1–29.5	0.73	Synergistic
HepG2	5	SF 3 μM	58–36	0.75	Synergistic
MSTO	3	PX 1 μM	60–42	0.78	Synergistic
SaOS-2	2.5	AF 3 μM	85.8–68.1	0.83	Synergistic
BxPC-3	3	DX 3 μM	59–37	0.81	Synergistic
SK-N-SH	2.5	ET 0.5 μM	0.43	0.51	Synergistic
SH-SY5Y	2.5	ET 0.5 μM	0.72	0.95	Synergistic
A-498	2.5	TM 12.5 μM	CI ≈ 1.8 at 24 h. CI < 1 at 48–72 h	1.87	Early antagonism due to mTOR feedback; synergy emerges as mitochondrial apoptosis overcomes survival buffering after prolonged exposure
K562	9	SF 5 μM	54–37	0.73	Synergistic
Z-138	12.5	SF 5 μM	19–11.8	0.61	Synergistic
NCI-H522	6.25	SF 6 μM	56–31	0.68	Synergistic
LNCaP-FGC	10	SF 0.6 μM	45-65	0.68	Enhanced apoptotic signaling, but survival feedback of MAPK, PI3K, and Wnt) limits final cytotoxic effect

Abbreviation: PX- Paclitaxel, AF- Afatinib, TM-Temsirolimus, BZ- Bortezomib, SF- Sorafenib, DX- doxorubicin; ET- Etoposide; CI- combination index.

Such findings hold significant translational implications. While the mechanistic potential of VC to amplify apoptotic signaling is well supported, *clinical benefit will depend on optimizing dose, sequencing, and co-targeting of feedback survival pathways* to prevent resistance. This nuanced interpretation forms the basis for the following discussion of *translational considerations*, where the promise of VC–enhanced therapy is evaluated considering pharmacokinetics, tumor heterogeneity, and patient-specific metabolic context.

Translational Challenges and Controversies

Although the laboratory findings presented here offer mechanistic clarity, translation to the clinic remains complex. The pharmacokinetic difference between oral and intravenous VC administration is substantial. Oral VC is saturable, achieving plasma concentrations below 0.2 mM, whereas intravenous infusion can transiently raise levels to 15–25 mM - within the range shown to be cytotoxic *in vitro*.

Clinical studies have produced mixed outcomes. Some early-phase trials have reported improved quality of life, reduced inflammation, and lower chemotherapy-induced toxicity. Yet survival benefits remain inconsistent. This discrepancy may reflect variations in patient selection, dosing schedules, cancer type, and co-administered drugs. For example, administering VC concurrently with certain redox-active drugs could either potentiate or quench desired oxidative effects depending on the intracellular milieu.

A related question concerns *timing and sequencing.* Should VC be given before, during, or after chemotherapy? The current experimental chapters provide insight: simultaneous treatment often enhanced apoptosis, but pre-treatment sometimes increased antioxidant defenses, temporarily protecting cells. Such findings emphasize that VC's therapeutic window is *dynamic, not static,* and may require individualized scheduling to optimize its synergy with antineoplastic agents.

The variability observed across the cancer models in this book reinforces this principle. In some systems, such as pancreatic, osteosarcoma, mesothelioma, and liver cancer, VC potentiated chemotherapeutic efficacy in a straightforward manner. In others, such as *renal carcinoma (A-498)* and *prostate cancer (LNCaP-FGC),* synergy was *conditional* - emerging only with *prolonged exposure or co-targeting of compensatory survival pathways.* These findings highlight that *VC does not act as a universal cytotoxic enhancer,* but rather as a *context-dependent redox modulator* whose therapeutic benefit depends on the *signaling state, metabolic condition, and adaptive capacity* of cancer.

This introduces an important clinical consideration: many cancer patients begin treatment *already in a state of chronic vitamin C depletion,* driven by tumor metabolism, systemic inflammation, stress, and poor nutritional intake. In this context, the first question may not be whether VC should be *added* to therapy, but whether *restoring physiological VC levels is necessary before any treatment can perform as designed.* If the baseline redox environment is unstable or deficient, cells may be primed for survival pathways rather than apoptosis. It is therefore plausible that *repletion of VC to normal physiological levels first, followed by the strategic timing of high-dose VC in combination with antineoplastic agents, may shift cellular momentum toward mitochondrial commitment and apoptotic sensitivity.*

In other words, *what we treat is not only cancer, but the terrain in which it exists.* The success of cytotoxic therapies may depend as much on *the metabolic state of the host* as on the potency of the drug. The work presented in this volume suggests that the path to synergy is *not merely additive*, but *chronobiological* - sensitive to timing, sequence, and the biochemical readiness of the cell to respond.

Future Directions: Bridging Bench and Bedside

The next phase of VC research must move toward *precision redox therapy* - integrating laboratory findings with clinical pharmacology and patient heterogeneity. Several key directions emerge from the bench to the bedside:

1. *In vivo validation and dosing studies:* Animal models should be used to confirm in vitro mechanisms under physiological conditions. Determining optimal infusion rates, dosing frequency, and tissue penetration will be critical for translating cytotoxic concentrations safely.
2. *Biomarker-guided patient selection:* Patients with low catalase activity, altered mitochondrial enzymes, or redox-sensitive oncogenic mutations (e.g., KRAS, p53, or IDH1) may respond more favorably to VC-based therapies. Identifying these biomarkers could personalize treatment.
3. *Combination scheduling and pharmacodynamic modeling:* Computational modeling could predict synergistic or antagonistic interactions between VC and specific drugs, minimizing trial-and-error in clinical settings.
4. *Clinical endpoints beyond survival:* VC's ability to reduce chemotherapy-induced fatigue, nausea, and neutropenia should not be overlooked. Improving patient tolerance and life quality are meaningful outcomes, particularly in advanced cancer stages.
5. *Expanding to immuno-oncology:* Emerging data suggest that VC may modulate immune function and T-cell activity via HIF-1α and TET-dependent epigenetic pathways. Combining VC with checkpoint inhibitors could represent a new frontier in integrative oncology.

By pursuing these directions, the scientific community can refine VC's role from experimental adjuvant to *rationally designed therapeutic component.*

Clinical Pearl for Physicians

Cancer patients frequently present *chronic vitamin C depletion* due to cancer metabolic consumption, inflammation, stress physiology, and decreased dietary intake. Because redox balance shapes mitochondrial susceptibility to apoptosis, restoring *physiological vitamin C levels first* may improve responsiveness to chemotherapy. High-dose IV vitamin C should therefore be considered *not as a one-time adjunct*, but as part of a *sequenced therapeutic strategy: replete* to baseline (normalize plasma VC), *then administer* concurrent or timed antineoplastic therapy. Effective clinical translation will require *not only determining whether to use vitamin C, but* when *and* how *to use it.*

Proposal Clinical Trial Design

The findings summarized across this book suggest that the therapeutic impact of VC is *not uniform across cancers*, but instead depends on *timing, dosing sequence, and the metabolic state of the tumor microenvironment.* To translate these observations into clinical practice, future trials should move beyond simple "add-on" administration and instead evaluate *structured treatment sequencing.*

This design *tests the hypothesis* emerging from this experimental data: *VC does not simply "assist" chemotherapy - it must be sequenced to shape apoptotic readiness.* If confirmed clinically, this would shift vitamin C from a perceived adjunct supplement to a *deliberate, timing-dependent therapeutic co-factor* capable of modifying the intracellular decision landscape between survival and apoptosis.

Phase I/II Adaptive Trial Design

Population: Patients with solid tumors or hematologic malignancies receiving standard-of-care therapy.

Intervention Strategy

- *Step 1: Physiologic Repletion Phase:* Oral or low-dose IV vitamin C administered for 1–2 weeks to *restore baseline redox homeostasis,* which is commonly depleted in cancer patients.
- *Step 2: Pharmacologic Augmentation Phase*: High-dose IVC administered *in coordinated timing* with the antineoplastic agent(s), guided by pharmacokinetics and target pathway dynamics.

Comparator Arms

1. Standard therapy alone
2. Standard therapy + high-dose IVC administered *concurrently*
3. Standard therapy + VC *after a defined lead-in repletion period*
4. Timing-shift arm (VC given *before vs. during vs. after therapy*).

Primary Endpoints

- Safety and metabolic tolerability
- Early changes in apoptotic markers (cytochrome c release, caspase activation)
- Modulation of major survival pathways (PI3K/Akt/mTOR, MAPK, Wnt/β-catenin), measured through plasma or exosome biomarkers.

Secondary Endpoints

- Cancer response rate
- Progression-free survival
- Patient-reported symptom outcomes and quality of life
- Immune activation markers, including PD-L1 modulation and T-cell function.

Final Reflection: Reclaiming Curiosity

The journey through this book demonstrates that even well-known molecules can yield new insights when revisited through modern lenses. The rediscovery of VC in cancer biology is more than a scientific story; it is *a lesson in humility and persistence*. Science evolves not by discarding old ideas but by refining them through evidence.

The data presented here - from altered mitochondrial potential to Smac/DIABLO activation, from changes in MEK signaling to modulation of oxidative stress - collectively assert that VC's effects are neither simplistic nor redundant. They invite a new phase of investigation, where VC is studied not in isolation, but as part of a networked therapeutic system that respects the biochemical complexity of cancer.

If the early 20th century witnessed VC's discovery as a vitamin, and the late 20th century saw its dismissal in oncology, perhaps the 21st century will mark its *rehabilitation as a redox therapeutic* - guided by mechanistic clarity rather than speculation.

Every molecule in medicine carries both data and story - and VC's story is particularly human. From Linus Pauling's early advocacy to decades of skepticism, VC embodies the tension between curiosity and convention. This work, situated at the intersection of biochemistry and oncology, contributes to bridging that divide.

This book does not claim VC as a miracle compound, but it restores *scientific balance* to the conversation. By grounding hypotheses in mechanistic evidence - mitochondrial dysfunction, apoptosis induction, oxidative modulation - it transforms anecdote into evidence.

Moreover, there is a broader message: innovation often begins with revisiting what we think we already understand. VC, once dismissed as merely an antioxidant, may in fact remind us that biology's elegance lies in duality - in how one molecule can heal or harm, depending on context and concentration.

In "*Vitamin C and Cancer: Mechanisms and Therapeutic Synergies,*" I offer data and direction. It shows that redox modulation is a viable strategy for influencing cancer cell survival and drug sensitivity. It also demonstrates that the bridge between nutrition and pharmacology is narrower than once believed.

My hope is that this work inspires others - clinicians, researchers, and students alike - to continue asking bold questions about simple molecules. For in that simplicity may lie the next generation of cancer therapeutics, shaped not only by chemistry but by the enduring human drive to understand and heal.

Selected References

[1] Du J., Martin S.M., Levine B.A., Wang S., Knudsen C.M., Cullen J.J. Mechanism of ascorbate-induced cytotoxicity in pancreatic cancer. *J Am. Assoc. Cancer Res* 2010 ; 16 :509-520.

[2] Chen Q., Espey M.G., Krishna M.C., Mitchell J.B., Corpe C.P., Buettner G.R., et al., Pharmacological ascorbic acid concentrations selectively kill cancer cells : action as a pro-drug to deliver hydrogen peroxide to tissues. *PNAS* 2005 ; 102 : 13604-13609.

[3] Chen Q., Espey M.G., Sun A.Y., Lee J.H., Buettner G.R., Levine M. Ascorbate in pharmacologic concentration selectively generate ascorbate radical and hydrogen peroxide in extracellular fluid *in vivo*. *PNAS* 2007 ; 104 : 8749-8754.

[4] Olney K.E., Du J., Van Erve T.J., Witmer J.R., Wagner B.A., Buettner G.R, et al., Inhibitors of hydroperoxide metabolism enhance ascorbate-induce cytotoxicity. *Free Radic Res* 2013 ; 47 :154-163.

[5] Bennett L.L. Potential synergistic interaction between curcumin and sorafenib enhances cytotoxicity in NCI-H5222 lung cancer cells. *OBM Genetics* 2025 ; 9, 4.

[6] Carr A.C, Cook J. Intravenous vitamin C for cancer therapy: Identifying the current evidence and quantifying ongoing clinical trials. *Front Oncol* 2018 ;8 :453.

[7] Rouleau L., Antony A.N., Bisetto S., Newberg A., Doria C., Levine M., et al., Synergistic effects of ascorbate and sorafenib in cancer models. *Free Radic Biol Med* 2016 ; 95 : 308-322.

[8] Böttger F., Valles-Marti A., Cahn L., Jimenez C.R. High-dose intravenous vitamin C, a promising multi-targeting agent in the treatment of cancer. *J Exp Clin Cancer Res* 2021 ; 40 : 343.

[9] Fan D., Liu X., Shen Z., Wu P., Zhong L., Lin F. Cell signaling pathways based on vitamin C and their application in cancer therapy. *Biomedicine & Pharmacotherapy* 2023 : 162, 114695.

[10] Li W.N., Zhang S.J., Feng J.Q., Jin W.L. Repurposing vitamin C for cancer treatment: Focus on targeting the tumor microenvironment. *Cancer* 2022 ; 14 (11), 2608.

[11] Hoffer L.J., Levine M., Assouline S., Melnychuk D. Systematic review of intravenous ascorbate in cancer clinical trials. *JNCI Monogram* 2012;(45) :17-24.

[12] Pawlowska E., Szczepanski J., Blasiak J. Pro- and antioxidant effects of vitamin C in cancer: Revisited. *Oxid Med Cell Longeval* 2019 ; 19 : 7286737.

[13] Ngo B., Van Riper J.M., Cantley L.C., Yun J. Targeting cancer vulnerabilities with high-dose vitamin C. *Nat Rev Cancer* 2019 ;19(5):271-282.

[14] Yun J., Mullarky E., Lu C. Vitamin C selectively kills KRAS and BRAF mutant colorectal cancer cells by targeting GAPDH. *Science* 2015 ;350(6266) :1391-1396.

[15] Polireddy K., Dong R., Reed G., Chen P., Williamson S., Pessetto Z., et al., High dose parenteral ascorbate inhibited pancreatic cancer growth and metastasis: mechanisms and a phase I/IIa study. *Sci Rep* 2017; 7: 17188.

[16] Schoenfeld J.D., Sibenaller Z.A., Mapuskar K.A. $O_2^{\bullet -}$ and H_2O_2-mediated disruption of iron metabolism causes differential susceptibility of NSCLC and GBM to pharmacologic ascorbate. *Cancer Cell* 2017 ; 31(4) :487-500.e8.

[17] Ma Y., Chapman J., Levine M., Polireddy K., Drisko J., Chen Q. High-dose parenteral ascorbate enhances chemosensitivity of ovarian cancer and reduces chemotherapy toxicity. *Sci Transl Med* 2014;6(222):222ra18.

[18] [18] Wei M., Cao Z., Dong L., Wang W., Wie M., Ji L., et al., The advantages and challenges of sorafenib combination therapy: Drug resistance, toxicity and future directions. *Oncol Lett* 2025; 526 :15272.

[19] Bennett L.L., Mondal A. Curcumin and afatinib synergistically inhibit growth of human osteosarcoma cells by inhibition of matrix metallo proteinases, mitogen activated kinases 1-4, and reactive oxygen species. *J of Pharmacy and Drug Devel* 2021 ; 3 : 1.

[20] Taira A., Palin K., Kuosmanen A., Valimaki N. Vitamin C boosts DNA demethylation in *TET2* germline mutations carriers. *Clinical Epigenetic* 2023 ; 15 :7

[21] Davis L., Recktenwald M., Hutt E., Fuller S., Briggs M., Goel A., et al., Targeting HIF-2a in the tumor microenvironment: redefining the role of HIF-2 for solid cancer therapy. *Cancers* 2022 ; 14 : 5.

[22] Doskey C.M., Buranasudja V., Wagner B.A., Wilkes J.G., Du J., Cullen J.J., et al., Tumor cells have decreased ability to metabolize H_2O_2 : Implications for pharmacologic ascorbate in cancer therapy. *Redox Biol* 2016 ;78(6) : 274-284.

[23] Chen P., Reed G., Jiang J., Wang Y., Sunega J., Dong R., et al., Pharmacokinetic evaluation of intravenous vitamin C: A classic pharmacokinetic study. *Clin Pharmacokinetics* 2022 ; 61 : 1237-1249.

About the Author

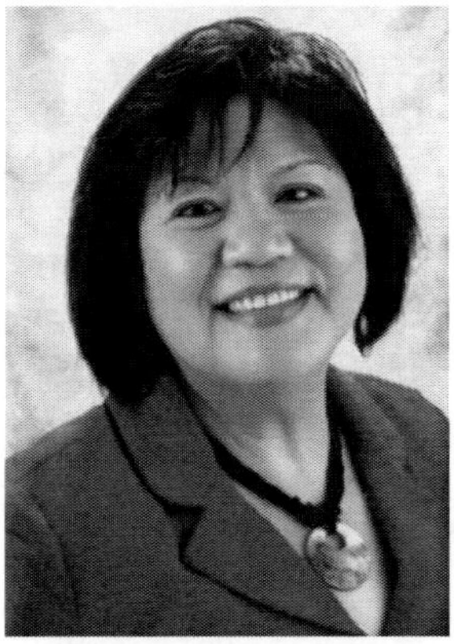

Lunawati Lo Bennett MS, MRE, PhD, PharmD, FACN, CNS
Professor of Pharmaceutical Sciences,
Union University, College of Pharmacy
Jackson, TN, USA

Dr. Lunawati L. Bennett is a tenured Professor of Pharmaceutical Sciences at Union University College of Pharmacy in Jackson, Tennessee, USA. She holds both a Ph.D. in Pharmaceutical Sciences and a Pharm.D. in Pharmacy, reflecting her integrated commitment to biomedical research, pharmacotherapy, and patient-centered care.

For nearly two decades, Dr. Bennett has taught pharmacology to future pharmacists, guiding students through the therapeutic use of medications across a broad range of disease states, including endocrine, gastrointestinal, respiratory, cardiovascular, and central nervous system disorders, as well as gout, rheumatoid arthritis, cancer, and infectious diseases. She is a member of the Rho Chi Honor Society of Pharmacy and is licensed as a pharmacist in multiple states.

Dr. Bennett has published extensively in peer-reviewed journals, with research focus on cancer pharmacology, particularly the role of nutraceutical, vitamin C and their interactions with antineoplastic agents. She is the author of several scholarly books, including *Frontiers in Lysosomal Storage Disease, Consumers' Guide to Prescription and Over-the-Counter Medications, Frontiers in Leukemia Pharmacotherapy, Caspase-3: Structure, Functions, and Interactions, and Gaucher's Disease: From Diagnosis to Treatment.* She also contributes to professional education through continuing education programs on topics such as Gaucher disease and enzyme replacement therapy.

Her research interests include antioxidant-based therapeutic strategies in oncology and the pharmacologic management of lysosomal storage diseases. Above all, Dr. Bennett is deeply committed to teaching and mentorship, with a passion for empowering students and patients to understand medications and apply pharmacologic principles wisely to improve health outcomes. She attributes her perseverance in scholarship and service to her faith in the Lord Jesus Christ.

Contributors

Ola Boateng MBA
PharmD candidate class of 2026
Union University
College of Pharmacy
Jackson, TN, USA
(Wrote Neuroblastoma background in chapter 1 under primary author's guidance).

Joanne Shen PharmD
PGY2 Post-Graduate Residency
Health System Pharmacy Administration and Leadership
University of Illinois
Chicago, IL, USA
(Wrote Breast Cancer background in chapter 1 under primary author's guidance).

Index

D

E

F

G

T

V

W

More books by *Lunawati L. Bennett* can be found at:

https://novapublishers.com/writer/lunawati-l-bennett/